Toward A Holistic Developmental Psychology

LIST OF CONTRIBUTORS

Sybil S. Barten, Natural Sciences Division, State University of New York at Purchase

Sandor B. Brent, Department of Psychology, Wayne State University

Robert A. Ciottone, Department of Psychology, Clark University

Leonard Cirillo, Department of Psychology, Clark University

Margery B. Franklin, Department of Psychology, Sarah Lawrence College

Joseph A. Glick, Department of Psychology, City University of New York Graduate School

Gail A. Hornstein, Department of Psychology, Mount Holyoke College

Bernard Kaplan, Department of Psychology, Clark University

Edith Kaplan, Boston Veterans Administration Medical Center

Jonas Langer, Department of Psychology, University of California at Berkeley

Ogretta V. McNeil, Department of Psychology, Holy Cross College

Ricardo B. Morant, Department of Psychology, Brandeis University

Angel M. Pacheco, Department of Psychology, University of Puerto Rico

Robert H. Pollack, Department of Psychology, University of Georgia

George Rand, Graduate School of Architecture & Urban Planning, University of California at Los Angeles

Seymour Wapner, Department of Psychology, Clark University

Toward A Holistic Developmental Psychology

Edited by
Seymour Wapner
Bernard Kaplan
Clark University

LEA LAWRENCE ERLBAUM ASSOCIATES, PUBLISHERS
1983 Hillsdale, New Jersey   London

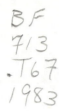

Copyright © 1983 by Lawrence Erlbaum Associates, Inc.
    All rights reserved. No part of this book may be reproduced in
    any form, by photostat, microform, retrieval system, or any other
    means, without the prior written permission of the publisher.

Lawrence Erlbaum Associates, Inc., Publishers
365 Broadway
Hillsdale, New Jersey 07642

Library of Congress Cataloging in Publication Data

Main entry under title:

Toward a holistic developmental psychology.

   Bibliography: p.
   Includes index.
   1. Developmental psychology.   I. Wapner, Seymour,
1917–   .   II. Kaplan, Bernard, 1925–   .
BF713.T67   1983   155   83-5548
ISBN 0-89859-262-3

Printed in the United States of America
10 9 8 7 6 5 4 3 2 1

Contents

Introduction   1

1. **Change in Structural Size and Change in Organizational Form: A Formal Model for the Relationship Between Growth and Development**

   Sandor B. Brent   7

       Introduction   7
       Steady-State Ranges of Population Size for
         Specific Forms of Structural Organization   10
       Steady-State Ranges for Seven Distinct Classroom
         Formats   11
       Upper-Boundary Phenomena of the Steady-State
         Range   17
       Extensions and Limitations   28
       Summary and Conclusions   32

2. **Piaget, Vygotsky, and Werner**

   Joseph A. Glick   35

       Introduction   35
       Piaget   39
       Vygotsky   43
       Werner   47

3. **Genetic-Dramatism: Old Wine in New Bottles**

Bernard Kaplan **53**

    Introduction   53
    Development: Genesis in Genetic-Dramatism   57
    Dramatism   61
    The Perspective of Genetic-Dramatism   68
    Conclusion   71

4. **A Developmental Approach to Systems Theory**

George Rand **75**

    Architecture and Psychology   75
    Comparative Mental Development   82
    A Theory of Practice   84

5. **Reflections on Culture and Personality from the Perspective of Genetic-Dramatism**

Bernard Kaplan **95**

    Introduction   95
    Development As Normative:
      Immanence and Transcendence   97
    Development as Descriptive (D–D):
      Who Shall Describe?   100
    Outsiders and Insiders: Vox Populi, Vox Dei   104
    Meditations on Genetic-Dramatism, Culture,
      and Personality   106

6. **An Examination of Studies of Critical Transitions Through the Life Cycle**

S. Wapner, R. A. Ciottone, G. A. Hornstein, O. V. McNeil, and A. M. Pacheco **111**

    Introduction   111
    Critical Transitions   112
    Developmental Analysis   116
    Four Person-in-Environment Transitions   118

7. **Regression Revisited: Perceptuo-Cognitive Performance in the Aged**

Robert H. Pollack **133**

8. **Process and Achievement Revisited**

   Edith Kaplan **143**

   > Introduction 143
   > Visuo-Spatial Exemplars 144
   > Naming 148
   > Immediate Memory 150
   > Gestural Representation 151
   > Summary 155

9. **Some Aspects of a Developmental Analysis of Perception**

   Ricardo B. Morant **157**

   > Introduction 157
   > Werner's Impact on Perception 158
   > A Developmental Approach to
   >   Sensory-Tonic Theory 159
   > Adaptation to Prism Rearrangement 160
   > Suggested Studies on Perceptual Adaptation
   >   and Aftereffects 165
   > The Results Briefly Related to
   >   Image and Flow Theories of Perception 168
   > The Audio and Oculogyral Illusions 168
   > The Phenomenological Unity of Perception 171
   > The Orthogenetic Principle: Development
   >   Versus Change 174

10. **The Aesthetic Mode of Consciousness**

    Sybil S. Barten **179**

    > Introduction 179
    > Aesthetic Versus Mundane Modes of
    >   Consciousness 180
    > Werner's Views on Aesthetic Phenomena 183
    > Object Description in Artists and Scientists 184
    > Conditions for Expressivity 188
    > Conclusions 191

11. **Play as the Creation of Imaginary Situations:
    The Role of Language**

    Margery B. Franklin **197**

    > Introduction 197
    > Language in Play: Three Paradigms 201
    > Concluding Comments 214

12. **Concept and Symbol Formation by Infants**
    Jonas Langer   **221**

> Operations   222
> Functions   224
> Representation   225
> Representational Cognition   231

13. **Figurative Action from the Perspective of Genetic-Dramatism**
    Leonard Cirillo and Bernard Kaplan   **235**

> Introduction   235
> Speaking Metaphorically   237
> The Therapy of Politics and
>   the Politics of Therapy   238
> The Powers of Figurative Action   240
> The Home Front   242
> Mundane Allegories   244
> Secular Rituals   246
> Figuratively Free   248

Epilogue   **253**

Author Index   **255**

Subject Index   **261**

Introduction

The main aim of this volume is to suggest new ways of conceptualizing human development and new domains of theorizing and engaging in practice for those who are vitally concerned with the nature and value of human beings. Toward this goal, colleagues and students of the late Heinz Werner, believing that Werner provided the schema for such a vision, here present modifications, extensions, and elaborations of his insights concerning the nature of development. These papers were presented in summary form and critically discussed in a round-table format at a conference held at Clark University in June 1981.[1] This volume contains most of the papers presented at the conference.[2] To orient the reader, we here present a brief synopsis of the papers making up this volume.

Sandor B. Brent (Chapter 1) tries to demonstrate some relationships between growth—defined in terms of physical increase in size or number—and development characterized in terms of the orthogenetic principle. He presents schematically some argument and evidence to suggest that changes in size of a structure (growth) may provide the impetus for change in the forms and functions of that structure. Brent's primary illustration, pointing to changes in form and function of a classroom group depending upon size of group, is extended by him to other content domains.

---

[1] The conference, "Developmental psychology for the 1980's: Werner's influences on theory and praxis," held under the auspices of the Heinz Werner Institute of Developmental Psychology took place on June 1-2, 1981 at Clark University.

[2] Several of the papers presented at the conference are not included in this volume. These are papers by Roger Bibace, Roger Bibace and Mary Walsh, and by Mary Walsh, Felicisima Serafica and Roger Bibace.

Joseph A. Glick (Chapter 2) explores the different conceptions of development utilized by Piaget, Vygotsky, and Werner. Distinguishing between the "natural object" (i.e., the subjects and specific subject-matter) and the "conceptual object" (i.e., the theoretical topics and aims of the investigator), Glick attempts to demonstrate that these three major developmental theorists have concerned themselves with different natural objects and different conceptual objects. He argues that Piaget's conceptual object is taken to be the relationships between life experience and the universal forms of rational thought. He sees two Vygotskys. Vygotsky I *(Thought and Language)* is taken as focusing on the relationship between socialized systems of mediation (e.g., language) and the individual's reconstructions of these in his/her own private world, as exemplified in the problem of "inner" and "external" speech. The conceptual object for Vygotsky II *(Man in Society)* is construed as the problem of identifying how representational systems transform person-environment relations, and how interpersonal relations are internalized in the course of socialization. Werner is taken as concerned with the manner in which the wholeness of organisms can be preserved and theoretically represented even when one is dealing with seemingly circumscribed areas of function. Glick sees Werner as stressing process-product distinctions and offering a vectorial, dynamic language which, when added to a structural language, could preserve notions of developmental change and organismic wholeness. On this basis, Glick argues that Werner's approach offers the clearest path to a theoretically and descriptively adequate account of psychological functioning and development.

Bernard Kaplan (Chapter 3) argues for a new yet ancient-developmental approach, which he dubs Genetic-Dramatism. He takes this approach as integrating the insights of Heinz Werner and the literary critic, Kenneth Burke. Kaplan maintains that "development" is a normative notion—a movement toward perfection, and that the job of a developmental approach is to facilitate the movement toward perfection in domains of action, in interpersonal relations and in the transformations of the Self. Such a task, he insists, involves an understanding of factors at every level of organization that might have a bearing on the development of human beings.

George Rand (Chapter 4) seeks to unite developmental theory and systems theory to examine environmental design and architecture. His aim is to offer a psychological view of the environment that has pertinence to the design of present and future settings. Toward this end, the paper explores a number of ways in which the transitional relationships are manifest in the history of architecture—e.g., viewed from a psychological perspective as discovering and creating of a series of "mind-built-forms." A process analysis is proposed of the dialectic between romantic/intuitive and the rational/deductive procedure in project planning. Comparative-developmental theory is used to create a psychologically salient view of systems analysis, which can be used as a tool in defining and creating an anthropology of planning and public policy. Toward this end, the core terms of a developmental approach (e.g., settings of relevance, role perceptions, etc.) and its contrasts with a Technicist/Systems approach to practice are described. He suggests that such elements of systems theory needs to be redefined with cogent examples that reflect the unique complexities of practical affairs. Rand's aim is to emphasize the self-definition of people in relation to technical systems, the importance of building a collective consensus, stimulating and liberating collective imagination, and, in general, facilitating a developmental process of mutual learning and discovery.

In Chapter 5, Bernard Kaplan considers two general notions of development, as this term is applied to individuals, socio-cultural groups, and individuals-in-society. Kaplan distinguishes between ''descriptive developmentalism,'' which claims to be value-free, and concerned only with the discovery of the ''facts'' and ''causes'' of change over the life span, and a normative developmental approach to which he subscribes. The normative approach takes development as a concept by postulation—a concept used to assess and evaluate performances and modes of functioning on socio-cultural and individual levels. The main thrust of the paper is to argue that descriptive developmentalism (as manifested in psychology or anthropology) is a sterile intellectual enterprise, which implicitly subscribes to two noxious doctrines, viz., whatever is is right, and whatever is later is better.

Seymour Wapner and his colleagues (Chapter 6) explore various critical person-in-environment transitions from a developmental perspective. Looking at transitions varying from first nursery school attendance to radical transition from one cultural setting to another, Wapner et al. examine how such transitions may be the occasion either for developmental regression or developmental advance. Critical transitions are taken to provide the opportunity to restructure the individual's world, including the self and its relation to the non-self in less mature ways (developmental delay or dedifferentiation) or in more mature ways (developmental advance or differentiation and hierarchic integration). Wapner, et al. not only deal with transitions from an organismic-developmental point of view but exploit the concepts of such phenomenologists as Alfred Schutz and ethnomethodologists influenced by Schutz.

Robert Pollack (Chapter 7) utilizes Werner's process-achievement distinction in his analysis of perceptuo-cognitive performance in the aged. Pollack questions the view that a breakdown in performance domains in middle and old-age is due principally to a loss or deficit in higher forms of cognitive activity—to a disintegration and dedifferentialtion of a hierarchically organized system. He offers evidence and argument to show that a reduced achievement in perceptual performance involving figure-ground articulation need *not* be accompanied by the breakdown of high level conceptual strategies and that problem-solving performance does *not* decline from youth to old age when figure-ground articulation is not involved. Pollack argues that while classical regression may occur, it is most probably a result of pathology that happens to accompany aging in some cases and not a result of the aging process itself. Elaborating on the practical implications of his work, Pollack suggests that prosthetic devices to improve the sensory-perceptual medium in which conceptual tasks are presented may restore adequate higher level performance.

Edith Kaplan (Chapter 8) also exploits Werner's distinction between process and achievement by focusing specifically on the understanding and diagnosis of pathology induced by brain injury. Contrasting Werner's perspective with the statistical testing approach that has long dominated research and clinical measurement of intellectual functioning, E. Kaplan seeks to provide a foundation for assessment of intellectual and cognitive activities that can more accurately and effectively differentiate the patient's abilities and deficits. She presents material drawn from observation of individual cases of patients with verified focal lesions as well as from research in normal and pathological development and aging. She also draws the implications of this process oriented mode of diagnosis for both theory and practice, including the suggestion of techniques of rehabilitation that might foster the developmental advance of patients with neurological insult.

Ricardo B. Morant (Chapter 9) examines some aspects of perceputal functioning both in ontogenesis and microgenesis. He illustrates some ways in which Wernerian theory can be used to study perceptual processes by applying an organismic point of view to the analysis of his experimental studies in space and form perception, including investigations of prismatic rearrangements in auditory and visual localization under labyrinthian stimulation, and on the ontogenesis of visual-haptic organization in infants reaching for virtual images of toys. Morant also raises the issue of whether development should be characterized in terms of an orthogenetic principle (e.g., movement to perfection) or taken as the outcome of causally induced changes.

Sybil S. Barten (Chapter 10) tries to remedy the relative lack of attention paid by developmental theorists to the aesthetic mode of consciousness in human functioning. Contrasting the characteristics of aesthetic consciousness with non-aesthetic modes, Barten presents evidence and arguments to the effect that an artist's typical orientation towards objects is one in which feeling, kinaesthetic experience and visual form are not kept rigidly distinct. She maintains that such an intentionality is not unique to artists, and proposes conditions for inducing and developing aesthetic consciousness in non-artists. The paper concludes with a plea for a psychology of art that takes as its starting point an analysis of aesthetic experience.

Margery B. Franklin (Chapter 11), exploring the metaphor of symbolic play as world-making, advances the thesis that play be viewed as the imaginal creation of possible situations. She argues that this metaphor—and the larger conceptual framework to which it belongs—not only provides a distinctive view of play, but holds implications for thinking about mental development more generally. Delineating three distinctive paradigms for conceptualizing the role of language in play (a self-guidance paradigm; a communicational paradigm; and a reality-creating paradigm), Franklin highlights how these different paradigms presuppose and imply different views of human development and of human functioning. She develops the reality-creating paradigm in relation to the more encompassing view of play as imaginative activity and offers a set of analytic categories with illustrative material. Franklin concludes with comments on the relations between play and reality and developmental lines in play.

Jonas Langer (Chapter 12) treats the relations between thought and symbolization with respect to two hypotheses. The first is that early cognitive development preceeds and informs early symbolic, including linguistic, development, and this is assessed with respect to findings on the relations between logic and symbolization as they develop between ages 6 and 18 months. The second hypothesis is that the structures of intermediate forms of symbolization, including the infant's first words, are partial developmental transforms of the structures of sensorimotor gestures. This hypothesis is evaluated with respect to findings on developmental transformations in infants' symbolization between ages 16 and 18 months.

Leonard Cirillo and Bernard Kaplan (Chapter 13) examine figurative action from the perspective of genetic dramatism. Figurative actions are defined as those symbolic acts which reorganize and reorient our visions of reality and our relationships to one another. The authors seek to highlight the constructive character of all symbolic activity by revealing that what is taken to be literal or real depends on the fixed orientation shared by the members of a social group. The ways in which figurative actions, verbal and nonverbal, are used to radically alter one's orientation are illustrated with examples from different domains: legal, political, literary, religious, and, especially therapeutic. The authors suggest that highly developed (perfected) figurative action expresses and fosters our human capacities to transcend limited visions and narrow identifications, to understand and to create multiple, systematically related meanings.

It will be clear from this synopsis that those educated in the Wernerian tradition are not bound by any specific methodology or content area. They are however, governed by the view that the development of human beings is a supreme value and that psychologists should seek to clarify the nature of human development and to understand conditions on all levels that promote and inhibit developmental advance. They also appreciate the fact that human development cannot be collapsed into, or represented in terms of cognition, intellection, conation, or any single set of human functions. The Wernerian approach, in origin and aim, is concerned with the development of the whole human being. The papers here are only a stimulus to provoke others as well as ourselves to a new, yet old approach, to human experience, thought, and action.[3]

We wish to acknowledge the support of Clark University's Heinz Werner Institute of Developmental Psychology and the efforts of many individuals who made the conference and this volume possible. In addition to the authors, we give special thanks to the discussants—Marc Bornstein (New York University), William Damon (Clark University), Rachel Falmagne (Clark University), Howard Gardner (Harvard University), Roy Pea (Clark University and Bank Street College), Ina Uzgiris (Clark University), Sheldon White (Harvard University), and Peter Wolff (Harvard University and Children's Hospital). We further express our appreciation to Arthur Rummel, to Shyamala Venkataraman and other Clark students who helped with conference organization and preparation, and to Emelia Thamel for her extraordinary managerial efforts in supervising the work connected with pre-conference planning, with day to day conduct of the conference, with help regarding transcriptions, typing of manuscripts and preparation of this volume.

REFERENCES

Kaplan, B., & Wapner, S. (Eds.) *Perspectives in psychological theory*. New York: International Universities Press, 1960.

Love, J. *Worlds in consciousness: Mythopoetic thought in the novels of Virginia Wolff*. Berkeley: University of California Press, 1970.

Sack, R. *Conceptions of space in social thought*. Minneapolis: University of Minnesota Press, 1980.

Shumaker, W. *Literature and irrational*. Englewood Cliffs, N.J.: Prentice-Hall, 1960.

---

[3]Werner's influence beyond the traditional academic boundaries of psychology is manifested in the writings of students of literature, anthropology, psychiatry, and geography. See, for example, Wayne Shumaker (1960), Jean Love (1970) and Robert Sack (1980). The reader might also consult *Perspectives in psychological theory* (Kaplan & Wapner, 1960) containing essays by Silvano Arieti, Solomon Asch, Jerome S. Bruner, Tamara Dembo, Kurt Goldstein, Roman Jakobson, George S. Klein, Norman R. F. Maier, Abraham H. Maslow, Gardner Murphy, David Rapaport, Martin Scheerer, Theodore C. Schneirla, and Herman A. Witkin.

Change in Structural Size and Change in Organizational Form: A Formal Model for the Relationship Between Growth and Development

1

Sandor B. Brent
Wayne State University

INTRODUCTION

The attempt to understand the relationship between quantitative change and qualitative change is one of the oldest and most recurrent issues in the history of developmental theory. This chapter is concerned with one specific aspect of that problem: namely, the way in which changes in the number of constituent parts of a structure at one level of analysis affects and is affected by changes in the organizational form of that structure at some other level of analysis.

The basic thesis of the present approach is that for any given form of structural organization there is a finite range of population sizes within which that structure will remain formally stable and continue to function with optimal efficiency. I refer to this as the *steady-state range* of population size for that form of organization. As the population size of a structure approaches the upper or lower limits of that steady-state range, stresses appear within the structure which decrease both the stability of its organizational form and the efficiency with which it serves its intended functions. Finally, when its population size exceeds the limits of its steady-state range, a spontaneous reorganization of the form of the structure takes place (cf. Brent, 1978b). This reorganization takes place in such a way as to increase once again both the formal stability of the constituent parts of that structure as a whole, thereby establishing a new steady-state range for that new form of organization.[1]

In this chapter I explore three aspects of this relationship between change in size and change in form: First I consider in some detail a concrete example that illustrates the notion of a steady-state range itself. Second, using this same example, I consider the kinds of changes that take place in the form and function of a structure as its population size first approaches and then surpasses the upper limit of its steady-state range. Third, I outline briefly a quasi-formal model for some of the processes that govern the destabilization and the subsequent restabilization of a structure as its population size passes into a new steady-state range associated with a new, emergent form of structural organization. Finally, I consider the generality and limitation of the proposed model. I begin, however, with a brief set of formal definitions for some of the basic concepts I use just to be sure that, as we go along, we are speaking the same language. A fuller exposition of these concepts appears in Brent (in press).

Some Basic Definitions

The term *structure,* as I use it, refers to a relatively invariant set of relationships among a set of constituent parts. The set of invariant relationships themselves is the *form* of the structure; the constituents which are arranged in those relationships are its *contents.*

Every constituent of a structure may itself be considered a structure in its own right with its own form and its own contents at some more *microscopic level* of analysis. Similarly, every individual structure may be considered a constituent of some supraordinate structure at some more *macroscopic level* of analysis. The *population size* of a structure is then the number of such constituents which that structure contains at some specified level of analysis. Thus, in speaking of the population size of a particular structure it is essential to specify the level of analysis at which the population of constituents is defined.

Developmental theorists have in general been primarily concerned with the development of organic structures. An *organic structure* is one which meets at least four criteria: functional unity, structural integrity, interdependence among parts, and subordination of the parts to the whole. These four criteria, while focussing attention of different aspects of an

---

[1]In the language of the levels-by-stage model frequently used by developmental theorists (cf. Brent, in press), the steady-state range corresponds roughly to a developmental stage—i.e., an interval of time during which the organizational form of the structure remains relatively constant. Similarly, the loss of stability in efficiency at the boundaries of each steady-state range correspond roughly to the regression which frequently mark the transitions between developmental stages.

organic structure, are nonetheless closely related. *Functional unity* refers to the fact that each organic structure functions as a single, unitary constituent within the supraordinate contexts of which it is itself a part. *Structural integrity* refers to the fact that an organic structure is highly resistant to the arbitrary addition and deletion of constituents from its content set. *Interdependence* refers to the fact that the form and function of each constituent as a constituent of any particular structure is determined to a significant degree by the form and function of the other constituents of that structure at the same level of analysis. Finally, *subordination,* refers to the fact that the form and function of each microscopic constituent considered individually is also highly dependent upon (and is, in that sense, determined by) the particular position it occupies in the collective form and function of the macroscopic structure as a whole.[2]

The relationships among these structural concepts are readily illustrated by a natural English sentence. The form of such a sentence is most commonly expressed in terms of a set of grammatical, syntactical, or semantic relationships amongst its constituent parts. Those constituents themselves (i.e., its contents) exist at several levels of analysis: the phrasic, the lexical, the morphemic, the phonemic, the phonic, and so forth. The population size of a sentence thus may be specified in terms of the number of constituents it contains at any one of these levels of analysis. At the same time each such sentence itself functions as a single, unified constituent of some larger sociolinguistic structure—a structure that includes both that sentence and other linguistic and non-linguistic elements in the context in which it occurs. Thus, a particular written sentence may simultaneously be a content element of a paragraph, a section, a chapter, a volume and a multivolume work.

Such a sentence also illustrates the four criteria for an organic structure. It possesses functional unity by definition: that is, a sentence is a group of words that expresses a complete thought. Empirical evidence (e.g., Brent, 1969) has shown that a meaningful sentence (in contrast to an anomalous or a nonsensical sentence) does in fact function as a single unit item in rote-learning and memory tasks as well. Similarly, a meaningful sentence possesses a high degree of structural integrity. The arbitrary insertion or deletion of a word, for example, is relatively easy to detect and correct compared with the same substitution or deletion in an anomalous or a nonsensical sentence (e.g., Brent, 1965, 1967, 1969). Interdependence is illustrated by the fact that the specific form and function of each word in a sentence—at both the phonic and the semantic levels of analysis—is

---

[2]The role of such positional information in determining the form and function of individual biological cells as the constituents of local specialized organs of more complex biological organisms is a matter of considerable interest in contemporary embryological theory (cf. Bryant, Bryant, & French, 1977).

modified by those of all or most of the other words in the sentence; subordination, by the fact that the form and function of each word in a sentence is at the same time modified by the intended macroscopic meaning-function of the sentence as a whole.

This then is a brief outline of the basic structural concepts underlying our present approach. Let us now return to the principal issue of the present paper: the relationship between changes in the population size of a structure and changes in its organizational form.

STEADY-STATE RANGES OF POPULATION SIZE FOR SPECIFIC FORMS OF STRUCTURAL ORGANIZATION

The basic postulates of the present thesis is the existence of a steady-state range of population sizes for each particular form of structural organization. In this section we compare in some detail the functional characteristics of this steady-state range for several different forms of one particular type of structure: the college classroom. This familiar example illustrates many of the general principles with which we are concerned.

A formal and a functional definition of a classroom structure.   For present purposes a "classroom" structure is defined by a specific set of functional relationships between a teacher and one or more students. Such a functional definition is essential here since the intended function of social and psychological structures frequently play an essential role in determining both their organizational form and their internal, microscopic processes. I assume here that each classroom structure is intended to serve three specific functions: (a) conveying to the student specific information already known by the teacher; (b) helping the student learn how to process this information creatively, from both a theoretical and a practical point of view; and (c) teaching the student efficient methods for gathering new information as it is needed. Therefore the functional efficiency of each such structure must be measured by either the amount of effort required to achieve these goals when the level of achievement is held constant, or by the level of achievement attained when effort is held constant.

Three fundamental processes are involved in achieving these goals: (a) a *transmission* process—information must be transmitted from the teacher to the students; (b) a *verification* process—both the student and the teacher must be able to verify the accuracy with which the information which the teacher intended to transmit was actually received by the students; and (c) a *correction* process—both the teacher and the student must be able to correct any errors which are known to have occurred in earlier transmissions. As we shall see all three of these processes become increasingly vulnerable to degradation as the number of students per teacher—hence the population size of the class as a whole—increases. Reorganization of the form of the classroom structure itself is then one method for upgrading the quality of the transmission once again, hence of increasing the efficiency with which it serves its intended function. We now look at these processes and their consequences in greater detail.

STEADY-STATE RANGES FOR SEVEN DISTINCT CLASSROOM FORMATS

Let us begin by imagining the simplest of all such classroom structures—one consisting of one teacher and one student—and then proceed to add to that basic structure one student at a time. With each new addition we allow the organizational form of the structure to readjust itself in such a way as to achieve the maximum possible efficiency with respect to its intended goal. Figure 1.1 summarizes the results of such a thought experiment based upon my own teaching experiences. The diagrams in Fig. 1.1 represent six different forms of classroom organization: the individual directed study, the tutorial, the seminar, the small class, the large class, and the small lecture, respectively. A seventh, the large lecture, is not shown here. It is, however, an elaboration of the small lecture, and will be described in the following section. Associated with each format in Fig. 1.1 is an indication of the steady-state range of population sizes (R) for that form of classroom organization—i.e., that range within which the number of students in the class can vary while the organizational form and the functional efficiency of the structure as a whole remains relatively constant. The upper and lower boundaries of these steady-state ranges are not fixed particular values but central tendencies of stochastic distributions of such limiting values. In actual practice in my own experience any particular value may vary 20% or more around the central tendency depending upon the nature of the subject being taught; the level at which it is being taught; the teaching skill of the individual teacher; the format preferences of the teacher, the department, and the university; and, in the case of the smaller class-sizes, the particular individuals who constitute the class. However, despite these factors (and, presumably many others), which may influence the specific value of the threshold for any given transition from one format to the next at any given moment in time, the occurrence of such transitions themselves are not matters of mere caprice. They are rather dynamic processes driven by the conflict between (a) certain functional changes that take place in macroscopic structures as a result of changes in the size of their microscopic populations at some particular level of analysis, and (b) the attempt to serve the intended, unifying function of that structure with the least possible expenditure of effort.

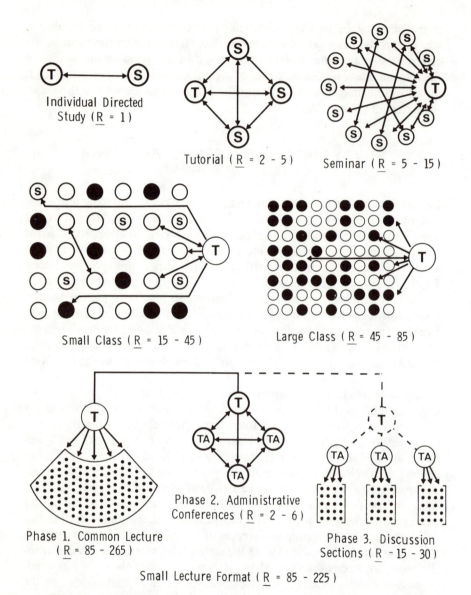

FIG. 1.1   Six formats for the organization of a college classroom (R = steady-state range of populations sizes for each format).

In the schematic representations shown in Fig. 1.1 a circle with the T represents the teacher. Circles with an S, empty circles, black circles, and small dots represent students. The relative size of the circles and dots in each diagram represents very roughly the relative power of each type of constituent—teacher and students—has to affect the macroscopic form and function of the structure as a whole. The change in the relative size of these symbols from one format to another represents the changes in these power relationships with each change in format. A circle with an *S* represents a particular student whose name is likely to be known to the teacher or to other students in the class; an open-circle without an *S*, a particular student whose face is likely to be known even though his or her name is not known; and a black circle or a dot, a student whose name and face are both unlikely to be known. The lines connecting constituents represent channels of communication. The solid lines represent channels which are frequently used; and the absence of lines, nonexistence of channels. A double-arrow represents a dialogue; a single arrow, a directed monologue. The burst of arrows from the teacher in the last two schematics represents the fact that in these two formats the teacher's communications are essentially scattered, shotgun fashion, in the general direction of the class as a diffuse whole, only occasionally being directed toward any particular individual in the class.

Let us now examine each of the formats shown in Fig. 1.1 focusing on four characteristics of the group process: (a) the nature of the communications exchanged amongst individual constituents within the group; (b) the processes by which procedural decisions are made; (c) the number of formal rules that are necessary for maintaining a given level of functional efficiency; and (d) the ease or difficulty of changing such rules once they have been promulgated.

1. Individual directed-study. The smallest population size in a teaching structure is an individual directed-study. This structure consists of a teacher and one student. Its processes are characterized by direct, at-will communication between the two. Communication is in the form of reciprocal dialogues. There can be relatively few formal rules. Decision-making can be collective and by consensus. Rules are flexible and subject to continual change as the need for such change arises. The distinction between the two roles is primarily functionally rather than formally determined.

2. Tutorial. With about 2 to about 5 students there is a shift to a new form of social organization. While direct, reciprocal, at-will dialogues are still common, there tends to be an increase in the number of rules necessary for the structure to function efficiently. While decision-making can still be collective and predominantly by consensus, it is more difficult to continually change the rules even when a need appears to arise. Since there are now so many possible channels open for dialogues between the various constituents the teacher begins to emerge as that nuclear center which not only disseminates stored information to the structure as a whole but also regulates the flow of communication when such regulation becomes necessary. It is however still possible for other participants to assume that role without reducing the functional efficiency of the structure as a whole.

3. Seminar. Once the number of students in a class exceeds about 5 or 6 there is a need to shift to a more complex form of classroom organization. In this new form dialogue between the teacher and each individual student is still possible. However dialogues between individual students is greatly reduced. Individual student-reports in such a seminar frequently provide a compromise—an intermediate form between the tutorial and the small class. Through this means each student has at least some period of time to serve as the integrative focus of the structure and to dialogue directly with all of the other students in the class in a way that is no longer possible in the general sense.

A still greater number of formal rules are required to coordinate the activities of the individual members of the group with respect to the collective function of the group as a whole. Decision making by consensus is however more difficult owing to the number and diversity of the points of view which must be reconciled in order to arrive at such a consensus. Collective decision making thus tends toward more complex formal procedures (e.g., a formal proposal, a discussion or debate, and a formal vote). Because these procedures are time-consuming and cumbersone they tend to reduce the functional efficiency of the group as a whole. As a result rules changes are infrequent and rules tend to remain relatively invariant. Those changes which do occur tend to be instituted by fiat of the teacher, although this fiat may be exercised with the advice and consent of the students.

4. Small class. The spatial form of a small class differs from that of a seminar in that the students and the teacher no longer sit in a circle. Therefore, students can no longer see each other's faces. They see instead only the teacher's face and each other's backs. The teacher, on the other hand, can see all of the student's faces. Although this new spatial arrangement still permits direct dialogues between the teacher and each individual student, the opportunities for such dialogues is markedly reduced. Similarly, although some dialogues between students do occasionally occur the frequency and duration of these dialogues is greatly reduced and at the same time tend to be more subject to regulation by the teacher. Many more rules are now required for the efficient functioning of this structure. Collective decision-making is very difficult and therefore proportionately rare. Almost all decision-making is now by the teacher's fiat, although an informal survey of student opinions may sometimes be taken for advisory purposes—e.g., "Shall we have a midterm exam on Monday or Friday?" However, major changes in procedural rules even by teacher's fiat are difficult since they tend to disrupt the organizational stability of the classroom, hence, to reduce its functional efficiency. As shown in Fig. 1.1 in a small class a teacher can still within a reasonable amount of time come to know the faces of most of the students in the class and the names of some significant proportion of those students.

5. Large class. The transition from the small to the large class is characterized by the fact that the teacher can no longer learn to recognize even the faces of any significant number of students in the class. Dialogues between the teacher and most students in the class is all but impossible. A few of the more aggressive students attempt to initiate such dialogues but these tend to be brief and fairly superficial in nature. Dialogues between individual students in class is now virtually impossible. All such communications tend to be mediated through the dialogues with the teacher. Both the number of rules and the difficulty of changing the rules increases once again. Even the teacher has great difficulty changing rules once they have been set without introducing major perturbations in the form of the structure and resulting in concomitant reductions in efficiency.

6. Small lecture. The distinction between the large class and the small lecture hinges upon the introduction of a new level of organization into the teaching structure—the discussion section. The teaching function now shifts from a monophasic to a triphasic process consisting of a lecture phase, a discussion-sections phase, and an administrative-meeting phase. During the lecture phase all of the students in the class meet simultaneously with the head teacher. During the discussion-section phase the total class is in effect divided into a number of smaller classes each of which is taught by a teaching assistant (*TA*). Finally, during the administrative-meeting phase the head teacher meets periodically with the TAs as a group for the exchange of information and the fine-tuning of rules, regulations, and procedures. Typically these three phases either alternate or are interlaced in some sort of complex temporal rhythm.

While dialogues between the head teacher and individual students and between individual students themselves is virtually impossible during the lecture phase, the possibility for such dialogues is reintroduced into the teaching process once again by the discussion-section phase. Now, however, the direct dialogue between a student and the head teacher is replaced by a dialogue between a student and the TA who is serving as a teacher-surrogate. The introduction of TAs thus constitutes a new hierarchical level in the organizational form of the teaching structure.

Within this more complex hierarchical form of organization are embedded analogues of some of the simpler forms of classroom organization. However, these simpler forms now appear not as functionally autonomous structures in their own right, but as functionally subordinated structures within the overall form of the larger lecture format. Thus, for example, the relationship between the head teacher and the TAs as a group is analogous in form to that of the simpler tutorial we considered earlier. Similarly, the form of the relationship between the individual TAs and the students in their discussion sections is formally analogous to that of the small class we considered earlier. However, the lecture format is not a mere agglutination of a previously autonomous tutorial with a set of previously autonomous small classes. Despite their similarities to these simpler forms these sub-structures within the overall lecture format are highly interdependent and subordinate constituents of that larger structure. The emergent nature of the lecture format is clearly illustrated by the fact that in this form of classroom organization the TAs serve a new function not previously re-quired of any of the participants in either the tutorial or the small class: namely, they become epicentric regulators of one of the principal channels of communication between the students and the head teacher. As such they have more power in determining the form and function of the macroscopic whole than they did when they themselves were students in a tutorial, and a different, more limited kind of power than did the head teacher when he or she was serving as the sole teacher of a functionally autonomous small class. Thus, for example, the TAs can now take an active part in the rule-making procedure through a process of dialogue and consensus with the teacher and the other TAs on the one hand, and with their own students, on the other.

Once again, however, most of the rules must be set before the structure actually begins to function. This is because once it begins functioning the structure has, owing to its sheer mass, a momentum of its own. Any signifi-cant change in direction may therefore result in a major perturbation that may markedly reduce the functional efficiency of the structure as a whole.

7. Large lecture.   The large lecture has all of the features of the small lecture plus one additional feature: Another hierarchic level is introduced into the organizational form of the structure—a chief TA who serves as an administrative assistant to the head teacher. All of the trends we have previously noted continue to this level. Here, however, the form of the rela-tionship between the head teacher and the chief TA is now formally analogous to that of the teacher to the student in the simpler individual directed student (cf. Fig. 1.1).

Two Provocative Questions

This detailed examination of the distinctive functional characteristics of various forms of classroom organization raises two provocative theoretical questions. First, what kinds of dynamic processes determine the upper and lower boundaries of the steady-state range of population size for any given form of organization? In other words, under what kinds of conditions or constraints should we expect such boundary phenomena to appear? Second, why is it that certain kinds of reorganizations of the form of a given structure result in an increase in both the functional efficiency and the formal stability of that structure, even when the content and the basic function of that structure remain the same? In other words, why does it help to shift from one form of structural organization to another? The following two sections address these two questions.

UPPER-BOUNDARY PHENOMENA OF THE STEADY-STATE RANGE

As we have seen, certain functional characteristics of the classroom structure changes as that structure shifts from one form of organization to another. From the dynamic point of view, however, the most interesting phenomena take place in the vicinity of the upper and lower boundaries of that range since it is these boundaries which, by definition, mark the points of transition from one form of organization to another. In describing these boundary conditions it is useful to begin by considering the concept of formal saturation.

The Concept of Formal Saturation

The concept of *formal saturation* derives from the basic assumption of the present work: namely, for any given form of structural organization with respect to any given function of the structure as a whole there exists some maximum number of constituent parts at a given level of analysis whose individual activities can be optimally integrated with respect to that function. If its population increases beyond that number then the structure begins to exhibit both a decrease in the efficiency with which it serves that function and a decrease in the stability of its organizational form with respect to that function.

A *saturated structure* contains exactly that maximum number of constituents; an *unsaturated structure* contains fewer than that number. An unsaturated structure therefore retains the capacity to absorb, incorporate, or integrate additional constituents at that level of analysis without undergoing significant change in its macroscopic form or function while a saturated structure cannot. A *supersaturated structure,* on the other hand, contains more than that maximum number of constituents. It absorbs the stress caused by these additional constituents by undergoing a distortion of its organizational form. This distortion results in a decrease in the efficiency with which it serves its function. Despite these distortions, however, its basic form, that form which defines it as a particular type of structure, remains unchanged. Finally, an *undersaturated structure* contains too few constituent parts for optimal functioning—its organizational form is too elaborate, or too complex for the number of constituent parts it is intended to integrate with respect to its intended function.

In summary then within each steady-state range there is a region within which the structure is unsaturated. In this region growth can take place without any concomitant process of formal development. In the regions of supersaturation and undersaturation, on the other hand, further increase or decrease in population size, respectively, will bring the structure to a developmental crisis point—that is, to a point beyond which any minor quantitative changes in the indicated direction (e.g., any further increase in population size) will result in a major, qualitative transformation in organizational form (cf. Brent, 1978b).

What kinds of changes take place in the form and function of a structure as its population first approaches and then surpasses the upper boundaries of the steady-state range? From the formal point of view, the most striking of these changes is a loss of cohesiveness.

The Concept of Structural Cohesiveness

The transition from mere saturation to supersaturation is characterized by the gradual loss of structural cohesiveness. The concept of *cohesiveness* refers to the degree to which the form and function of each microscopic constituent part of a structure is in fact interdependent with those of the other constituents and subordinate to the specific functions which that structure as a whole is intended to serve.

The concepts of functional unity and structural cohesiveness are of course closely related. The difference between them is primarily one of emphasis. When we speak of a loss of cohesiveness we emphasize the fact that although the unifying function of the macroscopic structure as a whole remains stable some of its individual constituent parts at some more microscopic level of analysis tend to exhibit a loss of interdependence and of subordination. Loss of unity, on the other hand, emphasizes a loss of that macroscopic integrating function itself. The relationship between loss of cohesiveness and loss of unity is thus one of degree. The degree of cohesiveness of a structure may be indexed by the proportion of its population that exhibits a loss of interdependence and subordination. When the loss of cohesiveness exceeds some critical value, the functional unity of the macroscopic structure as a whole is lost and the structure itself undergoes a process of disintegration.

Because supersaturated structures tend to exhibit both a loss in functional efficiency and a loss of cohesiveness, it is useful to distinguish between these two effects as well. Briefly, a *loss in efficiency* is indicated by the fact that the same amount of effort on the part of the teacher and the students results in a smaller amount of learning by the students; or, equivalently, a greater amount of effort on the part of the teacher and the students is required in order for the students to achieve the same amount of learning within the structure. *Loss of cohesiveness,* on the other hand, is in the simplest cases indicated by such facts as students coming late, leaving early, or missing class entirely; and the fact that while students are in class their attention tends to wander from the information the teacher is attempting to convey to them. A structurally more complex indicator of loss of cohesiveness is the tendency for epicentric subgroups to form within the overall classroom structure. In a large class or small lecture, for example, local groups of two or three students will begin talking to each other in audible whispers in such a way as to interfere with other students' ability to hear what the teacher is saying (cf. Fragmentation, below). This loss of cohesiveness characteristic of supersaturated structures can be partially counteracted by increasing the strength of those factors which help to maintain cohesiveness within such structures.

Factors that maintain cohesiveness. Cohesiveness is maintained by a variety of dynamic factors operating within a structure. Among the most important of these are those constraints which establish and maintain interdependence of the constituent parts of that structure with each other and their subordination to the whole. In the classroom situations for example, a constraint in this sense is any force, factor, or condition that restricts the range of activities exhibited by individual students when they are constituents of a particular classroom structure compared with the total range of activities they exhibit when they are functioning independently of any particular structure (cf. Brent, in press).

In classroom structures cohesiveness is generally maintained by two types of constraints: focalizing constraints and enveloping constraints. *Focalizing constraints* maintain cohesiveness by focusing the students' attention on the information the teacher is attempting to convey. *Enveloping constraints,* on the other hand, maintain cohesiveness by preventing students from leaving the classroom regardless of whether they are attending to the information the teacher is attempting to convey. Focalizing constraints include such factors as the students' interest in the subject matter itself, and the attractiveness of the teacher's particular teaching-style, and so forth. In addition, as we have seen in Fig. 1.1, various classroom formats increase the tendency of the students to focus upon the teacher. Enveloping constraints include such factors as closing the doors of the classroom once the class has begun; taking attendance; giving surprise quizzes; and so forth. We shall return to the significance of these distinctions shortly.

The Seminar-format under Saturated and Supersaturated Conditions

Let us examine once again the classroom structures we have just been considering. This time let us examine what happens when we hold the particular form of classroom organization constant while increasing the number of students in the class one student at a time. In so doing let us consider each of two cases separately: The first is the case in which there is no external limits on the maximum physical space available for expansion of that structure. The second is the case in which more and more individual students must fit into a fixed space so that population density as well as population size become critical factors in the evolution of the structure.

Let us consider next first the spatial and then the formal and functional characteristics of the seminar format under the saturated condition. How are those normative characteristics affected when population size is increased to a supersaturated condition?

The distinctive spatial characteristic of the seminar format as shown in Fig. 1.1 is a radially symmetrical closed form with all constituents—teacher and students—distributed more or less evenly around the circumference and facing "inward" toward the geometric center of the configuration. This spatial arrangement facilitates the efficient functioning of several distinctive characteristics of the seminar form: e.g., frequent face-to-face dialogue between the teacher and each individual student; frequent face-to-face dialogue between students; the ability of everyone in the class to know everyone else in the class by sight, and many by name; and active participation by all constituents in the process of deciding upon both collective goals and rules of procedure toward those goals. Let us imagine the kinds of changes that take place at both the macroscopic and the microscopic levels of analysis as we increase the number of participants in this seminar one at a time from 15 to 30 persons. First, in terms of its spatial configuration the sides of the closed spatial form become progressively flatter. As a result an increasing number of people can see the faces of those people who sit opposite them but not the faces of the two or three people on either side of them. Second all individuals sit farther from each other and farther from the teacher—i.e., across an increasingly wider open space—so that each participant must speak in a louder voice in order to be heard and move with larger or more intense gestures in order to be seen. Thirdly, because of the greater number of students in the class there is proportionately greater competition for the time available both to dialogue with the teacher and to dialogue with other students. All three of these factors, amongst others, serve: (a) to reduce the probability that any particular individual will have a chance to enter into a productive dialogue with anyone else in the class, (b) to reduce the amount of time that such a dialogue will last when it does occur; and (c) to favor more verbally aggressive students over those who are less so. In this seminar format dialogue between participants is the primary active form of functional interaction; listening to two other participants dialoguing or to one other participant—either student or teacher—present some organized body of material are the two most important passive forms of functional interactions. As the number of participants increases the ratio of passive to active interactions increases. Thus, as long as the seminar format is maintained an increasing proportion of individual students find it increasingly more difficult to focus attention on the processes taking place in the structure as a whole. Under these conditions loss of structural cohesiveness is, as we have already noted, manifested in such phenomena as students arriving late for class, leaving before the class has ended, doing homework for some other class while the seminar is in session, and carrying on local side conversations with some close neighbor while some other dialogue is being conducted by the class as a whole. Indeed, it is not difficult to imagine that if one attempted to maintain a seminar form of classroom organization with population sizes approaching 50 or more students such fragmentation would spread rapidly resulting in a concomitantly rapid drop in the functional efficiency of the structure as a whole.

Structural Responses to Supersaturation

A supersaturated structure is both formally unstable and functionally inefficient. Thus, still further increases in its population will eventually push it to a crisis point. At this point even a minor change in this quantitative characteristic may precipitate a major change in certain of its qualitative characteristics—i.e., its form, function, or contents (cf. Brent, 1978b). One means by which organic structures resolve this precarious condition and return to a higher level of stability is by partitioning the total population of the original supersaturated parent structure into two or more daughter populations, each smaller in size than the original population from which they all were derived.

Such a partitioning can be achieved by any one of several different processes. Each process results in a different final steady-state form of relationship between the daughter populations that it produces. Each therefore has different consequences for the subsequent development of the original population of constituents as a whole. In the present section we outline briefly four such restabilizing partioning processes: depopulation, fragmentation, fission, and differentiation.

Depopulation.   Depopulation is the simplest and the most form-preserving of the four processes we shall consider. Here the negative effects of supersaturation are counteracted by ejecting or in some way eliminating individual constituents from the structure until its population size is reduced to a level that once again falls within the steady-state range for its original form of organization. Thus depopulation in effect divides the original population into two subpopulations: those which are retained and those which are eliminated. Those which are retained assume once again the steady-state macroscopic form of organization characteristic of the original parent population. Those which are ejected are ejected as functionally autonomous individual microstructures with no stable formal relationship to each other or to the original parent population.

The population size of a supersaturated classroom, for example, may be reduced by encouraging or forcing some proportion of the students to "voluntarily" drop the class. A teacher whose class is greatly oversubscribed may, for example, give very difficult examinations or very heavy homework assignments during the first few class sessions in order to cull from the original population those students who are least talented or least motivated to do the intended work of the class. Once the population size has been reduced to within the steady-state range once again the teacher will then typically return to a form of classroom organization and a mode of classroom functioning that he or she originally intended for that class.

Fragmentation (disintegration). Depopulation consists in the intentional ejection of a certain number of individual constituents from the original parent structure. The form of that original parent structure is however maintained by those constituents which remain. Fragmentation, in contrast, consists in the spontaneous breaking up of that original structure into a set of daughter structures that are both smaller in population size and lower in the complexity of their organizational form than the original. Thus whereas depopulation is the most form-preserving of the four processes we shall consider, fragmentation is the least form-preserving. It is useful in this context to distinguish two functionally distinct types (or degrees) of fragmentation: fringe-area fragmentation and structural disintegration.

When a hierarchically integrated organic structure reaches a certain level of supersaturation some of those constituents furthest from its center of functional integration—i.e. those on the fringes or periphery of the structure—tend to form small, semi-autonomous, epicentric subgroups. These function within the boundaries of but are not entirely integrated into the organizational form and macroscopic function of the structure as a whole. I refer to this process as *fringe-area fragmentation* because it tends to occur most frequently near the periphery of larger structures. It can however in principle occur anywhere with such a structure. We encountered an example of such fringe-area fragmentation when we considered certain supersaturated classrooms in which students sitting at the back of the class began carrying on private conversations with each other while the class was in progress. In situations such as this the original parent structure continues to function with its original form in its normative way. The effects of fringe-area fragmentation, while disruptive, is not in itself destructive of the original parent structure. It thus tends to affect functional efficiency more than structural stability.

Structural disintegration, in contrast, refers to that process through which the functional unity and structural integrity of the original parent structure as a whole is entirely lost. This is most likely to occur when the center of functional integration itself (the nuclear core of the structure) is no longer able to serve its hierarchical, integrating function. In the classroom situation, for example, structural disintegration may occur when the teacher is, for some reason, no longer able to serve as an integrative focus for the class as a whole. In a college classroom, even a vastly overpopulated one, formal and functional disintegration would only occur under extraordinary circumstances—e.g., the unannounced failure of the teacher to appear in class for half an hour after the scheduled starting time of the class; or the intrusion into the classroom processes of intensely emotional but extraneous political debate and so forth. In some junior high school and high school classrooms, on the other hand, such fragmentation appears to occur frequently, even when the teacher is present and is attempting to serve his or her focalizing function within the structure of the classroom as a whole.

The result of such total disintegration is a heterogeneous collection of daughter structures that are smaller in size, simpler in organizational form, and (as a group) lower in functional efficiency than the parent structure from which they were derived. Indeed, owing to their loss of a stable macroscopic form, the resulting collection of fragments is most often no longer capable of serving those functions previously served by the parent structure as a whole. Therefore, disintegration is from the developmental point of view a regressive solution to the problems posed by the condition of supersaturation. Indeed, fragmentation represents a "resolution" of these problems only in so far as the resulting fragments tend on the average to be more stable in their form, function, and content than the original super-saturated parent structure from which they were derived.

Fission. Fission, on the other hand, is that process by which a parent structure divides into two or more daughter structures that, although also smaller in population size, are equivalent in organizational form to the parent structure. Thus, the distinctive feature of fission is that each new subgrouping of the original population is itself a functionally autonomous structure that, although at the same level of organization as its parent group, is smaller in population size—indeed, small enough to fall once again within the steady-state range for that original form. In times of economic well-being, for example, when teacher services are plentiful, it is common to set an upper limit on enrollment in a given seminar. When enrollment in the original seminar exceeds that upper limit then the student population of the original supersaturate seminar is subdivided into two or more formally similar but functionally autonomous seminars on that same topic. Each such daughter structure then has its own teacher, its own students, its own unity, its own integrity, and so forth. These autonomous seminars may then maintain some sort of loose functional relationship to each other or not, depending on the particular circumstances.

Differentiation.   Depopulation, fragmentation, and fission all cope with supersaturation by reducing in various ways the population of the over-populated parent structure. Differentiation, in contrast, attempts to cope with supersaturation by a structural reorganization and functional refocus-ing of the total original parent population, thereby maintaining the func-tional unity and structural integrity of that original macroscopic structure as a whole. In other words, the process of differentiation results in a for-mally new steady-state structure that, although identical in content, is within its steady-state range larger in population size and more complex in its organizational form than the original unsaturated parent population. In-deed it is specifically to this process that developmental theorists have tradi-tionally referred when they speak of the process of development (cf. Werner, 1957). It is useful in this regard to distinguish two basically dif-ferent types of differentiation: horizontal differentiation and vertical differentiation.

Horizontal differentiation results in the partitioning of the parent population into two or more subpopulations which then become reorgan-ized in such a way as to constitute formally distinct but functionally equivalent substructures within the basic organizational form of the original parent structure. For example, some teachers attempt to maintain the seminar format with supersaturated seminar structures by shifting from a single circular form to two concentric circles of students. This new form of organization effectively reduces the spatial dispersion of students, hence in-creases the functional cohesiveness of the total group. These two concentric rings, while formally distinct, play functionally equivalent roles within the overall function of the structure as a whole. This concentric-ring form of organization can be seen to be intermediate in its formal and functional characteristics between the simple seminar and the small class. A more com-plex form of horizontal differentiation occurs in the transition from a seminar to a large class form of organization (cf. Fig. 1.1).

Vertical differentiation, on the other hand, results in the partitioning of the parent population into two or more subpopulations that are functional-ly as well as formally distinct from one another. Vertical differentiation thus tends to result in more hierarchically organized daughter structures. Through vertical differentiation, the focalizing power of the functional focus of the structure is increased relative to those of the constituents. For example, the fragmenting propensities of a supersaturated seminar format may be reduced by increasing the concentration of attention-getting, focalizing power of the person conducting the seminar. This may be achieved by any one of several different formal means: for example, shifting from a circular to an oval or a horseshoe spatial-configuration with the focal person at the narrow or the opened end; the teacher standing up and pacing around while speaking; an increasing proportion of lecture over dialogue as a means of accomplishing the function of the group; and so forth. Indeed, any device that tends to give more power to one individual both as a focus of attention and as a source of functionally relevant information will tend to re-establish the cohesiveness of the class structure. However, with the emergence of this form of organization, the spatial configuration most appropriate to the seminar classroom format is no longer the most efficient. Since that arrangement allows the students to all face each other, it in fact detracts from the organizationally cohesive power now concentrated in the focal individual in the group. The transition from the seminar to the small class (cf. Fig. 1.1) is under these conditions both easy and natural. In the supersaturated seminar we have been considering, a form of organization intermediate between the true seminar and the small class is sometimes used. In this intermediate format the teacher as the integrating focus allows different individual students to occupy temporarily the position of attention-getting power (the narrow end of the oval) as a teacher-surrogate in order to present some portion of the information to be transmitted. Thus while only one individual at a time can occupy that position, the power resulting from that position is shared by the teacher with the other members of the class.

Elsewhere (Brent, in press) I've discussed in great detail the importance of the distinction between symmetrical and asymmetrical interactions for structural theory. Briefly, in the present context, one result of the increased inequality in the distribution of power among the various microscopic constituents in the class structure is a progressive increase in the number of asymmetrical relative to the number of symmetrical interactions that take place among constituents. More particularly, any person occupying the narrow focus of the oval will have a geographic positional advantage over all of the other constituents in the group. In addition, the teacher, who presumably possesses both the greatest amount and the highest quality of required and desired functionally relevant information about the subject, and, because of his or her social position as teacher, has a social positional advantage over all other potential occupants of that geographically dominant position, hence can usurp that position virtually at will.

Differentiation, fission, and fragmentation.   It is useful in concluding this outline of various kinds of reorganization to summarize the distinctions

I've made between differentiation, fission, and fragmentation. All three involve the attainment of greater efficiency and greater stability through the division of a previously homogeneous set of constituents within a supersaturated structure into a set of new, locally more cohesive subgroupings of those constituents. The distinctive result of the process of *differentiation* is that these new subgroupings remain subordinate in their form and function to the form and function of the same macroscopic structure of which their constituents were originally a part. That original supraordinate structure as a whole thus achieves a higher level of organization as a result of this process of differentiation. The distinctive feature of *fission* on the other hand is the fact that each new subgrouping is itself a functionally autonomous structure that is at the same level of organization as its parent group. They differ from that parent only in that each has a smaller and therefore presumably a more cohesive population for that original supersaturate form of organization. Finally, the distinctive feature of *fragmentation* is that the new subgroupings are by-and-large, or on the average, not only smaller in size but also at a lower level of organization than the parent group. In summary, then, differentiation results in formal and functional progression of the original structure; fission, in formal and functional reproduction of the original structure; and fragmentation, in formal and functional regression (cf. Brent, in press).

An Informational and Attentional Model of Classroom Cohesiveness and Efficiency

The primary function of the classroom structure as we have defined it above is the exchange of various specific kinds of information between the teacher and the students. The cohesiveness and the efficiency of each form of classroom structure is thus limited by both the amount and the quality of the information that can be exchanged between the two under various forms of classroom organization. These two parameters—amount and quality of information—depend in turn upon both the signal-to-noise ratio of the means used for the exchange of information between teacher and students, and the attentiveness of each communicant to that information being transmitted by the other.

Quality of information and attentiveness to it are closely related. This relationship derives from the fact that as the information being received becomes degraded in quality the receiver of that message must pay increasingly closer attention to the message in order to be able to extract the same amount of information from it. One of the limiting factors determining the maximum class size for any given form of organization may thus be presumed to be the ability of both the students and the teacher to pay enough attention to the messages being transmitted to them to extract an adequate amount of information from those messages. However, as the channels become more degraded in quality more and more attention is required to extract the same amount of information.

What then is the relationship between class-size and quality of information in the spatially-expandable structures that we are currently considering? In a classroom structure direct information exchange and cohesiveness are maintained primarily by means of two channels of communication: visual and verbal. Increasing class size increases the degradation of the information received over these two channels by increasing the average distance between the teacher and the students. Increasing distance contributes to a degradation of the information received in two ways. First, for any given level of energy (for example a given volume of speech) projected by the source to the receiver, the level of energy actually received by the receiver from that source will decrease approximately as a cube of the distance between the two. This rapid weakening of the transmission signal itself tends on the average to decrease the signal to noise ratio, hence the quality of the information received. As we have already noted, one means available to each listener to compensate for this loss of signal quality, hence to increase the quality of the information received under a given set of conditions, is to be more attentive to what is being transmitted. Ironically, however, as the average distance between the transmitor and the receiver increases, the number of distractors to the listener's ability to attend to the message being received also increases—in this case by about the square of the distance between them. In summary then these two factors—the quality of information received and the ability to attend to that information as it is received decrease with increasing size of an expandable class. The solution to both of these problems is then to find various means to increase either the quality of the signal being sent from the teacher to the students, or to increase the ability of the student to attend to the teacher, or both. A number of devices are typically used in a teaching situation to achieve these ends. In large lectures, for example, mechanical devices such as microphones and overhead projectors help to increase the intensity of the auditory and visual signals respectively, hence to compensate to some extent for the loss of quality owing to increased distance.

However, the central question of the present paper specifically concerns the relationship between growth (change in structural size) and development (change in organizational form). Therefore, from the point of view of developmental theory, the device that is of primary interest is the reorganization of the form of the classroom structure itself. Indeed it is specifically an attempt to understand the way in which increase in size drives the reorganization which has been the principle focus of our considerations in this paper. In these considerations we have focused on the format of college classrooms to illustrate some of the basic principles involved. We may now ask how general these principles are.

EXTENSIONS AND LIMITATIONS

The two basic tenets of the present model are, of course: (a) that as the size of a structure approaches the limits of the steady-state range of population size for a particular form of organization the means of *interconnectedness* amongst its constituent parts begin to decrease in efficiency; and (b) that the shift to a different form of organization is then driven by an attempt to regain both *a more stable form of organization* and *a more optimal level of efficiency* with respect to some particular function. Our examples so far however have been restricted to consideration of the effects of increases in population size on the organizational form of classroom structures. In those structures the primary means of interconnectedness among constituents is the visual and verbal exchange of information. In this concluding section I summarize briefly the extension of the basic model to other types of organized structures and to those modes of interconnectedness appropriate to each of those structures. I also indicate what I see as the limitations of such extensions.

Other Social Structures

Extension of the present model from the classroom structure to other types of social structures appears quite clear. The work of Steiner (1955, 1972), for example, suggests a direct and immediate extension to the task-oriented small groups traditionally studied by social psychologists as well as to the dimension of interpersonal perceptions amongst members of such groups. Steiner's argument is interesting in this regard in that it is based on the assumption that as groups increase in population size, it is specifically the degradation of the channels for the exchange of *interpersonal* information that drives the shift from an individualistic to a role-determined form of group organization.

On a still larger scale are recent models for the evolution of urban centers as a function of population size. These models are based upon the assumption that the interconnectedness among the individual constituents of such centers depends in part upon the movement of high energy resources into each center and the movement of low energy waste products out of the center (e.g., Allen & Sanglier, 1978; Brent, 1978c; Prigogine, 1980). When the population which depends upon this system of transportation increases beyond a certain size, an increasing strain is placed upon the carrying capacity of the system. It is then in part this degradation of the systems of transportation which necessitate the evolution of more complex forms of macroscipic social structure—neighborhoods, wards, cities, counties, regions, states, multinational corporations, and so forth. While these processes may differ in many mechanical details from those described for the simpler classroom structure many of the basic constraints govering the relationship between change in population size and change in organizational form appear to be similar in the two cases.

Enveloping Versus Focalizing Constraints

We noted earlier two basic types of constraints that help to maintain the cohesiveness of organized structures: focalizing constraints and enveloping constraints. The classroom structures we have explored in this paper were governed primarily by focalizing constraints. This meant that under pressure of increasing population size in addition to undergoing formal reorganization, the structure as a whole could also expand to occupy more space. As a result, while individual students within the structure had to change their external relationships with the teacher and with each other, those individuals themselves did not undergo any marked changes in their own individual forms or functions as a result of changes in population size. Enveloping constraints, in contrast, make it impossible either for the structure as a whole to expand or for individual constituents to emigrate from the structure to other regions of the environment. As a result one effect of increasing population in enveloped structures is to increase density of the microscopic constituents of the structure. Increased density increases the proximity of constituent parts to each other, hence increases both the frequency and the intensity of the interactions amongst those parts. This in turn results in increasing stress upon the formal stability and the functional efficiency of the individual microscopic constituents themselves. One limitation of the present model is, then, that it has not attempted to address the effects of increased population density, but only of increased population size, where density was assumed to remain relatively constant. Future work will have to expand the model in this direction.

It is interesting to note, however, that the research on the effects of overcrowding on animal and human social structures has thus far yielded ambiguous results. A classical animal study by Calhoun (1962, 1963) suggests that under such circumstances the social cohesiveness of communities of caged rats begin to break down entirely: Many individuals within such groups become extraordinarily anxious, aggressive, depressed, and generally maladaptive. Grooming, mating, and child-rearing become nonfunctional. From the developmental point of view such social fragmentation is of course a regressive change in organizational form. However, because of the special circumstance under which the animals were observed and the specialized nature of laboratory rats themselves, the generality of these results are unclear. Among humans, for example, it has been suggested that the Japanese adapted to the effects of increasing population pressure upon individuals with their social structure by both (a) increasing the restrictions upon each individual's physical and psychological life-space; and (b) developing a highly complex set of formal rules governing the relationships between individuals within this restricted space. The attempt to maintain the cohesiveness of a social structure by shifting to progressively more hierarchical structures, with more restrictions on each individual's freedom of action, and increasing reliance on fairly rigid formal rules is of course a phenomena we have already met with in our analysis of classroom structures, as well.[3]

The contrasting case to that of traditional Japanese society is North American society from the 16th through the middle of the 19th century. During this time when room for expansion appeared relatively unlimited compared with the rate of population growth, at the frontiers of expansion, there existed a relative absence of formal rules and of hierarchical structures empitomized by the proverbial "lawlessness" of the old Western frontier, in contrast with the growing formality of the increasing densely populated Eastern seaboard.

Undersaturated vs. Supersaturated Structures

While our general model postulates both an upper and a lower limit to the steady-state range for population size we have in this chapter given detailed consideration only to certain phenomena that occur in the vicinity of the upper boundary of each such range. An entirely different but equally interesting set of phenomena are associated with a structure characterized by a progressively shrinking population size. According to Tuchman (1978), for example, during the middle of the 13th century late Medieval Europe lost approximately one-third(!) of its entire population to the black plague in a matter of several months. The effect of this massive depopulation on the previously elaborate and formalized socioeconomic structure was so devastating as to mark the beginning of the end of feudal society throughout western Europe. A formally analogous situation would be that of attempting to use a lecture format (Fig. 1.1) to teach a class that had only 20 or 25 students. While we cannot explore the phenomenon of undersaturation in greater detail at the present time, one general principle seems quite clear: The relationship between population size and organizational form is, to some extent at least, a reciprocal one. Thus, just as a certain level of organizational complexity is required to maintain the cohesiveness of a structure that has a population of a particular size, so a certain minimum population size is required to maintain the cohesiveness and efficiency of a structure of some given level of organizational complexity.

---

[3]This was of course treated in some detail by Freud (1961). For a more recent ethological analysis cf. Leyhausen (1965/1973).

Extension to Non-Social Psychological Structures and to Non-Psychological Structures

Thus far we have focused upon the relationship between the population size and the organizational form of various kinds and levels of social structure. In concluding this chapter, I should like to indicate briefly the extension of these considerations to non-social psychological structures and to non-psychological structures.

One simple and classical non-social psychological example is provided by the traditional studies of masses-vs-distributed practice in skill learning. Massed practice may be taken as analogous to rapidly increasing population size, where population size is defined as number of times a skill has been practiced. During the early stages of practice, marked improvement appears (unsaturated structure), but gradually an asymptotic level is achieved (saturated structure). If practice continues beyond that point a decrement in performance can frequently be observed (supersaturated structure). If, however, a fallow period intervenes, then after the end of the fallow period a new level of competence is exhibited that involves a much higher level of integration of the previously practiced skill than was exhibited on the last practice (new, more complex level of organization). At this new level new practice sessions (additional population) can now be added.

At the linguistic level a given form of sentence structure—a simple sentence, let us say—can only contain a certain number of words. As the number of words in the sentence approaches some limit, the cohesiveness of the ideas that the sentence is intended to convey begins to break down; the interconnectedness amongst its constituent parts become progressively degraded. If, at the appropriate point, one switches to a new form of linguistic organization—e.g., two simple sentences, or a single complex sentence; then the cohesiveness of the whole can once again be established. (Katz & Brent, 1969).

Similarly, the same general relationship between increase in structural size and increase in organizational form can be observed with respect to various levels of cognitive structures—be they simple concepts or elaborate scientific theories. If we consider the population of such a structure to be the number of distinct empirical facts that it can integrate within a single explanatory framework, then we can readily see that any given concept or theory has only a finite number of such constituents that can be incorporated within its organizational form without exhibiting a loss for formal stability or a loss of functional efficiency. The reason for this seems quite clear. Each additional instance or fact includes two components: One component is that whose variance is accounted for by the existing structure; the other is that source whose variance is not accounted for. It is the latter, the residual variance, which tends to accumulate with increasing populations, and the accumulation of this residual, unaccounted empirical variation is the driving force for the evolution of new and more complex forms of cognitive organization.

One striking non-psychological example of the relationship between change in structural size and change in organization form is provided by the work of Eigen and others on the evolution of complex information bearing and information using molecules such as DNA and RNA (cf. Eigen et al., 1981; Kuppers, 1975). Here, too, we see that for given forms of molecular organization, there is a maximum length that a molecule can obtain without jeopardizing the reliability of its informational capacity. Increases beyond that maximum length become possible only with the emergence of new, more complex forms of organization.

SUMMARY AND CONCLUSIONS

For any given form of structural organization there is a range within which population size can vary while the organizational form and the functional efficiency of that structure remain relatively unchanged. I refer to this as the steady-state range of population sizes for that particular form of structural organization. As the population size of a structure approaches the upper or lower boundary of that steady-state range there is a tendency for the inconnectedness among its constituent parts to become degraded in quality. The net effect of this degradation is a gradual loss of structural cohesiveness and a concomitant loss in the functional efficiency of the structure. The kind of interconnectedness that exists among constituents and the kinds of degradation that occurs in those interconnections vary with the form and function the structure itself. Three general principles therefore define the present analysis of the relationship between change in populations size and change in organizational form: (a) the postulation of the existence of some such interconnectedness in all organized structures; (b) the occurrence of a degradation of that interconnectedness as population size approaches the limits of the steady-state range for a given form of organization; and (c) the regaining of formal stability and functional efficiency through a reorganization of the form of the structure itself.

REFERENCES

Allen, P. M., & Sanglier, M. Dynamic models of urban growth. *Journal of Biological and Social Structures,* 1978, *1,* 256.

Brent, S. B. Organizational factors in learning and remembering: Functional unity of the interpolated task as a factor in retroactive interference. *The American Journal of Psychology,* 1965, *78,* 403–413.

Brent, S. B. Linguistic and nonlinguistic processes in serial learning and in retroactive interference. *The American Journal of Psychology,* 1967, *80,* 133–137.

Brent, S. B. Linguistic unity, list length, and rate of presentation in serial anticipation learning. *Journal of Verbal Learning and Verbal Behavior,* 1969, *8,* 70–79.

Brent, S. B. Individual specialization, collective adaptation, and rate of environmental
change. *Human Development,* 1978, *21,* 21–23. (a)

Brent, S. B. Motivation, steady-state, and structural development: A generalization of
Stagner's homeostatic model. *Motivation and Emotion,* 1978, *2,* 299–332. (b)

Brent, S. B. Prigogine's model for self-organization in non-equilibrium systems: Its relevance for developmental psychology. *Human Development,* 1978, *21,* 374–387. (c)

Brent, S. B. *Psychological and social structure: Their organization, activity, and development.* New York: Springer Publishing Co., in press.

Bryant, P. J., Bryant, S. V., & French, V. Biological regeneration and pattern formation.
Scientific American, 1977, *237* (No. 1), 67–81.

Calhoun, J. B. Population density and social pathology. *Scientific American,* 1962, *206,*
139–148.

Calhoun, J. B. The social uses of space. In W. B. Mayer, & R. C. van Gelder (Eds.), *Physiological Mammology I.* New York: Academic Press, 1963.

Eigen, M., Gardiner, W., Schuster, P., & Winkler-Oswaitsch, R. The origin of genetic information. *Scientific American,* 1981, *244* (4), 88–119.

Freud, S. *Civilization and discontents.* New York: Norton, 1961.

Katz, E., & Brent, S. B. Understanding connectives. *Journal of Verbal Learning and Verbal
Behavior,* 1968, *7,* 501–509.

Kuppers, B. The general principles of selection and evolution at the molecular level. *Progress
in Biophysics and Molecular Biology,* 1975, *30,* 1–22.

Leyhausen, P. Social organization and density tolerance in mammals. In K. Lorenz & P.
Leyhausen (Eds.), *Motivation of human and animal behavior; an ethological view.* New
York: Van Nostrand, 1973. (Originally published as "The communal organization of soli-
tary mammals." *Symposia of the Zoological Society of London,* 1965, *14,* 249–263.)

Prigogine, I. *From Being to Becoming: Time and Complexity in Physical Sciences.* San Francisco, Ca.: W. H. Freeman and Company, 1980.

Steiner, I. Interpersonal behavior as influenced by accuracy of social perception. *Psychological Review,* 1955, *62,* 268–274.

Steiner, I. *Group processes and productivity.* New York: Academic Press, 1972.

Tuchman, B. *A distant mirror.* New York: Knopf, 1978.

Werner, H. The concept of development from the organismic point of view. In D. Harris
(Ed.), *The concept of development.* Minneapolis: University of Minnesota Press, 1957.

2 Piaget, Vygotsky, and Werner

Joseph A. Glick
CUNY Graduate School

INTRODUCTION

Developmental psychology is at an interesting period of its development. Transitions, or apparent transitions are everywhere. The Piagetian enterprise is under attack, Vygotsky is being vigorously rediscovered, while for much of the field, Werner, if he is known at all, is accorded a somewhat nostalgic and esoteric position. There are signs here and there that Werner's contributions to the analysis of symbol formation are increasingly cited (e.g., Bates et al., 1979), and equally significant signs of disappearance (e.g., the decision to drop the chapter on Werner from the upcoming edition of Carmichael's Manual). This chapter is motivated by the conviction that Werner's essential insights have yet to be assimilated by the field, and that, at least, another pass at exergisis and adapting the position to a changing field is warranted.

In order to accomplish this task it is essential to understand in some depth the essential nature of the intellectual currents in the field, and to readdress, in the same spirit, the unique contributions that those of us who have lived with and followed Werner can yet provide. There are a number of ways of approaching this task. The way chosen here is to seek out the "root metaphors' (Pepper, 1942/1970; Reese & Overton, 1970) or "epistemes" (Foucault, 1973) or "paradigms" (Kuhn, 1970) that current theoretical positions seem to be operating with, and to compare theories at the level of the presuppositions that they embody in their theoretical discourse. It is my conviction, and I hope it will be the readers by the end of this piece, that at the level of theoretical deep structure, Werner's unique message has not yet been heard.

The method adopted here is based on a conviction that current understandings of the competing claims of theories in developmental psychology (and indeed in psychological theory more generally) have failed to fully recognize fundamental facts about the ways in which theories operate. It is not until one sorts out the complexities of the relationship of theory to a field of concrete interest, that one can come to a clear evaluation of the importance of the theory for our understanding.

The most basic level on which theories exist is the claim to offer understanding about some process or set of processes that characterize some topic of interest. Thus, we can say that all competing developmental theories have some degree of relationship insofar as they propose to offer an account of the topic of "development." On some level we might inquire of such theorists as Piaget, Vygotsky, and Werner what news they have to offer us about the way in which development (whether it be ontogenetic, cultural historical, or more broadly orthogenetic) occurs.

Yet upon close examination of this standard of theoretical accountability, there is considerable uncertainty about whether this level of theory is more a concern of the consumer of theoretical knowledge than it is a concern of the producer of knowledge (the theorists themselves). As consumers of theory we often start with some "natural object" of interest, such as the child, and inquire of various theoretical positions what they have to tell us about the processes of the child's development, affective development, etc. And, to be sure, various theoretical positions seem to offer us more or less direct answers to these questions. One can collect the various theoretical propositions and address them to the topic of our concern. Yet one might fairly ask whether this process of collection (upon which the ability to compare the adequacy of the theory to the phenomena of interest is based) is fully warrented. Indeed we may question whether the "seeming" commensurability of theoretical enterprises is more apparent than real.

Theories of development are often the battleground for differing conceptions of the nature of man. They are motivated by questions that lie far beyond the attempt to gain descriptive adequacy with respect to the unselected empirical facts of development. More deeply, the "facts" that theories deal with are pieces of data that are produced by the theory. Thus, there are, in the experimental approach, operations that tap behavior within a narrow band of possibilities, and put constraints upon the responses that would be considered to be of theoretical relevance. Those theories that do not opt for a narrow experimental approach nonetheless similarly select just what in the range of the world's phenomena will be taken as matters of particular importance. The recognition of the selective nature of developmental theory invites an analysis that looks directly at the nature of the selection process, as a deeper level of understanding of what different developmental theories are all about.

When one examines developmental theories in this way, it becomes clear that differing theories are in some basic way incommensurate with one another. Different ranges of phenomena are taken as topical, and with the different phenomena different sorts of theoretical mechanisms adequate to their explanation come into play. Confusion is generated when theories are compared in terms of the mechanisms without at the same time understanding that the range of phenomena (the "facts") to which the theory applies is also different.

Consideration of theories at this level of analysis is an attempt to identify the "conceptual object" of the theory. It is an attempt to precisely identify just exactly what the theory is a theory about.

Piaget, Vygotsky, and Werner have been chosen as targets of this sort of analysis because the conceptual objects that these theorists deal with delimit quite nicely the current, and immediately future boundaries of developmental psychology. This should not be construed as a claim that these theories in total are adequate—rather only that they indicate directions at the heart of our inquiry. Nor, should the device of comparative analysis be interpreted as a direct comparison between the theories. For, indeed, if the conceptual objects of the theories actually differ, then the theories are in some fundamental way incommensurate.

But there is a way in which theories can be, and indeed often are compared. And this turns us to the other side of our discourse—that inquisitive news-seeking side of us. For after all, many of us want to know about the "natural object" of the theory. While theories do not totally converge on the same natural object, they may each come to rest upon one that suits our comparative interest as some portion (great or small) of their news-seeking activities. And it is here, at the perspective of the natural object that some comparisons might be made, and rival candidacies for our theoretical affections be sorted out. Since one of the premises of this volume concerns Werner's place in developmental psychology, it seems not unreasonable to begin our inquiry with respect to the adequacy of the various theories to be considered, to the investigation of the child.

Such a conceptual move may seem like heresy to those whose training stressed the ideal-constructive nature of developmental theory, and were always careful to differentiate between developmental psychology and child psychology (a stand—in for the distinction between the ideal-constructive nature of developmental theory and the mere empiricism of studying children in all of their manifestations). Werner too expanded his inquiry beyond the facts relevant to children in order to orchestrate (in the *Com-*

parative Psychology of Mental Development, 1948) evidence from a wide variety of sources to build the notion of a developmental theory not completely exhausted by child-lore.

To objections I can only answer in two relatively straightforward ways. First, I do not attempt to totally identify developmental psychology and child psychology. The two are indeed different. Yet in seeking a point of comparison between developmental approaches, some axis of comparison must be siezed or else we are forever proclaiming incommensurability (a la Pepper or Reese and Overton), solving our own needs for purity and helping anyone in the field who does not share our refined notion of the relation of developmental and child psychology, not at all. Second, and this is more directly on target, while developmental psychology and child psychology are not to be fused, they are not to be radically separated either. It would indeed be tragic news if a general developmental theory did not relate in particular to the development of children. To the extent that development is a more embracing conceptual category than child development, it should be richer than, but not different from the less embracing concept. To believe otherwise would be to reconstruct within our field the radical Platonic separation between the world of ideas and the world of experiences.

One further note on this issue. If it be grudgingly accepted that there is some relationship to be found between the child and the concept of development I would not expect that relationship to be post hoc or trivial. It is not merely that the child is another instance *to which* the concept of development might be applied. Rather, the child should be richly informative to the developmental theorist. For if one believes in the organismic assertions of Werner's thought, then all of the phenomena that are to be investigated are to be investigated in a richly contexted manner. By this I mean that the nature of the organism is of considerable concern to the comparative organismic theorist.

Stated otherwise, the concern here is that a theory embody in its conceptual approach some manner of recognizing and dealing with the phenomena of "completeness" that organisms show. The completeness condition is simply a way of recognizing that human organisms are multiform, multileveled beings, blending splendid rationalities and equally splendid incoherences. A developmental theory that attempts to meet the minimal criterion of descriptive adequacy would have therefore to embody concepts that can allow us to understand the variety of the human condition. Such a theory would fail to the degree that in its attempt to be clear and explicit, it proscribed its domain of interest to only a small and nether part of the organism's being in the world. On these monumentally simple premises much is to be built. Not the smallest edifice to be constructed is an enlivened and renewed sense of the importance and current relevance of Werner's thinking.

What follows is an attempt to identify the underpinnings of the system of developmental psychology constructed by Piaget, Vygotsky, and Werner, and their core colleagues. For each of these positions, some attempt is made to identify the conceptual object of the theory and to compare that conceptual object to what we would like to know about the child. My stand-in for "the child" is not a theoretically refined notion, but is rather one that should naively appeal to our intuitions about what knowing children might be like. To the extent that my appeal to "what everyone wants to know about the child" is theoretically biased, it is so in the direction of the picture of the child that emerges from Werner's comparative *and* organismic theory. I find that having roots, while somewhat an embarrassment for someone pretending to do comparative analysis, is nonetheless an inescapable and ultimately somewhat satisfying condition.

PIAGET

The conceptual problem that Piaget set out to solve has deep roots in the Western philosophical tradition. In many respects, his solution to this problem is brilliantly achieved on a theoretical level. Moreover, his work has generated an enormous amount of research and has served as one of the axes around which the developmental world has turned. Indeed there is almost no book in developmental psychology that does not touch down at some point or other on the seminal contribution of Piaget.

However, applying the rudimentary conceptual apparatus of separating the conceptual object of his theory from what may be our concerns about the natural object to which the theory has been applied, yields a rather surprising appreciation of this state of affairs. It seems to me that a great deal of the excitement has been generated for the wrong reasons. Piaget's conceptual problem solution has been taken by much of the community of theory consumers as a deeply informative description of the way that children are in the world. I am not sure that Piaget ever intended this to be so, but we must cope with it.

The problem addressed by Piaget is a critically important epistemological problem—the relationship between experience and the characteristic forms of rational thought. The particular conceptual problem was to solve the issue posed by Plato and Aristotle over the relationship between experience and ideas. As Plato posed the problem "how can we gain stable (eternal/necessary) ideas from experience which is contingent, changeable, and distorted." As Aristotle posed the issue "Accepting that Plato has identified the characteristics of ideas (eternal/necessary) how can we form a relationship between rather than just draw a line between, these ideas and experience." All of this is heady stuff; about ideas and experience, but is it necessarily about children? The child is, in a theory of this sort (or more precisely a theory that takes this sort of problem as its conceptual object) a *site* wherein the conceptual problems are located, rather than a topic of inquiry in its own right. The child is the natural object within which the conceptual object is located. We should not conflate the two. It may very well be the case that the conceptual problem may be brilliantly solved chez l'enfant, without at all informing us very much about the nature of the child that the conceptual problem is visiting.

In Piaget's theory the child is a stand-in, for a stage whereon a drama relating experience and form is played out. Piaget was attempting, as did Aristotle, to reconcile two antagonistic concepts; contingent experience and logical form. As did Aristotle, he held the fundamental Idealist position of accepting form as the problem to be explained, and as did Aristotle posited that experience and form must somehow be linked—rather than radically separated.

This constraint shows up well with regard to Piaget's notions of evoluly to a conceptual tactic of subordination of the facts of development to a critique which seeks their candidacy for explaining the primary problem, viz, the development of logic. In this spirit then, the Piagetian discourse always returns to its basic question format. Distinctions between organismic functional systems are made (e.g., between perception and cognition or language and cognition) in the service of attempting a developmental explanation of the growth of logic; and more particularly the growth of logically necessary judgments. The basic point, made in almost any part of the theoretical discourse that one engages (save the earliest works where a more naturalistic, descriptive approach is taken), is that a separate system (the organizational function) is required to account for the development of logical necessity, and is to be distinguished from those systems which give us merely adapted empirical or figurative knowledge of the world. While in the later works some relationship between figurative and operative aspects of knowledge is sought, the ultimate problem that remains is to find that class of mechanisms that will account for logical form. Experiential inputs to the process, in even the later theory, seek relationships of similarity of form (morphisms) between empirical experience and logical forms.

The theory then, in sum, puts selection pressure on the range of phenomena that it considers as relevant to its enquiry. The selection pressure leads to a narrowing of the range of phenomena to those that seem most capable of relating to the development of logically necessary judgements. Thus, only determinate systems can be addressed (e.g., those systems having sufficient internal connectedness so that their logical form is manifest) and this from the point of view of how the ostensive "contents" of these systems are transcended by a mind that reflectedly abstracts its own underlying order and goes beyond the simple abstractions that reflect the surface organization of content. Mind is seen as perennially disengaging concrete experience from its "underlying form."

If the problem is to provide for the conditions of the possibility of transcendent forms of thought that surpass intuitions at every turn, the Piagetian model of inquiry is quite successful. The bridge between experience and form is neatly handled by the notion of reflection operating upon action. Since action can be the same while the contents differ, it has the required characteristic of being something that is engaged with the world of experience and yet importantly goes beyond it (as it was for Plato, perception is rejected as a source of knowledge because it was "too related" to empirical knowings). Reflection on the patterns of action then could account for the growing transcendent properties of thinking. This is a brilliant solution to the classic idealist problem. But it is not a brilliant solution to the enriched descriptive, or ethnographic knowledge of the child.

In an actual world, for an actual actor, action is thick with its meaning (Geertz, 1973). It is constrained, working within a field of perceptual, cultural, and symbolic differentiation. Some combinations are routinized and preferred, and it is a matter of considerable importance for people to do things right in culturally acceptable ways. Thought and action in culture are not free—they are constrained—precisely by those things that give us some tangible sense of culture, and social life. Thus, in some important way, the transcendent notion of mind developed within the idealist tradition is fundamentally acultural. With Hegel we can, through such an idealist history, only aspire to God through history (the idealist problem) and paradoxically never to history itself. As with history, so with development.

This constraint shows up well with regard to Piaget's notions of evolutionary change. While some have likened Piaget's position to Lamarck's, this is an overdrawn likening. In rejecting classical Darwinian-Mendelian theory, Piaget was fighting against the idea of a history for the organism that was truly open to historical (and hence unconstrained) influence. For Piaget it was essential to fight against the idea of random variation perpetuated by ecological selection. Such a process would not allow for the development of stable "logically necessary" forms. Hence there must, in the account of evolution, be some essentially conservative forces that keep the process in a steady line of development toward an ideal end state. The steady engagement of behavior and its physical constraint provide just such a mechanism for Piaget.

Where this all differs fundamentally from Lamarck is in the conception of the experiential history in universal rather than particular historical terms. An historically particular account would seek some particular behavior, constructed for some requirement at hand (at a particular point in time and in a particular context), which would be perpetuated intergenerationally. This conception would of course, not lead to universal logical forms. Piaget preserved the notion of organism-environment interaction as a central aspect of his account of development, but gave it the sort of twist necessary to meet the Idealist requirement. For Piaget the environment interacted with is constrained by Universal laws (e.g. those of physics), which operate through all possible encounters. Thus history is given a universalized interpretation that aligns it more with the laws of physics than with particular experiences. If this is Lamarck, it is so in a totally unusual sense; past experience does not differ from present experience in any appreciable way. Accordingly, Piaget can treat historical factors in a manner quite consistent with the need for an epistemological absolute that could guarantee a universal logical development, historically conditioned.

This view of historical interchange serves to differentiate the Piagetian view from the Marxist view as well. For Marx, history was to be differentiated in terms of particular arrangements of production relations. For Piaget there are no significant qualitative differences between modes of production, since all production is ultimately contrained by an eternal, law-governed nature. Thus, in Piaget we can find a surface commonality with both dialectical notions of either the idealist (Hegel) or materialist (Marx) genre. But the treatment of the primitive terms of the dialectic serve to differentiate it from either of these views. A dialectical relationship between universalized forces (physics/the nervous system) is ultimately compatible to the idealist position—with the caveat of an interactional history added. The upshot of all of these considerations is that Piaget has constructed a theory of what he had set out to construct a theory of. But, most importantly that theory must be differentiated from the sorts of theories that attempt to deal with the qualitative variations among actual individuals. Piaget's individual is treated from the standpoint of epistemology of a particular sort, alternate epistemologies, or alternate non-epistemological standpoints on the life and times of children do not fall within the main purview of Piaget's work.

If a developmental theory is needed that can account for the possibility of there being a "transcendent" rationality, then Piaget's account of development is eminently satisfying. The human mind does, to the extent that science connects us via rational processes with underlying and non-intuitively available features of an actual world, subordinate ordinary experience to intellectual construction. A developmental psychology, focusing on that monumental achievement of human thought is clearly a part of what we should want to know about. Yet scientific achievement is to some extent a rarified actuality, coexisting with (often in the same individual), human processes of a fundamentally different sort. A theory of the organism that does justice to the forms in which we find human organisms will have to introduce terms that have a different characteristic than those developed by Piaget. For transcendent though we (some of us) might be, we are, at the least, more than that.

VYGOTSKY

The work of L.S. Vygotsky is known to us mainly in the form of two books: "Thought and Language" and "Mind in Society." Unfortunately for the sort of analysis that I am attempting here, these books are sufficiently different from one another so as to make the problem of conceptual analysis quite difficult. There are indeed some overriding conceptual notions that unite the two books, but there are as well sufficiently strong differences to lead to some tension. While all of the writing in the books is Vygotsky's (and hence written in the 1920s and 30s) the construction of the first book ("Thought and Language") is Vygotsky's own (though assembled from separate papers as he was terminally ill). The second book is a construction from several sources, skillfully orchestrated by editors, but accordingly with no warrant that the whole of the book fulfilled Vygotsky's criteria of wholeness. It may then be that the tensions of focus between "Thought and Language" and "Mind in Society" reflect the somewhat mixed provenance of the pieces that construct the books. Indeed, it may even be argued that the second, constructed book is a selection designed to make the book maximally compatible with current trends in the fields of education and cognitive developmental psychology. It is perhaps the case that in this process several of the underlying generative ideas have been muted.

This interpretive uncertainty is of some importance here in that the distinction between Vygotsky I and Vygotsky II is important for assessing the relationship of Vygotsky's thought to Werner's. Indeed the comparison of Vygotsky I and II is in part a measure of the conceptual distance that the field has traversed (if the Vygotsky II reconstruction is taken as symptomatic of the current field), and hence provides a measure of the distance that we must traverse in recognizing the position of Werner vis a vis current trends in the field. I shall, in fact, argue that Vygotsky I and Werner are quite close in some respects, and that the distance increases immeasurably by the time that Vygotsky II has been reconstructed.

In "Mind in Society" (Vygotsky II), the underlying conceptual object appears to be the identification of the manner in which sign systems transform organism-environment relations and the means by which mind becomes socialized. This is depicted by the editors (and by Vygotsky in embedded quotes) in the following manner (Vygotsky, 1978):

> The specilization of the hand—this implies the tool, and the tool implies specific human activity, the transforming reaction of man on nature...the animal merely uses external nature, and brings about changes in it simply by his presence; man, by

his changes, makes it serve his ends, masters it. This is the final, essential distinction between man and other animals.'' Vygotsky brilliantly extended this concept of mediation in human-environment interaction to the use of signs as well as tools. Like tool systems, sign systems (language, writing, number systems) are created by societies over the course of human history and change with the form of society and the level of its cultural development. Vygotsky believed that the internalization of culturally produced sign systems brings about behavior transformations and forms the bridge between early and later forms of individual development. Thus for Vygotsky, in the tradition of Marx and Engels, the mechanism of individual developmental change is rooted in society and culture (Introduction p. 7).

This influence is at first interpersonally inculcated and later "internalized.'' Thus, we emerge with the fundamental picture of development as the importation of socially constructed representational systems and other instruments via processes of learning that are initially interpersonally guided (as in schooling and parent-child and peer interactions).

In addition, we are exposed in "Mind in Society" to important insights with respect to both method and evaluation of capacities. The editors point out, and Vygotsky exemplifies, the importance of "process oriented" approaches. With this sort of method, which the editors point out shares deep similarities with Werner's genetic approach, the objective is to place the child in a situation beyond his or her current capabilities and to document the manner in which the child assembles him- or herself to meet the demands of the task. In this process, both the child's intrapersonal efforts, and interpersonal seekings for help are included in the data base. This notion is extended with profound consequence to the issue of capacity evaluation, wherein a process oriented approach (Zone of Proximal Development testing) is substituted for standardized approaches to the evaluation of capacity (e.g., IQ tests and the like).

This version of Vygotsky selects and reinforces some portions of Vygotsky's approach already visible in the "Thought and Language" book. Without yet focusing on the differences between the two books, it is important to see what the selection process has done in placing Vygotsky at the center of current psychological inquiry.

There are, I believe, several main currents in the field today. First, there is a fundamental rejection of what might be called the "fixed capacity" model. This model views development as the progressive acquisition of abilities that are somehow possessed by the organism under investigation. Development then would be seen as the march (either orderly in the Piagetian sense or unorderly in the Empiricist sense) of these capacities through ontogeny. Under the aegis of this model, developmental investigation becomes the uncovering of these capacities and then asking questions about their orderly or non-orderly relationship to one another.

As these questions have been asked we have received only muddled and confusing answers. Accordingly, there have been vigorous attacks on this model. Some of the attacks have attempted to supplement the notions of capacity (understood as some underlying structure) with the notion of skill or metaskill that governs the application of capacity to a problem at hand. The hope is that by distinguishing the two levels (skill at application, and structure to be applied), some greater order can be introduced. As this strategy has been increasingly adopted, the burden of experimental performance shifts from the child alone (confronted in splendid isolation with a task) to a more interactive or shared responsibility between investigator and child—where it becomes increasingly the problem of the experimenter to alter features of the testing procedure so as the tap into the child's skill level (or what some have called the child's cultural knowledge) to more fairly reveal what there is to be revealed. This view of the problem, initially articulated at a methodological level, has come increasingly to alter our notion of development. The unit of analysis shifts to the interpersonal level, to the problem of "negotiated sharing" of the culture of the experiment, and the theoretical items that enter into this equation become things that are called, "world knowledge," "cultural knowledge," "interpersonal exchange," "skills," and possibly "structures" (now understood as at least entering into some compound with the other terms of the analysis).

In opposition to the idealist view of things, this new approach represents a fundamental paradigm shift. In many respects this shift is, in my own opinion, salutary. The notion of method becomes more dynamic, more sensitive to ethnographic surround, more process and context oriented. And indeed, many of these features of method lie within Werner's approach albeit in underveloped form.

The problems, however, to which these methods are beginning to be applied are perhaps as dry as those addressed by the more idealistically oriented theories. For in many respects the modern version of the application of these methods (as represented perhaps in the work of leading "cognitive developmentalists" and "information processing analysts") seems to be framed within the context of the kind of questions raised by Piaget and his school. The target of the analysis seems largely to be the sort of issues raised by Piaget concerning intellectual structure considered from the point of logic. What has merely happened is that the tasks (or their variants) have been taken over, and readdressed with a new armament of concepts and terms for analysing performance on these tasks (e.g., Siegler, 1981). Thus, in some fundamental way methods of approach have changed, but the underlying topic of the method remains stable. We have shifted from structure to task, and its socialized nature.

In "Thought and Language" we find Vygotsky asserting the same sorts of methodological issues as in "Mind in Society," but the focus of the inquiry is fundamentally different. In "Thought and Language" the underlying conceptual problem is the relationship that exists between socialized systems of mediation and the individual's reconstruction of these in an interior, and perhaps not fully socialized way. The major conceptual problem is the relationship between "inner" and "external" speech (a topic that receives little explicit consideration in "Mind in Society").

The driving idea behind the "inner speech"–"external speech" differentiation is that the individual develops from an initially undifferentiated state (egocentric speech) to one where there is increasing distance between thought (inner speech) and communication (external speech). If this relationship is taken as topic, then it becomes clear that there can be no simple socialization of the mind. While environmental input initially provides mediational systems, the organism operates upon these by progressively matching *and by progressively mismatching* to those systems. Indeed, if the message of "Thought and Language" is heard clearly, it follows that there must be some input to the developmental equation that allows for the private constructions of the organism to stand in an essentially dialectical relationship to the socialization pressures on thought and action. This is heard all the more strongly when we listen to Vygotsky's repeated assertions that the unique "private" characteristics of thought progressively develop their uniqueness in the course of development (Vygotsky, 1962):

> In our conception, egocentric speech is a phenomenon of the transition from inter-psychic to intrapsychic functioning, i.e. from the social, collective activity of the child to his more individualized activity. . . . Since the main course of the child's development is one of gradual individualization, this tendency is reflected in the function and structure of his speech (p. 133).

> Our investigation established that the traits of egocentric speech which make for inscrutability are at their lowest point at three and at their peak at seven. They develop in a reverse direction to the frequency of egocentric speech. While the latter keeps falling and reaches zero at school age, the structural characteristics become more and more pronounced (p. 134).

It is also clear from the surrounding text that Vygotsky is not arguing for a disappearance of the structurally different private organization at the age of seven. It is only the external form that allows us to see (in egocentric speech) the structural peculiarities of internal speech, that disappears. The implication of this is that our private meanings remain problematic throughout development, and may even increase in their internal peculiarities throughout development.

The upshot of these considerations is that the Vygotsky of "Thought and Language" does not fully use a socialization model of mind. Rather, there are developing antagonistic strains that serve to pit internally organized private meanings and thoughts with publically available means of expression in an essentially dialectical relationship. These strains come together in Vygotsky's treatment of the development of word meanings.

> The leading idea in the following discussion can be reduced to this formula: The relation of thought to word is not a thing but a process, a coninual movement back and

forth from thought to word and from word to thought. In that process the relation of thought to word undergoes changes which themselves may be regarded as development in the functional sense. Thought is not merely expressed in words; it comes into existence through them. Every thought moves, grows, and develops, fulfills a function, solves a problem. This flow of thought occurs as an inner movement through a series of planes. An analysis of the interaction of thought and word must begin with an investigation of the different phases and planes a thought travels before it is embodied in word (p. 125).

Without belaboring the point it seems clear to me that the conceptual object of Vygotsky's treatment of development is not a socialization model of development. Rather the conceptual object of "Thought and Language" is the dialectical relationships that exist between individuals and societies. The focus is on the relationship between internal organization and external form in the creation and realization of meanings. This view bears deep affinities to the work that Werner and Kaplan have pursued in "Symbol Formation."

However deep the affinities, there are equally deep differentiations between the approaches. It appears to me that when Vygotsky gets down to cases he is really after that array of abilities that we now call "cognitive." Accordingly, the hints that he gives us about the nature of internal organization (e.g., his representation of individuality) are somewhat murky. On the one hand, he seems to talk of expressive, affect laden, ineffabilities, and on the other he uses predication as the model of our innerness. The predication model suggests that our innerness is made up of predicates without their surrounding sentences. This view is compatible with a notion that inner experience is a truncation of, but not a different sort of thing than, outer experience and expression. If inner speech is predication, then it is perhaps not a fully adequate model of the internal organismic state of affairs.

It appears to me, naively now, as a consumer of theories about children, that there is much more in a child than his or her cognitions. While the theory of predicates may be bent to dealing with more than coding operations in cognition, that thrust is not fully developed in Vygotsky's own writings. The "what more there is in the child" has to do with emotions, perceptions, even convincing irrationalities, that are, for me, more the province of the child as a fully ethnographic subject; and is a topic that could be developed from the Vygotsky of "Thought and Language."

It is on this point, more than any other, that despite the deep affinities between Werner and Vygotsky, they divide as distinguishable theorists.

WERNER

Formalizations of Werner's theory may be found in several sources, so I will not try to repeat them. Rather, I would like to focus on what I believe to be the generative ideas within the theory. What follows is a compendium of reading, memory (both academic and personal), and a rechewing of ideas as I have tried to locate them in my own, different looking, psychological work. This treatment may, perhaps, be at variance with various formalizations of Werner's system. My feeling is, however, that though Werner's thought was indeed systematic, it is not the sort of system that is brought neatly into formalization without considerable loss of insight.

It is the part that escapes formalization that is perhaps the most interesting. What is underrepresented in all of the formalizations of the theory is the identification of its criterial feature—its standpoint for analysis. It is the standpoint that serves to most profoundly differentiate Werner's thought from most others.

Throughout Werner's seminars on language development, an important distinction kept reemerging; the Humboldtian distinction between language as Ergon and language as Energaia. Roughly translated this distinction refers to the differences between looking at the problem of language from the viewpoint of analyzing it as a structure (with corresponding lists of semantic features, syntactic devices, pragmatic types, or whatever) and analyzing language as an embodied moment of meaning located both in the organism and in the medium that the organism uses for expression. Language as Energaia is language at the moment of its use, at the moment when it is shaped as the bearer of an intended meaning in a medium that can display that meaning in public. It is language alive, in an actor.

This distinction, so important in Werner's treatment of language, is what I find characteristic of Werner's psychology as a whole. His conceptual object is not something that can be held "out there" and studied merely as either "form" or "code." It is rather an attempt to represent in one dramatic moment the innerness and shaping characteristics of psychological organization.

This fundamentally fluid and dynamic view of the nature of psychology represents enormous problems of relating to a field that is organized in other terms—a field that is organized, and organizes its seeking for information in terms of things that can be held "out there," disembodied from their generating internal and external contexts.

The depth of this chasm can be sensed by examining Werner's treatment of the proper way to look at the development of various psychological functions. The separable categories of function, e.g., language, perception, cognition, etc., are seen by Werner as having achieved separableness in the course of both ontogenetic and microgenetic development. They are forms of functioning that have been "autonomized". _made_ separate—in the course of development. They do not exist in earlier form as things already separate. Thus, in seeking a developmental analysis of such things as language, perception, cognition, etc., the standard tactic of looking for earlier manifestations of the separated function is denied. Thus, what for the field are topics, such as "early language development" or even "language development" are for the Wernerian approach non-topics. The topic has been inverted. It is rather the separation of language from a more primordial soup of affect, perception, and the like that serves as the theoretical topic. And, inevitably, along with the problem of differentiation comes the problem of accounting for the preserved connection between the separated functions and their organismic base.

The connection is preserved within the theory by focusing on the dialectical process of moving through planes that Vygotsky talked about in "Thought and Language." For even at more advanced levels of autonomization the autonomization is achieved through a microgenetic process. In a manner analogous to Vygotsky's treatment of the dialectical relationship between inner and external speech in a process of shaping in a medium, one can preserve both the notion of autonomization and the notion of a rich organismic grounding. Even autonomized forms are worked through in a process linking surface to base, product to process, in a moment of organization, with the materials at hand. This conceptualization radicalizes our view of psychological processes so that they must always be understood in their process terms; as Energaia rather than in their product terms, as Ergon.

The task of uniting process and product, and orchestrating the various organismic strands that coalesce into a process, required a fundamentally new theoretical language—a language that did not freeze itself into a mold appropriate only to a segregated function. The theoretical medium is found in a language that is amenable to cross-modal and cross-functional relationships, belonging to none and appropriate to all; the language of dynamic, vectorial forces, and a structural language that was not composed of entities of structure (e.g., operations), but of states of connection and organization (differentiation and heirarchic organization).

Throughout his writings, in almost any sphere of inquiry (from sensoritonic field theory, to the dynamics of binocular depth perception, to the work on symbol formation), there is a consistent opting for a vectorial language; a language of forces, of dynamic tendencies. This sort of language functions in much the same manner as Gibson's language describing stimuli in terms of functions and transformations, it allows for the development of an amodal, functional treatment which can have general intrapsychic (and extrapsychic) application. A dynamic, physiognomized language is the necessary tool of the organismic theorist. Not uninterestingly it is also the language of intimate experience, art and metaphor. Our inner speech is not only predicative, it is dynamic and physiognomic as well.

It seems to me that the theoretical task that Werner most often set for himself was to deploy the physiognomic, vectorial language as a tool to analyze the relationship between various functions and their organismic basis, in process terms. It is this feature which perhaps makes the Wernerian insight so elusive—difficult for the field to assimilate and difficult sometimes to communicate. For this approach offers no less than a paradigm shift from a language of separated functions, analyzable in ordinary and/or clear technical terms, to a language of organismically interacting systems analyzable in a special physiognomized language necessary to the purpose. In this world of theory, developing functions do not have clearly segregatable histories. Segregation and connection are taken as the problem, and history re-writes itself at various levels of connection within the organism.

In a similar manner, the structural claims of Werner's theory are only loosely specified. The general notions of increasing differentiation and hierarchic integration exist as loosely specified notions. Their function in the theory is heuristic. The precise specification of differentiation (what is differentiated from what) and integration (what precisely are the modes and manners of subordination) are left to be specified in the particular case. The adherence to the loose form of the theory is clearly intended to allow developmental formulations to embrace a wide variety of phenomena without being overly specified or too closely adapted to any kind. However the structural language also reinforces the organismic language within the theory. The intent is to represent wholeness, and as well, to point out clearly that the later developed organized and separated functions are achieved in development rather than pre-existing.

Looked at in this way, Werner's theory is not a theory at all. It is rather an heuristic stance toward phenomena. It remains in all cases to be specified as the heuristic is applied to a set of phenomena at hand. The particular terms of explanation will of needs be particularly adapted to individual cases. The general theory is an assertion that a wide ranging set of considerations will apply to that specification, and that the theory cannot be identified with structures (e.g., operations) of a particular sort. If the structural language was to be specified in the manner that Piaget did, for example, then the theory would itself constrain the kinds of developmental phenomena that it could deal with. There is a trade-off here between precision of particular description and an heuristic looseness.

All of this difficulty is accepted because of the attempt to keep preeminant the notion of organismic wholeness. This is, indeed, the tactic by which Werner attempted to align the conceptual object of his theory with the natural object within which it resides. For, at heart, the organismic assertion is an assertion that there should not be a distinction between the two.

There is a very deep irony in all of this. The theoretical tactic that makes the representation of wholeness in relationship to parts the theoretical problem to be solved, involves the organismic theorist in a stance that serves no separate him from the field, which is eager to know about the "whole child" but is only prepared to listen to the news as a catalogue of its parts. Perhaps this explains why Piaget, who has, perhaps, the least to say about the child as a natural, ethnographic, or "whole" being, is so much listened to; why Vygotsky, when treated as a stand-in for the socialization theory of mind, is listened to, and Vygotsky when he is grappling with the organism's relationship between public and private parts of self is not; and finally, why Werner, who took the problem of organismic wholeness as the center of his inquiry, has to be rediscovered.

As partisans, the task before us is one of mounting an attack on the category structure of the field that we wish to have listen to us. We must begin to turn traditional formulations on their head. As an example, there are a number of people who are concerned with the splitting off of our understanding of the child. They express this concern by asking questions about the relations of affect and cognition, cognition and perception, culture and mind, and the like. These questions deserve organismic answers, but require reformulation. We might begin to pose the issue as "how, out of global experience, do such things as affect and cognition seem to become separate, and how do they preserve their developmental connection?" If these questions are turned on their heads we shall be able to reassert that the problem is really the linkage between the whole and its parts, and not the linkage between already segregated parts.

There is work along these lines already. While it may not yet use an organismic or recognizably Wernerian language, it nonetheless shares the essential perspective. We can recognize our allies, and potential allies, by asking about any piece of work, "What standpoint does it take?" "Does it share the view that the proper place to begin is with an organism in the process of acting, and does it share the view that the categories for analysis of that action are achieved, and segregated in the course of the action itself?" "Does it share the view that the proper view of the child is as "Energaia-ist" and not a child divided Ergon-ically into one that can only live in the taxidermist's shops that our current books and journals are?"

Our friends are those who are beginning to understand the importance of context as a determinant of behavior. We must extend our notion of context to include external context (whether it be an expressive medium, an historical era, a social organization) in clearer terms than we have heretofore. And we may enlighten our allies about the considerable insights that the analysis of interfunctional relationships at different developmental levels can give to the analysis of the effects of context (inner context).

These tasks are not easy. In writing this chapter, I convinced myself again that whatever the difficulty the job is well worth doing. It is refreshing to think again of a child with some confusion in it, with a task before it somewhat like ours; to find a place for our wholeness in a world, and to make our meanings clear.

ACKNOWLEDGMENTS

This chapter was initially presented in somewhat altered form at Clark University, June 2, 1981.

REFERENCES

Bates, E., Begnini, L., Bretherton, I., Camaioni, L., & Volterra, V. *The emergence of symbols: Cognition and communication in infancy.* New York: Academic Press, 1979.

Foucault, M. *The order of things.* New York: Vintage, 1973.

Geertz, C. *The interpretation of cultures.* New York: Basic Books, 1973.

Kuhn, T. S. *The structure of scientific revolutions.* 2nd ed. International Encyclopedia of Unified Science, Vol. 2 no. 2, Chicago: University of Chicago Press, 1970.

Pepper, S. C. *World hypotheses: A study in evidence.* Berkeley, Calif.: University of California Press, 1942/1970.

Reese, H. W., & Overton, W. F. Models of development and theories of development; in Goulet, and Baltes (Eds.) *Life span developmental psychology: Research and theory.* New York: Academic Press, 1970.

Siegler, R. S. Developmental sequences within and between concepts. *Monographs of the society for research in child development,* 1981, 46 (2 Serial No. 189).

Werner, H. *Comparative psychology of mental development.* Chicago: Follett, 1948.

Vygotsky, L. S. *Thought and language.* Translated and edited by E. Hanfmann & G. Vakar. Cambridge, Mass.: MIT Press, 1962.

Vygotsky, L. S. *Mind in society.* In M. Cole, V. John-Steiner, S. Scribner, & E. Souberman (Eds.). Translated by M. Cole and M. Lopez-Morillas. Cambridge, Mass.: Harvard University Press, 1978.

3 Genetic-Dramatism: Old Wine in New Bottles

Bernard Kaplan
Clark University

INTRODUCTION

In his magisterial work, *Metaphor and Reality,* the philosopher, Philip Wheelwright, commenting on an observation by Remy de Gourmont, says:

> To speak forth honestly is to report the world as it is beheld (however precariously) in one's own perspective. Things have contexts, but only a person has perspectives. The essential excuse for writing, then, is to reveal as best one can some perspective that has not already become ordered into a public map (1962, pp. 15f).

Were I to abide by Wheelwright's rationale for writing, I would in one sense, stop here: The perspective I shall advocate is already on the public map, and has been on it at least since the time of Aristotle. Indeed, one might almost say that it is the public map. It is, I submit, the perspective almost all of us adopt in our daily lives: when we participate as agents or actors in various social settings; when we seek to understand and assess the actions of others and to justify our own; when we drop our specialized, limited and transient role of the impartial value-free observer, and catch ourselves as we actually live our lives in society. On the analogy of the "perennial philosophy," one might say that what I here call Genetic-Dramatism is the "perennial perspective."

Why then write about it for this occasion in a paper directed towards developmental psychologists when everybody, or almost everybody, uses a variant of the genetic-dramatistic perspective in everyday transactions? My rationale for such an exposition here is three-fold. First, the fact that one adopts a perspective does not entail that one is reflectively aware of doing so; I want to make psychologists aware of the fact that they do so use it. Second, many who call themselves "developmental psychologists" explicitly promote "theories" of human action and human development (especially the action and development of others than themselves) that they implicitly repudiate in their everyday life transactions in society, even in laboratories where they collaborate with others; I want to call attention to this inconsistency (see Kaplan, 1982; Kaplan, this volume). Third, through this and other papers, I hope to contribute to a fundamental, a radical, re-orientation of developmental psychology in the United States and elsewhere; a re-orientation that will make human development the central concern of all psychologists and will lead to the dissolution of artificial political and cultural boundaries between developmental psychology, social psychology and clinical psychology.

Before I outline my interpretation of the perennial perspective, the interpretation I have dubbed Genetic-Dramatism, I would like to allude briefly to some of my sources of information and inspiration, both recent and ancient. Only subsidiarily, as far as I am aware, do I do this to identify myself with potent voices from the near or remote past.[1] My principal reason is to *orient others* to these sources: first, to enable them to get a much fuller treatment of developmentalism and/or dramatism than I can possibly offer here, or might be able to offer, even with world enough and time; second, to suggest rich treasures of information, insight and subtlety for those who are stimulated by my formulation of the approach to go beyond it and *develop* it; and third, to absolve those whose ideas I use in my exposition from any responsibility for the ways in which I interpret their ideas, while yet crediting them with the general ideas I have borrowed from them.[2]

Among the sources of which I am focally aware, the most recent are Heinz Werner and Kenneth Burke. It was from Werner (1957) that I took over the genetic or developmental perspective, and with him that I worked to modify it so that the idea of development was disentangled from ontogenesis, phylogenesis, etc., and elevated to a standard for assessing events in time. It is perhaps of some interest that one of the factors that led to the formulation of "the orthogenetic principle" (Werner & Kaplan, 1956) was Kenneth Burke's animadversions on the "temporizing of essence" (1945/

---

[1]My discussions with Leonard Cirillo, especially with regard to the significance of Burke's writings, have made me painfully aware of the extent to which academicians (including myself) invoke the "names of gods" to inflate and "legitimize" undertakings that may have little to do with those "gods." Projects that might be regarded as trivial or inconsequential on their own merits are endowed, or intended to be endowed, with an aura of sanctity and significance through the invocation of the names of power.

[2]Although we may all be doomed to "misprision" in interpreting the work of others, or perhaps *because* we are, I want explicitly to distinguish my interpretation and use of someone's work from the work itself. I have been sensitized to this issue in recent years through reading radical misrepresentations of Werner's work by some who seem to have arrived at their views of Werner by being the last person in a rumor experiment.

1969, pp. 430 ff)—the tendency on the part of anthropologists, psychologists, psychoanalysts and others to take for granted that formal or structural differences in modes of mentation are manifested as a rule, or through necessity, in some fixed sequence of stages over time.[3] The intent of the "orthogenetic principle" was to disentangle "essence" from "existence," and to suggest that the idea of "levels" or "stages" pertained to the *meaning of development,* and was neither derived nor derivable from the vicissitudes and contingencies of actual existence.[4] Once "development" as ideal was distinguished from ontogenesis as actual, it was apparent that whether, and under what conditions, specific individuals developed or regressed in the course of ontogenesis were empirical questions.[5]

It was also through my association with Werner that I began fully to appreciate that the concept of development ought to be taken to apply to the ways in which agents[6] utilized or constructed "means" for the attainment of "ends." Only those beings who could be construed as capable of utilizing different means for the attainment of invariant ends could be said to have the possibility of development.[7] Beings whose motions and alterations of motion were construed as determined or determinable solely by extrinsic

---

[3]The "temporizing of essence" is, of course, closely linked to the "temporalizing of the great chain of being" in the 17th and 18th centuries (see Lovejoy, 1936; also my paper *Strife of systems* in Kaplan, 1967/74/82).

[4]The failure to realize the distinction between the idea of development and the actualities of ontogenesis has led some psychologists to conclude on the basis of a limited number of studies that "there are stages" followed in ontogenesis; others, likewise on the basis of a limited number of circumscribed studies, that there are no stages in ontogenesis; and occasionally the same individual at different times to conclude now that there are and now that there are not stages. For a critique of the thesis that actual history or actual biography is "progressive" or follows a fixed series of stages, see Mandelbaum, 1971, Chaps. 11 and 12.

[5]Thus, there is no necessity that individuals will regress after a certain age, or for that matter, advance developmentally with age. In this life, contingent factors may occasion transient regressions even in those who are as a rule quite advanced in their functioning, and may allow for developmental advances in those who may otherwise function quite primitively (see Pollack, this volume).

[6]"Agent" is used here to refer to any being, individual or collective, that is taken to act and to utilize means in the service of ends. It is as legitimate or as illegitimate to talk of collectives as agents as it is to talk of so-called individuals as agents. Talking about any entity as an agent stems from the use of a perspective, a "metaphor," or what Burke (1966) calls a "terministic screen." There are, of course, psychologists whose terministic screen obliges them to deny agenthood to individuals, including themselves (see Lovejoy, 1922; Thurstone, 1960). And, of course, there are also some who would claim that what certain people call individuals are usually really warring collectivities of "roles" or "nuclear egos" or "mes."

[7]Werner and others have sometimes written as if acts or the products of acts could be characterized as relatively primitive or advanced in themselves. I have explicitly taken the position that "primitivity" etc. were terms applicable only to *means-ends relations,* and could not be predicated of an act, response, or production without a consideration of means-ends relations (Kaplan, 1966).

"causes" or "antecedent conditions" did not and could not develop; they could merely change.[8]

Within the Wernerian framework, therefore, we have development pertaining to the ways in which agents utilized means in the service of ends. If one differentiated the generic notion of means into acts and instrumentalities, and made explicit what was tacit for Werner, viz., context or scene, we had the famous pentad of Kenneth Burke's *Grammar of Motives:* agent, act, scene, agency (or instrumentality), and purpose. Now, obviously, it was not Burke's pentad, in its nudity, that interested me. As such, the pentad merely corresponds to the familiar questions of the reporter, "Who, What, Where-When, How, and Why." It was rather Burke's scintillating handling of his "grammar of motives" to illuminate and clarify the most complex human behavior, not only as represented in the works of literature but as exemplified in everyday life.[9] Despite the divergence in their specific interests, there was no doubt in my mind that there was a close kinship between Werner's enterprise and the Burkean undertaking. Unwilling to admit impediments to the marriage of true minds, I have for more than two decades wedded Burke to Werner in my teaching and insinuated Burkean notions in some published articles (see Kaplan, 1967; Wapner, Kaplan, & Ciottone, 1981; Wapner, Kaplan, & Cohen, 1976). In here suggesting a new title, Genetic-Dramatism, for the integration of the Wernerian and Burkean points of view, I explicitly give Burke a status equal to Werner in my vision of a developmental psychology for the 1980s.

From the less recent past, there are other major sources: the Chicago school of John Dewey (1929, 1934, 1938) and George Herbert Mead (1934, 1936, 1938), on one hand, and Ernst Cassirer (1946, 1953, 1955, 1957, 1963) on the other. And, from the nineteenth century, both the critical idealists and the critical (dialectical) materialists (see Bernstein, 1971; Hughes, 1977; Mead, 1936; Taylor, 1979). Behind these 19th century movements, the Renaissance neo-Platonic tradition, so brilliantly explored by Cassirer (1963) and by Jackson Cope (1973) with regard to its emphasis on the theatrical or dramatic model for comprehension of human existence. And

---

[8]It is fascinating to observe how many psychologists, even those who take themselves to be "developmentalists" in a Wernerian, Piagetian, or psychoanalytic sense, strive to show that "ontogenetic changes," that is, historical changes in individuals, are strictly determined by extrinsic "causes" or conditions, and can, in principle be predicted. Such extrinsic determination is characteristically reserved for others; the investigator himself/herself takes his/her beliefs, modes of reasoning, etc., as the results of autonomous acts of an agent (See Bakan, 1965). It is as if the First Critique of Kant is applicable to others, while the Second and Third apply to oneself. A subtle treatment of this complex issue is provided by L. W. Beck (1975).

[9]See Burke, 1972. (Also, H. Dalziel-Duncan, 1968a, 1968b; Hyman, 1964.) For works explicitly indebted to Burke, see F. Fergusson, 1953; 1957; 1961; 1968. See also Brissett and Edgley (Eds.), 1975. Burke's influence is clearly apparent in a wide range of works in sociology, ethnolinguistics, and sociolinguistics.

behind them all, remote and yet ever-present, the "master of those who know," the progenitor both of "developmentalism" and 'dramatism'—Aristotle—who, in Burke's terms, was "anima naturaliter Dramatistica" (1972).

I shall, in what follows, discuss first development; then dramatism; and finally the unitary perspective of Genetic-Dramatism.

DEVELOPMENT: GENESIS IN GENETIC-DRAMATISM

Although the notion of "development" that I propose here may seem strange to those enmeshed in contemporary developmental psychology, it is not at all a strange conception to many throughout the world, nor is it a novel one. In many societies, the process of *development,* in contradistinction to the process of mere change, is a movement towards *perfection,* as variously as that idea may be construed. Among hermeticists and occultists, this view of development is embodied in the maxim, "Become what you are." One is said to develop only insofar as one moves in the direction of realizing one's full potentialities. "Development," so to speak, is the "curse" or obligation placed upon "souls" or "selves" incarnated in bodies to become the God, in whose image they were made. Had we not had to suffer incarnation, there would be no need for "development." Once embodied, however, we are under the obligation to struggle *in time* to attain whatever degree of perfection we can. Not that the passage of time or the events occurring in time insure development. In this struggle to become what we are, we all suffer contingencies of various kinds—physical, chemical, biological, interpersonal, social, etc.—that do work or may work to prevent us from moving in the direction of perfection, and that may even lead us to fall from whatever level of perfection we have attained. These "contingencies" may block us from enlarging our perspectives, our ways of envisaging the world; they may block us from increasing our knowledge, of ourselves as well as of what is not ourselves; they may set limits to our power, circumscribing our autonomy; they may incline us to malevolence towards others, rather than 'good will' and love for others. On the other hand, some of these "contingencies," in providing obstacles we have to confront and overcome, may provide the stimulus by which we become transformed; they may function as "ordeals" which, if we pass through them, enable us to advance toward higher levels of perfection.

Surely, some of you will find what I have just said too theosophical for your taste. Such views may be music for mystics, but have little to do with the way we scientific moderns view development. Well, let us see if that is so. Let us see if our implicit theory of development is so far removed from this perennial way of looking.

Do I assume rightly that all of us admit the possiblity that some individuals are more advanced than others: either as full-blooded persons, or considered in terms of some abstracted aspect of human functioning? Do we not all acknowledge, in our practices if not in our preachings, that one individual may function in toto at a higher level than another? May attain a higher level of cognitive development than another? A higher level of language development than another? A higher level of moral development than another? Do we not also speak as if a specific individual may, during one period of life as compared with another, manifest a higher stage of development with regard to personality formation as a whole; or with regard to any one of the abstracted and hypostatized aspects of human functioning to which we are inclined to attribute an independent reality?

I submit that most, perhaps all, of us acknowledge not only the *possibility* of such holistic or partitive development, but the actual occurrence of such progressions. To be sure, we may forcibly restrain ourselves from *talking* in this way, especially when we adopt the role, in circumscribed settings, of disinterested spectator or detached scientific observer; when we limit ourselves to recording and reporting "what happens and how"; when we anesthetize ourselves to differential values of different modes of thought and action (Schutz, 1973; Beck, 1975). But, in less guarded moments, when we are participants in research, teaching, therapy and a multitude of other activities, we cannot help *thinking* in developmental terms. In our very acts of criticizing our own work or that of others, we presuppose that certain modes of thinking are more advanced, more perfect, than others. In assessing the social transactions and interpersonal involvements of human beings—ourselves as well as others—we cannot escape assumptions—dogmas if you like—that certain modes of relating to persons are more advanced, closer to perfection, than other modes. Even if we jettison the received dogmas—doctrines if you like—with respect to higher levels of moral action and social interaction, we do not generally reject the idea of development in these domains; rather we engage in a transvaluation of all values, a *bouleversement complèt*. Thus, we may dismiss "mutuality" or "the categorical imperative" as representing a higher stage of sociality or morality than egocentric hedonism, but only to suggest that thought and action dominated by one's self interest, and irrespective of an impact on others, is now a higher stage of development. To be sure, we may not go quite that far in tilting the tablets: We may retain the usual notions of lower and higher forms of morality for the ordinary, average individual, introducing a new, higher stage to accommodate our own special transactions with others.

Again, in our pedagogical activities, surely we believe that the ways of thinking we try to inculcate in, or evoke from, our students are more advanced than, or at least on a par with, those the students bring with them. Our aim is not merely to change their ways of thinking, irrespective of direction, as if change per se were a value. Nor is our aim to induce an alteration in their modes of thought and action so that they will conform to the ways of thought and action of the majority of actual others in the society who happen to be older than they are, as if an increment of age had some intrinsic connection with development. Surely no one will deny, in our teaching and training activities that our aim is to maintain advanced modes of thinking in our charges or to facilitate the transformation of their ways of thinking so that they progressively approximate what we take to be the most *advanced* or perfected modes of thought.

I will cut the litany short. The same point can be made with regard to many domains of human action and transaction. In sum, my thesis is that even those among us who explicitly seek to determine the nature of "development" from empirical or experimental research tacitly presuppose, in their own transactions with others and attempts to change themselves, ideas of development in the sense of movement toward perfection; ideas that are in no way derived or deduced from empirical research or experimental inquiry. However these ideas have come to be instilled in us—ideas of lower and higher, less advanced and more advanced, regress and progress—they surely cannot be derived from the mere facticity of what is observed or from any knowledge of conditions under which phenomena come into being and pass away in the course of time. They belong to a different order than empirical or experimental inquiry. Their home, I submit, is primarily in the domains of axiology and eschatology: values and final ends.

In other words, I suggest that "development" in our actual practice, in our own transactions with the world, is a value, policy or normative notion, a *concept by postulation* rather than a *concept by intuition* (see Northrop, 1947). It is, if you like, a mythos in the sense formulated by Kerenyi (1963), or, *horribile dictu,* a dogma.[10] It is in terms of such a mythos, dogma, theory, perspective, etc., that we evaluate, assess, and seek to regulate human actions and transactions, including those we call inquiry. And it is in the name of such ideas of "perfection-development," however dimly held or vaguely apprehended, that we ostensibly advocate different forms of education, different forms of therapeutic intervention, different forms of inquiry, different forms of governance, etc.

Now, if the ultimate telos of human beings is to "become God," to become the perfected being, then it is obvious that no embodied individual has come even remotely close to attaining perfection. In the sub-lunar

---

[10]Myths like dogmas are foundational and cannot be further grounded. I use the term "dogma" to stress that many psychologists who express an aversion to dogma, dogmatically assume certain perspectives and methods. What they reject as dogma is that which builds on a different foundation than they do. See also S. White, 1978.

sphere, one can only speak of relative perfection, or less advanced and more advanced stages or levels of development.[11] Moreover, no single individual—even a Da Vinci or a Goethe—can expect to attain a relatively high level of development in more than a few of the various modes of action that human beings are capable of. Specialization, so important to the attainment of relative perfection in any one domain, works at the same time, within the human context, to abort the realization of the possible others we might have been. These relatively perfected others we might have been are incarnated in other bodies, not only within the circumscribed socio-historical order in which we participate, but also in other socio-historical communities located elsewhere in space and time, world without end.[12] The only way we can transcend the curse of specialization is to participate, imaginatively, cognitively, and affectively in these other perspectives or roles which might have been ours; through such participation in the diverse roles of members of our own social groups and the varied social groups outside of our time and our place are we able to come closer to the telos of development—albeit always at an infinite distance. Through bodily action, but mainly through the symbolic imagination and cognition, we can adopt an ever larger number of perspectives or roles while somehow yet remaining one. Some will be able to read in here the "orthogenetic principle," *defining* development as (ever) "increasing differentiation and hierarchic integration."

I trust it is clear from all this why I take ontogenesis to be neither coterminous with "development" nor likely to manifest development in any uniform or unilinear way. Ontogenesis—the actual life course of individual agents—is rather one field to which "development" as a normative notion may be applied.[13] And, with regard to this field, whatever time scale one uses,[14] the evidence is overwhelming that actual human beings manifest regressions as well as progressions, and often more of the former than the latter. Surely there is evidence from "billions and billions" (to use Carl Sagan's phrase) that inner or outer circumstances may lead even the most saintly among us to lapse into egocentric hedonism; even the most adept at formal operations to engage in "magical thinking;" even the relatively most perfect in any sphere to miss the mark. I return to this issue later, after my discussion of Dramatism.

---

[11]The metaphor of "stages" or "levels" is of course a component of the larger metaphor of ascent toward the highest. See E. Bevan, 1938.

[12]For a more subtle treatment of this issue than I am able to offer, see Yves Simon, 1980.

[13]The concept of "development" can be, and has been, widely applied to societies and nations construed as "agents."

[14]That is, whether one examines what takes place over a minute, an hour, a day, a week, a month, a year, a decade, a life time. For a discussion of time-scales in development, see Collingwood, 1957.

DRAMATISM

If the central theme of "development" is the *actualization of the ideal,* the main thrust of "dramatism" may be taken to be the *idealization of the actual:* The full interpretation of body movements, vocalizations, cries and whispers, as embodiments of meanings and values invisible to the corporeal eye.[15] Dramatism is, of course, only one method or one "terministic screen" for characterizing what takes place in human existence. Surely as the behaviorists and physicalists, from most ancient days, have demonstrated one can reduce all of the phenomena of the human world to matter in motion or some modern variant of that "metaphor."[16] But "dramatism" is the "screen" we are all likely to use tacitly, even in the process of seeking to persuade others to adopt a more astringent model or "metaphor" for the representation of human behavior. In utilizing "dramatism" to characterize the vicissitudes of human life, one employs analytic categories akin to those that inform the dramatist's art in his/her attempt to "imitate"[17] human action. One finds oneself living by the extended metaphor[18] implicit in Shakespeare's line: "All the world is a stage/And all the men and women merely players."[19]

Now, some of us may question whether "dramatism" is the model[20] or

---

[15]In writing this way, I do not intend to give either ontological or phenomenal priority to that "terministic screen" which leads to viewing all that happens in the universe in terms of matter in motion. This perspective or metaphor, partly derived from Hobbes' and Descarte's materialist epigones, leads to the dismissal of all higher orders of reality entertained by human beings as fictions or illusions, epiphenomena of material particles or physical energeis, the latter alone taken to constitute the way the world is. For critiques of this view, see Cassirer, 1946; 1953; E. Straus, 1963; Burke, 1966; N. Goodman, 1978; C. Turbayne, 1962.

[16]That it is a "metaphor" and not an unmediated reading of what there is has been emphasized by Turbayne, 1962. See also Kaplan, 1962; Black, 1962.

[17]I take over here Aristotle's conception of the function of drama. See Fergusson's (1961) edition of the *Poetics,* including commentary. Also R. McKeon, 1951.

[18]The idea that we live our lives in terms of myths and/or metaphors is a key thesis in Burke's perspective. It is also found in the work of Jung and his followers, in the writings of the exponents of myth-criticism and is implicit in Cassirer's work. One might seek Kant as the modern source, mediated through von Humboldt and the Romantics. See Burke, 1966; Cassirer, 1946; 1953; 1955; 1957; Vickery (Ed.), 1969. For a recent treatment, see Lakoff & Johnson, 1980.

[19]W. Shakespeare, *As You Like It,* Act II, Sc. 7. On the widespread use of this perspective or metaphor during the Renaissance and Elizabethan periods, see Cope, 1973. For more recent use of the metaphor in the human sciences, see Brissett & Edgley, 1975. Also Sapir & Crocker, 1977.

[20]I use "model" here only grudgingly, since it is now often used rhetorically to suggest something austere, precise, and scientific. It is important to recognize that the "limits of one's model are the limits of one's world." Models or "metaphors," like prisms, are valuable instruments as long as one recognizes them as instrumentalities for a certain purpose. It is when one takes the "facts" mediated through one's model as "the way things are" that models, etc., become hazardous to one's head. See Turbayne, 1962; Black, 1962; Whitehead, 1938; Burke, 1966.

metaphor we "naturally" or naively use for describing, representing and/or interpreting our *Lebenswelt*. Allow me, therefore, to put us through a catechetical exercise analogous to the one I used in exploring our tacit commitment to an idea of development entailing movement toward perfection. Do we, I and you, "mon lecteur, mon semblable," in our transactions with others, at least sometimes experience ourselves and others as *agents* engaged in certain *acts* for the achievement of certain *ends?* Sometimes in cooperation with each other? Sometimes in conflict? And do we not see these actions in the service of ends mediated by *agencies, instrumentalities, or means?* Ways or means of embodying the action? Do we not, further, see these actions or transactions occurring in, or with respect to, contexts or *scenes?*[21] Scenes sometimes visible, sometimes invisible or "imaginal?" Sometimes, perhaps rarely, a single, circumscribed scene; sometimes, perhaps often, several different, overlapping and conflicting contexts?

Moreover, are we not aware, on reflection or in adopting the spectator-at-a-distance role, that there is a dialectical relationship among the differentiated components of a situation: that how one interprets the goal affects how one interprets the agent, actions, instrumentalities and scenes? How one interprets the actions (or "defines" them) is interconnected with how one characterizes the agent, the goal(s), the scene(s), the instrumentalities? That the "same" pattern of movements for one agent and/or with respect to one scene signifies a different action than for another agent and/or with respect to another scene? That, as our conception (interpretation, representation) of the agent, scene, and/or goal changes, the "same behaviors," present or recollected, may be seen as different "actions"?[22]

---

[21]One may argue that every scene is symbolically constituted. Many scenes are tacitly defined, and one may lose track of the fact that they are constituted as thus and such a scene by symbolic action. Within such taken-for-granted scenes, one may, through symbols, establish scenes on heaven and earth impenetrable to those who insist that their own limitations of vision are canonical for all humankind.

[22]To spell this out somewhat: A certain pattern of behaviors (vocal and otherwise) may be taken as one action if the agent is construed as a con-man, another if the agent is construed as an upright citizen, a third if the agent is taken as an inebriate, and so on. Conversely, an individual may be construed as a different kind of agent depending on how his/her action is characterized. Both the nature of the agent and the nature of the actions will be conceived differently depending upon the end or goal assumed or posited, and the instrumentalities used; and the goal or goals posited will depend on how one conceives the agent and actions. And so on, round the horn. Moreover, in all of this, one cannot assume an "ideal observer;" a psychologist, sociologist, or anthropologist investigating human action is himself/herself one (or more) agent(s) in a scene acting in the service of his/her ends. The ambiguity and uncertainty inherent in this dialectical relationship may lead some, using a special terministic screen, to dispense with agents, acts, scenes, purposes, and retreat to bodies or "organisms" in motion, a move that seems to allow for precise measurement and quantification. Alas, there is no solution of continuity between motion and action. "Behavior," a hybrid term, is often used by "motorists" to fudge the distinction between motion and action.

Again, have we not observed, in others if not in ourselves that human beings are likely to manifest different "selves" in different scenes, incarnating different "roles," wittingly or not, in different contexts?[23] Selves, sometimes so seemingly disconnected from each other, that we may consider the individual a split-personality, a Dr. Jekyll and Mr. Hyde, a Miss Beauchamp, an Eve, a Sybil? Conversely are we not aware, in ourselves if not in others, that an individual may manifest selves in a closet or in Fantasy Island, a la Walter Mitty, that are never publicly manifested?[24]

Once more, do we not, often, see (describe, represent, interpret, understand)[25] the behaviors of others as manifested to secure approval, prestige, reputation, respect, love, power, cooperation, revenge, restitution, etc., [26] vis a vis others (present or absent, "real" or "imaginal")[27] irrespective of ends, goals or values those others insist on as governing their behaviors?[28] And do we not, sometimes, on reflection or retrospection, acknowledge that this might be the case for us as well? Even as we participate in a scientific society, devoted solely to the pursuit of truth and the advancement of knowledge? Even as we try to cajole others, invoking their interest, the community interest, the national interest, the cosmic interest, to pursue one course rather than another? Even when we try to get others to adopt a model for the representation and explanation of human action that omits

---

[23]See E. Goffman, 1959, 1971, 1974.

[24]See the cases, presented from an object-relations, psychoanalytic point of view by Masud Khan. The psychoanalytic and depth-psychological literature is, of course, a thesaurus for such cases. One should be skeptical, however, about the "terministic screens" used in describing such cases, "screens" sometimes taken as diaphanous by those who use them.

[25]I use these terms here to suggest how often they overlap. Description and representation already involve a "seeing as" (Wittgenstein) or a perspective, and are not theory-neutral. As Gombrich points out (1960), we do not see (or describe) with an innocent-eye. Indeed, it may be argued that we do not "see" in one sense of "seeing" with our eyes at all, but rather through our eyes. See Agnes Arber, (1964) and W. Werkmeister, (1951).

[26]The role of these "motives" and others in human actions and transactions is generally conceded, and yet human action is sometimes investigated by psychologists as if such "motives" had no role at all in affecting the kinds of actions, the manner of executing actions, etc., that individuals manifest or the kinds of scenes that individuals take themselves to be operating in. This is, of course, more likely to be true of "laboratory psychologists" than of "clinical psychologists." See Thurstone, 1960.

[27]Again, it is perhaps more likely that the "clinical psychologist" rather than the "academic psychologist" will realize that individuals sometimes act with respect to scenes and agents that have little connection with the scenes and agents the psychologist believes they are confronted with.

[28]The dangers involved in attributing motives to others that they do not recognize themselves is as great as the dangers involved in accepting an individual's motives as he/she represents them. Especially dangerous are the claims of specialized groups who presuppose an ontology of real "motives" and reduce all other motivational claims to these "real ones." See Burke, 1935; Ricoeur, 1970.

any reference to categories akin to those of the dramatistic model?[29]

To be sure, one does not always represent one's self and others as "agents" engaged in goal-directed action. Often—for some speculators, always—human beings are described (defined, interpreted) as "patients;" entities, whose motions, bodily or vocal, public or private, are taken to be determined by the "action" of something external to themselves—something human, non-human, inhuman, or super-human.[30] In such cases, such "somethings" take on the character of "agents" and human beings are taken as "scenic products" produced by those agents or "instrumentalities" through which those agents work. Have you not, on occasion, seen (described, interpreted) the behavior of others, and even yourself, in these terms? If not, nowadays, by invoking solar, lunar, or astral "agents" who shape human beings and use them as vehicles, then by invoking supra-individual or intra-individual "agents"—social, political, historical, economic, and/or infra-conscious—working cooperatively or competitively to determine human destiny, mold human character, and cause human behaviors?

Now, if we hold in abeyance any *ontological dogma* that only individual human beings can be agents who carry out actions in pursuit of ends,[31] and if we further bracket our concern for the "way things really are," do we not find, for ourselves as well as others, that human beings may be taken on occasion to function as any one of the generic components of situations? Not only as agent or instrument, but also as scene, act, or end? Correspondingly, is it not also the case that a certain aspect of a situation taken as scene by one individual may, by others, be construed now as agent, now as instrumentality, now as act, now as end (see Wapner, Kaplan, & Ciottone,

---

[29]Whitehead (1929) has called attention to those who seem to be obsessed with the purpose of demonstrating that there is no purpose in human affairs. The recognition that we are all agents in the pursuit of ends and that we try to influence others in order to attain our ends has led Burke to emphasize the importance of "rhetoric." See Burke, 1969; 1961. See, too, W. Booth, 1961, 1974a, 1974b. A most interesting area of analysis is the rhetoric of those who seek to occupy in their society the social role of men and women of knowledge. See Znaniecki, 1940.

[30]There are, of course, many psychologists who take it as indisputable that human beings, like other bodies on the earth, are always patients: puppets moved hither and thither by circumstances of conditions (tacitly taken as the benevolent or malevolent agents) inside or outside the bodies. Intoxicated by hubris or a passion for inconsistency, these psychologists usually include themselves out of the human condition.

[31]For those who maintain this dogma, the description or representation of inanimate things as engaging in action for the achievement of ends involves the commission of the "pathetic fallacy," or the violation of linguistic rules, a merely metaphorical or figurative way of speaking-thinking, or the insidious effects of mental illness. Those afflicted are often lovers, lunatics, lyricists, and little children.

1981). And so on, around the ring: Any feature or aspect of a situation taken as one of the components of a situation by someone may be apprehended by someone else as any other of the components. One man's scene is another man's purpose. One woman's agent is another woman's instrumentality. What would be taken as an instrumentality or tool by one is, by another, construed as a scene; by still another, as a goal.[31] And even when there is apparent agreement on the generic category to which an aspect or feature of a situation belongs, specific interpretations may differ for those participating in that situation, or for those participating in the role of detached observer in a larger situation including the original one. Perspectives doth make double-, triple-, or multiple- entendre makers of us all (see Cirillo & Kaplan, this volume). For illustrations, I refer the reader to the corpora of world literature, horror movies, and his/her own memory banks. For analysis and commentary to Aristotle, Burke (1935, 1966, 1969), Frye (1957, 1963, 1970), Fletcher (1964), Fergusson (1968), Booth (1961), 1974a, 1974b), and Shumaker (1966).

Now, not only does our latent and naive dramatistic perspective lead us to structure the human world, and often the non-human world, in terms of the aforementioned "categories,"[32] but it also leads us to entertain the idea of the relativity of means to ends (actions and instrumentalities to purposes).[33] Do we not see that "actions" and "instrumentalities" relevant to a drive or a transient motive may have little resemblance to, or influence on, the actions and instrumentalities pertinent to the struggle to attain long range

---

[32]There are surely cultural and sub-cultural differences as to the allocation of what there is to the different generic categories: What members of one group typically take as scenic, members of another group may take as agentive or instrumental. There are also individual differences within a culture or sub-culture: Where one sees the agent responsible for his/her action outside the self, e.g., Society, another sees his/her action as generated by the self, i.e., takes oneself as the responsible agent. And surely, through introspection or retrospection, each of us can become aware of a transient or enduring experience in which otherwise instruments became agents and other time agents were construed as instruments; where sometime scenic factors became ends, and sometime ends became parts of the scene; and so on, and so on, and so on.

[33]The problem of "the categories" is at least as old as Aristotle. Still in dispute is the issue of the universality of certain categories, the question of whether categories are "in things," "in the mind," "in the linguistic system," or in any combination of these. See Burke, 1966; Pepper, 1942; Whorf, 1956; von Bertalanffy, 1955. Burke seems to assume the universality of his categories, while acknowledging, indeed exulting in, the relativity of their application. One may take Burke's work as an attempt to arrive at the fundamental categories of the human social-emotional world. Jung, of course, took himself to be undertaking the same kind of "Kantian" task. There is, it seems to me, some overlap between Burke's and Jung's enterprises, but this is not the place to discuss their convergences and divergences.

goals or realize fundamental values?[34] And once this is recognized, may it not also allow us to entertain the unthinkable hypothesis that the manner in which an infant or child deals with the tasks of infancy and childhood may have little bearing on the manner in which the "same" adolescent, adult, or middle-aged person deals with the tasks and goals of later life?[35]

Again, may not our cognizance of the relativity of means to ends open up to us the possibility of variable durations and complexities of actions—durations and complexities determined by the goals wittingly or unwittingly pursued?[36] Does not the purpose of writing a play or a paper have different action-units and action-components (as well as different scenes and different instrumentalities) than the goal of solving a conservation problem or the value of perfecting oneself as a human being? Does not the goal of doing a traditional piece of "developmental research" involve different action-durations, action-units and action-components than the goal of helping others in a clinical setting?

Now, you may have assented to all of the "rhetorical questions" I have put to you, and may have even agreed with all of my assertions, and yet not feel that you know what *Dramatism* is. Like Burke, I have beat around the

---

[34]Whether or not ends justify means (Trotsky, 1969), it seems clear that ends determine the sphere of relevant means. Actions without ends, expressed or attributed, become mere motions, and instrumentalities lapse back into the status of scenic things. The positing of different "teloi" leads one to search for different "means." The implications of this point for developmentalists concerned with the steps or stages precursory to, or leading up to, different teloi should be obvious: Where the teloi are different, the kinds of actions of individuals relevant to the teloi are different. Is it possible that what Dewey calls an "occupational psychosis" had led many "cognitive-developmental" psychologists to presuppose formal operations or intelligence as *the* telos of development, and to represent ontogenetic changes solely in terms of those actions-instrumentalities pertinent to logical thought? In this connection, it should also be remarked that the witting or unwitting choice of a telos by an investigator may influence the description of what children do before attaining the telos; one may easily see precursors of any telos in every movement of the young child or adolescent. One may thus "read back" into earlier actions directed toward other ends prefigurations of the actions manifested in the attainment of the telos. One may refer to this tendency, to which historians, biographers, religious apologists, and developmentalists are addicted as "Clio's curse;" the assumption that there is (must be) a continuity between the earlier and the later. (See Kaplan, 1982.) To maintain this "dogma," we have the apparatus of "precursors," "transformations," etc. On some of the problems involved in constituting or representing "history," and by extension, "biography," see H. White, 1974, and D. H. Fischer, 1970. One need not reject the dogma; one should only be aware that it is one.

[35]The assumption put in question here is to the effect that what an individual does with respect to one task or goal must necessarily influence or affect what the individual does with respect to some other task or goal. Once again, I do not question that this presupposition may be employed. One should only recognize that it is a postulate.

[36]Since "actions" are ideal constructions, not reducible to motions, it is possible for certain actions to last a life time, and other actions to last a fraction of a second. Paradoxically perhaps, actions may be manifested in the absence of movement, and movements may not be construed as actions.

bush instead of going straight to the roots. Well, here are the roots. *Dramatism is a critical and self-critical method for making us aware not only of the remarkable range of "worlds" we inhabit,*[37] *but also of the symbolic ways in which we constitute such "worlds" and ourselves within those worlds.*[38] It insists on the fact, without denying our physicality and animality, that we are primarily symbol-users, symbol-makers, and symbol-misusers. Our "symbolicity" is constitutive of ourselves as human. Symbolic action penetrates all human activity including the activity of establishing a "self" or "selves" and a "world" or "worlds." Without symbolic action, we would not *know* any reality, but merely live in an environment animalistically, suffering transient experiences, incapable of any kind of reflection or contemplation, unable to communicate to our congeners *about* certain states of affairs not directly connected to the here/now.[39] Symbolic action—of which linguistic action is the dominant but not the only form—enables us to "store information;" fix the flux along certain lines rather than others; remember and generalize a transient episode; define, identify ourselves with, and disidentify ourselves with individuals, groups, nations, causes, movements; define the scenes in which we live; alter and try to persuade others to alter conceptions of what there is, what is happening, what has happened, what will happen.[40] Through symbolic action, we seek to regulate and direct not only others but ourselves. Dramatism as a method seeks to make us aware of the extent to which our sensuous experiences are, paradoxically, the "signs" of symbolically constituted concepts.

Now, although *dramatism* shares with other perspectives an emphasis on human symbolicity, it is not merely one more twist on the "symbolic turn." Perhaps because of Burke's concern with concrete cases, whether "real" or "fictional," the dramatistic method is often employed to show how individuals in social situations operate on each other through symbolic action. In so much of human action, individuals representing different interests struggle over how a situation shall be named because they implicitly realize

---

[37]The "worlds" we inhabit include worlds we may inhabit only for a moment or worlds we may inhabit only in our dreams; the worlds of people of archaic societies and of other times and places; the alternate "realities" of fiction and fantasy, and so on.

[38]The emphasis on symbolic action in constituting worlds is, of course, not peculiar to Burke. See Cassirer, 1953. Also Whorf, 1956; Langer, 1942; Urban, 1939; Goodman, 1978; Bryson et al., 1954, 1955; Werner & Kaplan, 1963.

[39]See Burke, 1961, 1969; also Cirillo and Kaplan (this volume). One might note that, through symbolic action, we define not only who and what we and others are, but also the actions, "visible" and "invisible," that we and others carry out, "externally" or "internalized." There are obvious links here to what is called "attribution theory."

[40] See Burke, 1961, 1969. Also Cirillo and Kaplan (this volume). In many works on sociolinguistics, anthropological linguistics, and child language, the "rhetorical aspect" is referred to as "pragmatics."

that the "definition of a situation" determines how one acts toward it and in it. Think of how people have tried to persuade us that what we would call an *invasion* is really a *protective reaction;* that our *planned economy* is really *regimentation;* that our *firmness* is really *stubbornness* or *obstinacy.* And consider how we have tried to persuade others that their *science* is really *superstition;* that their *minds* are really *ghosts* or that their *ghosts* are really *minds;* that their *mainstreams* are really *puddles;* that they are really complicated *machines* (see Cohen, 1954).

Thus, where others may focus on the relation of symbolization, linguistic or otherwise, to *logic,* the dramatistic perspective stresses the *rhetorical* aspects of symbolic action. Human beings use symbols to persuade, to convince, to establish identities and identifications, to exhort, to malign, to exclude, to plead, and to placate at least as often as they use symbols to reason. Indeed, one may argue that even the rules of right reasoning are established rhetorically, especially in domains where one is talking about some content (see Perelman & Olbrechts—Tytecha, 1969; Wheelwright, 1962; 1968).

One final point: Unlike many other points of view in psychology, the dramatistic perspective is both "reflexive" and conducive to self-reflection. It applies equally to those who use it as to those upon whom it is used. It therefore demands, although some of its practitioners may fall far short of realizing the telos, that one look at one's own symbolic actions and transactions with the same passionate dispassion as one looks at the symbolic actions and transactions of others. Embedded in it, therefore, is a variant of the categorical imperative: "Do unto yourself as you would do unto others." Or perhaps more pertinently: "Speak about yourself as you would speak about others."

THE PERSPECTIVE OF GENETIC-DRAMATISM

I have already hinted at the enormous difficulties involved in trying to bring "developmentalism" and "dramatism" into a single integrated perspective, that of Genetic-Dramatism. How often in the past have attempts been made to bridge the eternal and the temporal, the transcendent and the immanent, the ideal and the actual, the perfect and the imperfect, the normative and the positive, the ought and the is!? How inevitable that these attempts, in subsequent periods, have appeared partial and parochial? How inescapable that these "failures" have not forestalled later attempts, but indeed have acted as a stimulus for a never-ending quest?!

If the ultimate telos of development entails living the "divine life upon earth" (Sri Aurobindo), of attaining the "perfection" of the diety, then no human being has achieved that mode of living or attained that status to the satisfaction of all other human beings. In the immortal words of a current cliche, "Nobody's perfect."[41] Given our own inevitable finitude, our own inescapable blindnesses and limitations, how can we know what it *means* to be "perfect," either with respect to "the whole person," or to any of the activities of a person in his/her relations to nature, society or self? And yet, without such inchoate knowledge or claim to knowledge, what can it mean when we speak of "the development of the person," "the development of cognition," "the development of morality," "the development of skill," etc? (see Kaplan, 1981).[42]

And if, out of affection for modesty or aversion to elitism, we deny the possibility of such tacit knowledge to ourselves and others, averring that development has nothing to do with perfection but merely with change, then what grounds do we have for suggesting that people (including ourselves) ought to (learn to) think one way rather than another, (learn to) act towards others in this way rather than that, etc? Even more radically, what grounds do we have for *intervening,* as we inevitably do, in the lives of others—our children, our students, our clients, our peers—seeking to change the course of their actions, their current ways of being-in-the-world?

One might, of course, facetiously (or even seriously), incarnate the role of the disinterested "dramatist," adopt the posture of the pure scientist, and claim that the suggestions or interventions are simply intended to secure the widest range of information one can about the ways in which human beings act under the widest range of conditions. One is not concerned in the slightest with development in the sense of perfection; only with the knowledge of the ways things change under various conditions, or as a function of varying values of different variables. One will leave it to weak-minded activists to use such information for whatever ends they see fit; and one might even study such policy-makers to get more information about the variegated versions of the human comedy for other policy-makers to use.

But even this gambit, this attempt to escape from commitment to some ideal, turns out to be illusory. The most ardent "cultural relativist," the most passionate positivist-scientist, still claims tacitly or explicitly that his/her ways of arriving at such information are more advanced, "closer to the ideal," than ways that others use to arrive at knowledge. Otherwise, it is all full of sound and fury, signifying nothing.

---

[41]See Burke, 1973. "Perfection," like development, differentiation, integration, assimilation, accommodation, etc., is an analogical concept, taking on a different application in different contexts. For a rigorous analysis of such concepts, see D. Burrell, 1973.

[42]The "struggle" to develop different aspects of ourselves—logical competence, professional competence, motor dexterity, linguistic competence, communicative competence, etc.—are by some taken to constitute self-perfection. By others, they are taken to be marginal, secondary, or even inimical.

I will not argue the point further, but henceforth assume it: In Burke's phrase, "human beings are goaded by a spirit of perfection," and this spirit permeates everything we do. We struggle to develop (perfect) ourselves, and in this process, we struggle to develop different aspects of ourselves. Ideally, we would be "the totality," everything that is, was, or will be. Practically, as embodied beings, we are limited at most to relative perfection in a very restricted number of enterprises. Ideally, we would occupy all scenes, engage in all actions, master all instrumentalities, pursue all ends. Practically, as embodied beings, we are drastically limited to but a very few. Ideally, we would relate to other human beings in the infinity of ways in which human beings are capable of relating to each other. Practically, as embodied beings, we enjoy and suffer a finite range of relationships and engage in a limited number of transactions, often of a stereotyped and repetitive nature. Ideally, we would comprehend and eliminate all of those factors militating against "development-perfection." Practically, as embodied beings, we are individually, and even collectively, limited in our knowledge of those complex factors that interfere with the attainment of even relative perfection; and even with that knowledge, we are, individually and collectively, limited in our potency.

Yet, restricted as we are by our corporeity, we can through heart, mind, and spirit—love, empathy, science, and the symbolic imagination—at least partly transcend our local and parochial limitations. We can incarnate other selves and dwell in other scenes that those we have ever been able to enjoy solely as embodied beings. We can envisage ends and embody actions undreamt of by those who preceded us, and entertain visions that will be embodied or materialized by later generations. We can adopt perspectives other than those we have inherited, and experience the mysterious universe in ways that remain hidden and mute to us, unless we can free ourselves from our identifications with our bodies, with our roles, with our transient selves, with our habitual actions.

"The greatest thing by far," Aristotle observed, 'is to be a master of metaphor" (*Poetics,* xvii, p. 9). This famous phrase takes on a new significance if one equates "metaphor," as Burke does, with "perspective by incongruity"; the capacity to see the familiar in a new light, to break out of one's customary ways of seeing, doing, believing, and being. But even here there are obstacles, resistances, difficulties: inabilities to engage either in the willing suspension of disbelief or the painful suspension of dogmatic belief; inabilities to differentiate Self from social roles; ends from particular actions; actions from particular instrumentalities; self and others from embeddedness in particular scenes; and so on. There is implicit here a never-ending program of research, on all levels of analysis, to ascertain not merely in general, but *in specific instances,* the factors that militate against that *flexibility* and *stability* that characterize "development" in early domain. And, indeed, with a slight rotation of perspective, one might see that studies already done have some bearing on our understanding of factors inhibiting and conducing to development. I hope to elaborate on this point in another place, since I anticipate that some may see Genetic-Dramatism as antipathetic to experimental research.[43]

CONCLUSION

It is built into the perspective of Genetic-Dramatism that its program is impossible to attain; it is impossible to exhibit and exhaustively describe all the ways in which human beings symbolically constitute their worlds; it is impossible to gain a knowledge of all of the circumstances that militate against an individual's self-perfection or even perfection in any area of human endeavor; it is impossible to intervene in the cases of ourselves and others to remove these noxious conditions. Our project is an infinite project, and however close we get to attainment, we are always an infinite distance away from reaching the telos.

Despite this state of affairs, I am nevertheless heartened and hope you will be uplifted by a vision of the world, expressed by some anonymous Everyman on the walls of the Sorbonne: "Be realistic. Demand the impossible."[44]

REFERENCES

Arber, A. *The mind and the eye.* Cambridge: Cambridge University Press, 1964.
Aristotle. *Rhetoric.* Ed. by Weldon. New York: Macmillan & Co., 1886.
Bakan, D. The mystery-mastery complex. *American Psychologist,* 1965, *20,* 186–191.
Beck, L. W. *The actor and the spectator.* New Haven: Yale University Press, 1975.
Bernstein, R. J. *Praxis and action.* Philadelphia: University of Pennsylvania Press, 1971.
Bevan, E. *Symbolism and belief.* London: George Allen & Unwin. Ltd., 1938.
Black, M. On the definition of scientific method, *Problems of analysis.* Ithaca, New York: Cornell University Press, 1962.
Booth, W. C. *The rhetoric of fiction.* Chicago: University of Chicago Press, 1961.

---

[43]As Max Black and others have suggested, terms like "science," "experiment," and "research" are often used rhetorically to suggest that what one does is the proper thing to do. On the history of the idea of experiment in the early periods of Western thought, see Thorndike, 1958. See also Madden (Ed.), 1966; Black, 1962; P. Feyerabend, 1978. The concept of method is also given a detailed analysis in J. Buchler, 1961. See also A. Kaplan, 1964, on "methodolatry."

[44]Cited in O. B. Hardison, 1972.

Booth, W. C. *The rhetoric of assent.* Notre Dame: University of Notre Dame Press, 1974. (a)

Booth, W. C. *The rhetoric of irony.* Chicago: University of Chicago Press, 1974. (b)

Brissett, D., & Edgley, C. *Life as theater.* Hawthorne, N.Y.: Aldine Publishers, 1975.

Bryson, L., Finkelstein, L., Hoagland, H., & MacIver, R. M. (Eds.) *Symbols and values.* New York: Harper & Bros., 1954.

Bryson, L., Finkelstein, L., Hoagland, H., & MacIver, R. M. (Eds.) *Symbols and society.* New York: Harper & Bros., 1955.

Buchler, J. *Concept of method.* New York: Columbia University Press, 1961.

Burke, K. *Permanence and change.* New York: New Republic, Inc., 1935.

Burke, K. *Grammar of motives.* Berkeley: University of California Press, 1945/69.

Burke, K. *Rhetoric of religion.* Berkeley: University of California Press, 1961.

Burke, K. *Language as symbolic action.* Berkeley: University of California Press, 1966.

Burke, K. *Rhetoric of motives.* Berkeley: University of California Press, 1969.

Burke, K. *Dramatism and development.* Barre, MA: Clark University Press, 1972.

Burke, K. *Philosophy of literary form.* Berkeley: University of California Press, 1973.

Burrell, D. *Analogy and philosophical language.* New Haven: Yale University Press, 1973.

Cassirer, E. *Language and myth.* New York: Dover Press, 1946.

Cassirer, E. *Philosophy of symbolic forms.* Vols I, II, III. New Haven: Yale University Press, 1953; 1955; 1957.

Cassirer, E. *The individual and the cosmos in Renaissance philosophy.* New York: Harper & Row, 1963.

Cohen, F. J. Hidden value judgments. In L. Bryson, L. Finkelstein, H. Hoagland, & R. M. MacIver (Eds.), *Symbols and values.* New York: Harper & Bros., 1954.

Collingwood, R. G. *Idea of nature.* Oxford: Clarendon Press, 1957.

Cope, J. *The theatre and the dream.* Baltimore: Johns Hopkins University Press, 1973.

Dalziel-Duncan, H. *Communication and social order.* London: Oxford University Press, 1968. (a)

Dalziel-Duncan, H. *Symbols in society.* New York: Oxford University Press, 1968. (b)

Dewey, J. *Experience and nature.* Lasalle, In.: Open Court Press, 1929.

Dewey, J. *Logic: The theory of inquiry.* New York: Holt, Rinehart & Winston, 1938.

Dewey, J. *Art as experience.* New York: Minton, Balch & Co., 1934.

Fergusson, F. *Dante's drama of the mind.* Westport, CT: Greenwood Press, 1953.

Fergusson, F. *The human image in dramatic literature.* New York: Anchor Books, 1957.

Fergusson, F. (Ed.) *Poetics.* New York: Hill and Wang, 1961.

Fergusson, F. *Idea of theater.* Princeton, N.J.: Princeton University Press, 1968.

Feyerabend, P. *Against method.* London: Verso, 1978.

Fischer, D. H. *Historian's fallacies.* New York: Harper & Row, 1970.

Fletcher, A. *Allegory: The theory of a symbolic mode.* Ithaca, N.Y.: Cornell University Press, 1964.

Frye, N. *Anatomy of criticism.* New York: Atheneum Press, 1957.

Frye, N. *Fables of identity.* New York: Harcourt, Brace & World, Inc., 1963.

Frye, N. *The stubborn structure.* Ithaca, N.Y.: Cornell University Press, 1970.

Goffman, E. *The presentation of self in everyday life.* New York: Anchor Books, 1959.

Goffman, E. *Relations in public.* New York: Harper & Row, 1971.

Goffman, E. *Frame analysis.* New York: Harper & Row, 1974.

Gombrich, E. H. *Art and illusion.* Bollingen: Princeton University Press, 1960.

Goodman, N. *Ways of world-making.* Indianapolis: Hackett Publishing, 1978.

Hardison, O. B. *Toward freedom and dignity.* Baltimore: Johns Hopkins University Press, 1972.

Hughes, H. S. *Consciousness and society.* New York: Vintage Press, 1977.

Hyman, S. E. (Ed.) *Perspectives by incongruity*. Bloomington: University of Indiana Press, 1964.

Kaplan, A. *Conduct of inquiry*. San Francisco: Chandler Publishing Co., 1964.

Kaplan, B. Radical metaphor, aesthetic and the origin of language. *Review of Existential Psychology and Psychiatry*, 1962.

Kaplan, B. The study of language in psychiatry: The comparative developmental approach and its application to symbolization and language in psychopathology. In S. Arieti (Ed.) *American Handbook of Psychiatry*, Vol. 3. New York: Basic Books, 1966.

Kaplan, B. Strife of systems. *Rationality and irrationality in development*. Worcester, MA: Clark University Press, 1967.

Kaplan, B. *The development of language in relation to mental health*. Paper presented at Cornell University Medical College, September 15, 1981.

Kerenyi, K. Prolegomena. In C. G. Jung, & K. Kerenyi. *Essays on a science of mythology*. New York: Harper & Row, 1963.

Lakoff, G., & Johnson, M. *Metaphors we live by*. Chicago: University of Chicago Press, 1980.

Langer, S. K. *Philosophy in a new key*. Cambridge: Harvard University Press, 1942.

Lovejoy, A. O. The paradox of the thinking behaviorist. *Philosophical Review,* 1922, *31,* 135–147.

Lovejoy, A. O. *The great chain of being*. Cambridge, Mass.: Harvard University Press, 1936.

Madden, E. (Ed.) *Theories of scientific method*. St. Louis: Washington University Press, 1966.

Mandelbaum, M. *History, man and reason: A study in Nineteenth Century thought*. Baltimore: Johns Hopkins University Press, 1971.

McKeon, R. Literary criticism and the concept of imitation in antiquity. In R. S. Crane (Ed.), *Critics and criticism*. Chicago: University of Chicago Press, 1951.

Mead, G. H. *Mind, self & society*. Chicago: University of Chicago Press, 1934.

Mead, G. H. *The philosophy of the act*. Chicago: University of Chicago Press, 1938.

Mead, G. H. *Movements of thought in the Nineteenth Century*. Chicago: University of Chicago Press, 1936.

Northrop, F. S. C. *Logic of the sciences and humanities*. New York: Macmillan, 1947.

Pepper, S. C. *World hypotheses*. Berkeley: University of California Press, 1942.

Perelman, C., & Olbrechts-Tytecha, A. *New rhetoric*. South Bend: University of Notre Dame Press, 1969.

Ricoeur, P. *Freud and philosophy*. New Haven: Yale University Press, 1970.

Sapir, J., & Crocker, C. *The social use of metaphor*. Philadelphia: University of Pennsylvania Press, 1977.

Schutz, A. *Collected papers: The problem of social reality*. The Hague: Martinus Nijhoff, 1973.

Shumaker, W. *Literature and the irrational*. New York: Washington Square Press, 1966.

Simon, Y. *A general theory of authority*. South Bend: University of Notre Dame Press, 1980.

Straus, E. *The primary world of the senses*. London: Free Press of Glencoe, 1963.

Taylor, C. *Hegel and modern society*. Cambridge: Cambridge University Press, 1979.

Thorndike, L. *History of magic & experimental science*. Vols. I–VIII. New York: Columbia University Press, reprinted 1958.

Thurstone, L. L. The stimulus-response fallacy in psychology. *Nature of intelligence*. Paterson, N.J.: Littlefield, Adams & Co., 1960.

Trotsky, L. The moralists and sycophants against Marxism. *Their morals and ours*. New York: Merit Publishers, 1969.

Turbayne, C. *The myth of metaphor*. New Haven: Yale University Press, 1962.

Urban, W. *Language and reality*. New York: Macmillan & Co., 1939.

Vickery, J. (Ed.) *Myth and literature*. Lincoln, Neb.: University of Nebraska Press, 1969.

von Bertalanffy, L. An essay on the relativity of categories. *Philosophy of Science,* 1955, *22,* 243–263.

Wapner, S., Kaplan, B., & Ciottone, R. Self-world relationships in critical environment transitions: Childhood and beyond. In L. Liben, A. Patterson, & N. Newcombe (Eds.), *Spatial representation and behavior across the life span*. New York: Academic Press, 1981.

Wapner, S., Kaplan, B., & Cohen, S. B. An organismic-developmental perspective for understanding transactions of men in environments. *Environment and Behavior,* 1976, *5,* 255–289.

Werkmeister, W. On describing a world. *Philosophy of Phenomenological Research,* 1951, *2,* 303–326.

Werner, H., & Kaplan, B. The developmental approach to cognition: Its relevance to the psychological interpretation of anthropological and ethnolinguistic data. *American Anthropologist,* 1956, *58,* 866–880.

Werner, H. *Comparative psychology of mental development*. New York: International Universities Press, 1957.

Werner, H., & Kaplan, B. *Symbol formation*. New York: Wiley, 1963.

Wheelwright, P. *Metaphor and reality*. Bloomington: University of Indiana Press, 1962.

Wheelwright, P. *The burning fountain*. Bloomington: University of Indiana Press, 1968.

White, H. *Metahistory*. Baltimore: Johns Hopkins University Press, 1974.

White, S. Psychology in all sorts of places. In R. A. Kasschau, & F. S. Kessel (Eds.), *Psychology and society: In search of symbiosis*. New York: Holt, Rinehart & Winston, 1978.

Whitehead, A. N. *Function of reason*. Princeton: Princeton University Press, 1929.

Whitehead, A. N. *Modes of thought*. New York: Macmillan & Co., 1938.

Whorf, B. *Language, thought and reality*. Cambridge: MIT Press, 1956.

Znaniecki, F. *The social role of the man of knowledge*. New York: Columbia University Press, 1940.

4 A Developmental Approach to Systems Theory

George Rand
Graduate School of Architecture and Urban Planning
University of California at Los Angeles

The created product is not less than the creating mind.

Goethe

The most glorious poetry ever communicated to the world is but a feeble shadow of the original conception of the poet.

Shelley

ARCHITECTURE AND PSYCHOLOGY

In his recent book, Rudolph Arnheim[1] (1977) convincingly explores the hypothesis of a close kinship between psychology and architecture throughout history. All good and rational thinking aspires to the condition of architecture. For example, Immanuel Kant's conception of architectonics, or the "art of systems" as proposed in the Critique of Pure Reason, depended on available imagery drawn from Gothic Cathedrals and the structural discipline they exhibited. "A unity of purpose to which all parts refer and in view of which they also relate among themselves." These Cathedrals were approached by their designers like the Creator was alleged to have divined organic form. There are no wasted elements. From a section of any column or beam[2] (like a histological section), the designer could

---

[1]Arnheim's (1977) book applies principles of Gestalt psychology to architecture in much the same manner as earlier books on film and art. He cites liberally from 19th century aesthetic theories (Theodor Lipps, Alois Riegl, and Willhelm Worringer) as a reminder of the historical relationship between earlier theories of Einfuhlung (empathy) in art and architecture and modern theories of perception.

[2]An impressive history of the biological metaphor in architecture is presented by Philip Steadman (1979). Steadman reviews the organic analogy, early taxonomic theories, and ecological ideas that influenced both the history of architecture and ideas of evolution. The Gothic ideal was expressed as structural integrity; the ideal was later abandoned as Cartesian rationality and Jansenist thinking took hold in France. This led to a radical split between rational and emotive approaches to architecture in the 18th century that paralleled philosophical expressions of the same dualism.

75

discern the rational structure of the whole building. The procedure is the same combination of induction and deduction used to date a pottery shard or build an image of a prehistoric animal from fossils.

What is so interesting about this notion is that the early Rationalist philosophers borrowed so heavily on the Cathedral metaphor in constructing images in their minds about what it meant to have a rational order. Human references to systems and structure in mental life continue to be difficult to separate from images of buildings, bridges, mines, and pumps, which form the metaphorical substrate for many critical ideas we have about the inner "workings" of our minds. For Marcel Proust, architecture was such an attractive metaphor for the "work" that he apparently contemplated naming parts of his books by such titles as "porch," "stained-glass windows of the apse" and gave up these titles as too pretentious. Nonetheless, the organization of themes across the "body" of his work suggests the ordered majestry and paradoxical simplicity of the Cathedral. To carry forward the metaphor, is it an accident we speak in terms of "high hopes" and "deep thoughts?" Our conception of our interior life and the levels of existence we assign to it can be virtually interchanged with the words of the architectural critic spotting the existential roots of architectural transitions from one historic period to another, from the reverential orientation of the Gothic to the framed, delimited, articulate objectivity of the late renaissance: from living and guileful displays of the Baroque to the stark neoclassicism of the late 18th century.[3]

It is equally clear that when we interact with buildings and other environmental forms on the conetmporary landscape we are not responding to them de novo any more than the words we use to communicate can be viewed as empty abstractions devoid of historical significance and cultural meaning.

The "psychological fallacy," if I can refer to a term that I know must already exist, is to view mental development as if it exists outside a context—a system in its own right. All languages are seen as differing only in the way they cloak the same meanings with different (and 100% translatable) sounds.

An alternative approach is to imagine that the particular expressions chosen to represent a meaning, and their history, reveal something about the psychological underpinnings of a culture and its members—at the same time there may be universal types or forms.[4]

Beneath an expression like "high hopes" is a process of dynamic struc-

---

[3]A basic source of psychologically sensitive architectural history is Nikolaus Pevsner (1974). A less profound but more directly psychological approach can be found in Christian Norberg-Schulz (1971).

[4]A wonderful example of this analysis of psyche in the cultural context is presented by Adrian Stokes (1958). He pulls out various notions of the body and its humours present in common Greek thought and shows how they serve as the basis for ideals expressed in Greek art.

turization of space in Western European thought that helps to fund the expression with meaning. The Japanese notion of space is totally different (as in the Indian, etc.) even though the "objective content" of the expression may be translated from one language to the other. Contemporary language theories have come to recognize the limits of objectification of language. That is, language to language translation is incomplete unless it can convey with the words the underlying presuppositions, spatial metaphors, and folk theories that ground their meanings. "High hopes" qua Gothic cathedral means something different from "high hopes" qua the dialectics of "distant mountain-lake-island" images in Japanese landscapes.

In architecture, as opposed to language theory, these underlying "primitives" are more evident. The issues of architecture, for example, regulation of public-private relationships by spatial-gestural forms, are today the same as they have been since the literal beginnings of time. Buildings that we see all round us, even rather undistinguished ones, tend to use facades. These are walls which face the street, and employ a relatively formal composition of elements, saving informal features for the rear or side. What do we mean by the formal-informal dimension? It has something to do with traditions of mind that are matched to regularly encountered environmental "gestures"—architecturally expressed differences between front and rear or side—that have emerged in interaction with one another over the course of many generations. Mental manner and environmental gesture are very difficult to tease apart even at the simplest level. If we did not create parallel dimensions in the world of "mind" and the world of "matter," environments would not feel as familiar as they do; nor would they be as legible or readable as they are.

What can we say about the origins of these linkages between mind and matter (or more properly, dialectical distinctions that are made in the world of mind which find their parallel in dialectical distinctions that are apparent in the world of matter)? These dimensions do not come automatically. Typically they are invented by ordinary mortals and like other discoveries in the world of science, philosophy, and technology can be dated and traced to particular people and places. In some sense the distinction between front and side of buildings can be traced to Andrea Palladio, the early Renaissance Italian master architect who "invented" ideas of composition in his villas and chapels that later came to be thought of as "formal" designs inasmuch as they embodied the dialectic contrast of formal and informal.[5]

---

[5]Andrea Palladio was an oft-cited Italian architect from Padova/Venice in the 16th century who made many projects in Venice and nearby Vicenza. He was venerated by the famous critic Rudolf Wittkower (1952, 1974). Palladio represented the full expression of Renaissance (classical) rationality separated from residual Gothic and Romanesque themes present in the 15th century. In the Villa Rotunda, built for a renegade cleric in Vicenza, the "dome" was used for the first time as the centerpiece for a secular building. In Villa Foscari (1958–60), Veneto, Palladio created a side facade with a large garden window that contrasted with the ceremonial, formal front facade. A. Palladio (1570).

What I mean is the following. Palladio invented the idea of a formal facade by working on buildings that could be seen from one vantage; the canals of Venice. He was the first architect to truly secularize the architectural use of forms that had previously been reserved for serious meditative and religious use. Buildings now became "signs" of their contents rather than inexorable reflections of their intrinsic content. In other words, with Palladio comes a significant step in the separation of symbolic sign and referent to which it refers. Palladio, for example, lifted the "dome," previously reserved in the Christian world for religious use, and applied it to a villa for a rich private sponsor (Villa Rotunda in Vicenza). The client was not only using the domical form for private use but he also built the villa in what was then a rural landscape, appropriating an urban religious image for use in the countryside.

It was Palladio then, who vigorously explored what it meant to have a facade, multiple facades, square and rectangular shapes, etc. Just as Villa Rotunda experiments with this theme by having all four sides equal, so Villa Malcontenta utilizes a completely different vocabulary to express the appearance of the front and sides of the building. It becomes a theory-piece on how to embody the dialectics of public-private in a building.

Of course designing and building a few northern Italian villas does not etch into the minds and hearts of a whole civilization a certain and distinctive sensuous concept of formality. How does it come about?

In brief, I am suggesting the need to explore the dialectics of organism and environment revealed in the history of architecture and environmental design. I will try to explain the meaning of the words recognizing in advance the inordinate complexity of the issue I have raised and acknowledge that this is the subject of a longer work in preparation.

I am suggesting that architectural history is the discovery and creation of a series of "mind-built-forms." I am using this shorthand expression in the same way that physicists have, in frustration with the separation of mind and body, come to use terms like "body-mind" and "space-time." "Mind-built-forms" are really "living symbols." A building like Palladio's Villa Rotunda, when viewed today, embodies within it countless generations of architectural quotation. Design discoveries are incorporated into buildings and then passed on to subsequent works in which they are quoted. Palladio had spent time in Rome so that his understanding of Classical forms was not directly based on visits to Greece; he incorporated in his work the "distortions" that several generations of Roman emperors introduced into original Greek temple forms. From a psychological perspective, of course, it was not a distortion at all. Greek classicism is taken to be closer to the "source" (pure Platonic forms) although all architecture, including Greek temples are particular buildings. In short, they all tend to decay and crumble, leak in the rain, etc.

So Palladio's notion of front and side depended to a great extent on the observable "tricks of design" that were present in Roman ruins. These in turn, doubly distorted by the fact that they were in ruins, were dependent on early Roman constructions at the conquered Athenian Agora, built by Roman soldiers in the shadow of the Acropolis. The influence goes on, passed down by people designing in the shadow of or alongside other buildings. How then does a building like the Villa Rotunda get to be selected to define the mood of an era, or become a hallmark of the beginning of the Renaissance?

Again, the answer is a bit complex. In architecture, plans, sketches, and descriptions of buildings have always enjoyed wide circulation even before books were commonly available. Palladio had read Vitruvius[6] and in turn his own books were read by countless following generations of architects. The substance of these books is a corpus of buildings. They grow and differentiate over time. The original drawings are reported, redrawn and taken apart in various ways to make key theoretical arguments about their intrinsic geometries or the principles of design that inhere in their organization. Palladio then "invented" the notion of "formal-informal" in our culture to the extent that architects and designers used his documents as a "source" for their own designs and passed on his experimental discoveries through new buildings.

Another side of the issue is that through the course of history, the problems addressed in architecture have become increasingly focused on the creation of experienced "space." Architecture became the vehicle for the discovery of the intuition of space in much the same way that other disciplines—like music—became modes of manifesting significant dimensions of human experience. In this respect, Palladio stands above other architects because visits to his villas evoke an experience of "awe" that is evokable only in the presence of his architectural objects. The embodied work of architecture with its unique materials, circumstances, and conditions of observation can never be experienced in drawings or plans alone. Here the work becomes the subject of a pilgrimage. Just as Palladio visited Rome to see ancient ruins, so later generations of British architects travelled to Venice to see, experience, measure, and document his work. They then took this home to translate the experience of Palladiana into their own neoclassical Manor houses and churches.[7]

Finally, for the mood to invade the unconscious of an entire civilization, few of whom ever knew about these great buildings, the message had to be

---

[6]Vitruvius was the foremost Roman interpreter of Greek and Roman antiquity used as a source of authentication in the Renaissance by Sebastiano Serlio (1537) to define classical architecture by a series of rules based on Greek and Roman ideals (the "orders") for producing good form.

[7]This vastly oversimplifies the issues of "source" in architecture. Originally, there was no notion of mere formal resemblance and therefore equivalence. Classical buildings were thought to be handed down from the Temple of Solomon and therefore evolved from the founding sources of western society. For a more complete and truly elegant portrayal of this topic see Joseph Rykwert (1980).

reinforced in countless ways, in dress, manner, customs, belief systems . . . and be consonant with other structural forces in the society such as economic, political and technological paradigms that came to being at the same time.

Palladio "invented" the notion of "formal-informal" in our culture to the extent that other architects and designers used his buildings and designs as source for their own designs and passed on this expressive mode of structuring space with its half-hidden metaphorical baggage that dates back to classical Greece and Rome. So-called "powerful" buildings like the Pantheon interior or the dome of St. Sophia can be shown to produce unfiltered emotional responses. The form of these feelings is ambiguous—with membership in the Western culture it is interpreted as "awe." For example, Islamic architects historically used domes as normal roof systems and used them with abandon. These forms were reserved for the culminative spiritual experiences by European architects.

In similar fashion, Michelangelo can be said to have "invented" the idea of the cornice through the abstraction of the "form" of the Greek column (base, shaft, capital) and applying it to ordered Pallazzo facades. This theme was picked up by Sullivan who used it to organize the late 19th and early 20th century office and commercial towers of Chicago according to the same principles—rusticated base with shops, tiers of office floors separated by horizontal lines and capped by a large cornice above.[8] The same story can be told (and all can be sharpened in historical accuracy and detail) about the history of the "idea" of setbacks, walls, screens, plans. When we respond to a building as a member of a culture, we are perceiving by means of a set of primitives that give it inner form in addition to its ostensive form.

In the present century, architectural geniuses like Le Corbusier[9] tried to abstract these forms still further by inventing a language of design based on the response capabilities that had been discovered by modern psychology. Psychoanalysis allowed us to have emotions and feelings disembodied from the past, freely invented in the so-called "here and now." Perceptual and Gestalt psychology suggested to some architects and theorists the possibility of a functional language of design that depended only on autochthonous, form-perceiving capacities of people—the ability to see basic circles, squares, compositions—and did not need to rely on images of the past to provide order in the environment.

---

[8]Currently, new appreciation for these combinations of classical and modern are described as "Free-Style Classicism" in a special issue of *Architectural Design,* (Jencks, 1982).

[9]Jenneret, Charles Edouard (1971). Historically all architects have used proportions to scale buildings. Medieval architects used measures derived from the masonic arts and related to musical scales. Le Corbusier used a similar metric with the goal of deriving a single module which could allow all building to be systematized under an abstract language of design while retaining its humanistic spirit.

The proportions used by Palladio in his formal facades were translated and abstracted to serve as the basis for a modern aesthetic theory in Le Corbusier's *Modulor*. The dream at the time was of a universal style of architecture (a style that later became known as the International Style). This style espoused the need for consistency and regularity of volumes, spaces enclosed by planes and surfaces, elegant, technically perfect materials with fine proportions. It eschewed the individualism of Frank Lloyd Wright's organic architecture, or the references to history in the ornamental architecture of the late 19th Century. There was an idea of an objective language of design, freed of the shackles of history that could be used to house the institutions of a new, unified industrial world society which transcended and embraced all cultures in a kind of environmental Esperanto.

I will not labor over the relationship of this aesthetic theory to the concept of imperialism and the conception that the expansion of the U.S. and European economy could be supported by its internationalization. Suffice it to say the theory landed with a bang on American shores because it made practical sense. It allowed for expression of the U.S. entrepreneurial style by simplifying the building process (this was already being done in the U.S. with its traditional lack of concern for European canons of taste). The new canons were opened to broad judgment and subjective opinion and not rooted in traditions that relied on knowledgeable interpretations of historic precedents or appreciation by an educated eye. The allegorical contents—references to Biblical history, Solomon's temple, the tower of Babel, the holy grail and the gardens of Babylon—all of which had been implicated in design choices made throughout history—dropped out of the sight of the modern movement. It was conceived to be a qualitative breach with the history of mental life. The dawn of a new international culture comprised of the infinitely plastic psyches promised by Progressivists like Dewey and Mead, and inspired socialists around the world, was as shattering to the history of mind as was "relativity" to astronomy and physics.

In hindsight, we now know the argument for infinite plasticity of the human mind or of the material environment to have been overly optimistic.[10] Each increment in plasticity produces secondary effects that increase the costs of plasticity. In the environment, it is possible to turn arid regions into fertile zones, but it can produce social and political conflicts

---

[10]For a review of the history of the modern movement in architecture from a social perspective see, Tom Wolfe (1981). This review is popular and tainted, but gives the spirit of the polemic against modernism. Also, the final chapter in Oscar Newman (1980) explores the history of the international style in social perspective. This is not a simple issue inasmuch as the modern idea infatuated and later disappointed revolutionary socialist countries as well as capitalist cultures. See Alvin Toffler (1980) for an excellent review of the early Renaissance ideas that established the notions of modernism as far back as the 15th century, and an evenhanded condemnation of centralizing, hierarchizing, maximizing, and corporatizing cultures independent of political persuasion.

that threaten the future of society. We may rationalize these processes of planning by declaring they will produce a more logical system of distribution and location of food-production, land, and human habitation. Third World citizens, however, have a different view of rational order from their perspective. Without history to rely on, we become subject to the limits of human intelligence. Or, we begin to look to biology and instinct for principles of order that are deeper than canonic logic, the principle of clear reason used by the Greeks and Romans trying to do the same things in relation to the facts of their own societal histories.

COMPARATIVE MENTAL DEVELOPMENT

The context in which I wish to view these issues stems from Heinz Werner's notions of comparative mental development. Throughout history there has always been a conflict—a dialectical relationship—between the ecstatic and the ordered, the romantic and the rational. The way a culture manages this dialectic and makes distinctions of the sort, contributes to important political-economic choices that shape its main themes and qualities.

In Werner's espoused fondness for Goethe, his interest in expressive forms, I see a likeness to an understanding of the dialectic between the romantic and the rational that was present in Germany in the 19th Century—the Romantic classicism of Schinkel in the early years of the century and later Otto Wagner and others.

Romantic classicism, or Symbolic Realism as it is called by Richard H. Brown, (1977)[11] embodies this notion of harmony of opposites. Werner's concern with mental development expressed a balanced view of history and culture that kept him forever poised between the rational certainty of science and the intuitive choice-process of art. The discovery of "forms," Goethe insisted, is a matter of choice no less than a matter of understanding. Like Goethe's "transcendental zoology," a way of combining intuition and deduction into an understanding of nature and art, Werner's study of comparative mental development was a classical-romantic approach to patterns of mental life. Like Goethe, Werner used himself as a source of the forms—an objective awareness of his own subjectivity. To describe the psychological processes we take to be change or "development" we have to use some finite set of mental images of transition or change in state, no matter how abstract or complex the description. For example, time-lapse photography probably shaped intuitions about develop-

---

[11]Richard H. Brown (1977) describes an engaging approach to poetics similar to work of Jurgen Habermas in history. For Brown, consciousness makes it possible to have choice in a political sense; to assume an extra-historical attitude means to create a breach with the conditions of ordinary reality. This is perforce a radical artistic act.

mental transitions at the early part of this century. Computer simulations are used frequently as a model now. Werner never denied the lasting significance of the model in shaping the rational order and rigor of logic and mathematics served by the model.

The tension between the romantic and the rational was kept alive by Werner's *Comparative Psychology of Mental Development*.[12] His organismic theory was not a formal analysis of perception in the biological tradition of Gestalt psychology. It embodied the erratic, artistic intuitions of Kandinsky. Werner appreciated the virtues of the cool, rational tradition, but not as the expense of the ecstatic, emotional, natural sources of mental life. In light of later uses of his theory, Werner might be accused of being a systems-theorist, like Parsons in sociology or Von Bertalanffy in biology. There are strains of his having attempted to bring the primitive, aboriginal impulse under the rule of rationality, to make primitive perception, thought, and feeling seem to operate according to their own logics. I do not believe this was his intent. He was the appreciator of the "forms" underlying nature's diverse and disorderly appearances. The search for morphological forms that are manifested in diverse domains is not the same as the Positivist tendency to impose a rational order upon nature. These are forms that are at the same time objective and subjective. They express the choice-process of the artist and the selection and abstraction process of the scientist.

In architecture it is a constant theme and painful struggle to strike the balance between individual creation and collective evolution of buildings and artifacts. The conflict is most extremely portrayed in Ayn Rand's *Fountainhead*[13] and most eminently in Frank Lloyd Wright's (1957) organic architecture. The concept that buildings could be designed on the basis of abstract, scientific functional descriptions (needs for protection from the environment, etc.) was paralleled by attempts to built a soul-less psychology based on abstract needs, e.g., affiliation and achievement. Clearly there were people at the turn of this century that thought the science of society would advance to the point where we would deduce the shape and character of buildings and then build the people to occupy them (cf. Gropius, 1970).

We are now discovering in a number of fields that the forces which generate structure (from buildings to regions in architecture, from particle physics to astronomy) are not amenable to purely objective analysis. We are

---

[12]Heinz Werner's (1940, 1957) theory was an attempt to translate much of 19th century German aesthetics into a coherent psychology. Herbert Spencer's ideas of "systems" clearly serve as a model of this attempt at systematization.

[13]In *The Fountainhead,* Ayn Rand (1975) includes incredibly revealing quotations about the individual, libertarian spirit that steamed the passions of the modernist breach with historicism.

pattern-making creatures and what we take to be "order" in any domain depends on a combination of subjective and objective mental processes. In the generated structure of the human environment, the definition of structure also entails a considerable amount of choice based on values (unlike the structures of physics or chemistry). It is inadequate to elect either a rational approach based on the facts of social development (Durkheim, 1947) or an intuitive approach based on the episodic and atemporal choice process of the artist or mystic (Garfinkel, 1967). Werner's framework for the study of mental development encompasses both these concerns.

Werner's focus on mental development assures the persistence of the Platonic eidos. Buildings and other artifacts each have a "core" idea associated with them. Beethoven's Fifth Symphony cannot be reduced to a four-note theme any more than the Pantheon can be reduced to a grand dome. The ontological status of these themes, types, and forms could not be readily explained by Werner, but gratefully he was not willing to dismiss them by pushing for undue epistemological order.

A THEORY OF PRACTICE

In my practical, applied projects I have tried to use this orientation as consistently as possible, at least always grappling with its implications for policy and planning. I have worked on projects ranging in size from new-towns associated with resource developments (mines in Guatemala, West Africa), redesign of a large industrial complex for IBM, development of plans for low-cost residences for the elderly and disabled in Los Angeles, designing group homes for special populations, and individual homes for families. In all these instances my main concern has been for the mental grasp of the process and its outcome by participants. My colleagues and I refer to this as a "developmental approach" to planning and design although it may be different from the exact meaning development has in Heinz Werner's psychology and the elaboration and modifications of the theory by Wapner, Kaplan, and their students. Of course, many other fields have theories of development that bear similarities to Werner's theory of mental development (cf. Chodak, 1973, on societal development and Jantsch, 1975, which explores the same issues in systems engineering). Werner is never cited in these works and his work is not antecedent to theirs. None that I have found, however, deal explicitly with the notion of "mental development."

When I approach a planning or design project, I focus on the psychological "mapping" of the problem by participants and try to use this understanding in monitoring and facilitating the process. Typically, I have a partially formed theory of how the process should proceed, but like an artist, need to be open to the kinds of intuitive leaps that occur in any human activity.

Initially I was drawn to the *systems-approach* to problem solving because of its open-endedness. Generally speaking, systems-theory in engineering and planning conceives of a generic design process that goes through successive cycles of analysis' synthesis and evaluation. To deal with a complex object like a building, which today has as many as 500,000 parts that are worth cataloging, one has to be systematic. The problem-set has to be divided into subsets at a number of levels, and then a process needs to be established for cycling through these sets from the large to small scale and back, to see the implications of one scale or one aspect of the problem for others. The process needs to be rigorous with many checkpoints and benchmarks so that steps are coordinated and kept in phase, goals and objectives changed as needed.

In general I think it is fair to say systems-theory is not mere unenlightened positivism. General systems theory on which it is based (or GST as I will refer to it) is a theory about "ways in which entities in the world are adaptively and purposively related to each other." "A science of integration and synthesis, a science of complexities, of organized constraints and resources, of unified diversities." Basically GST provides a metaperspective by which points of analogy can be discovered across disciplines, then coherently described, examined, and synthesized into patterns.

GST is a very important and undeniably useful way of perceiving analogies among the systems properties of otherwise disparate structures. The U.S. government, the process of fermentation of wine, and the operation of an automobile all require information and transform it, waste energy, have output. They all have some means of keeping the process dynamically stable and goal oriented. They find ways to balance external demands with internal constraints by anabolic and catabolic means.

There is, however, something questionable about the equilibrial model that underlies systems-theory. It always ends up producing objects and human processes that are overly weighted in the direction of science and rationality. Artistic intuition is invariably compromised by the process.

Now this need not and should not be the case. Buckminster Fuller was reportedly fond of saying, "rational rules of nature are just as likely to produce a butterfly as a Sherman tank." Yet there is something about the systems-approach, as formulated, that has this stultifying effect on imagination. The alternative approach I propose is based on an anthropological grasp of processes involved in human problem solving. The categories we use, the way we divide problems into subsets, determine to a great extent the kinds of settings we create. I would contend that rational and intuitive designers set loose on the same problem would take totally diverse routes and come out with radically different products. The approach I would recommend exploits the dynamic tension produced by these divergent perspectives to arrive at a synthesis.

Take a relatively simple example. I recently studied a series of wineries in order to learn how to design one. Wine making is amenable to systems-theoretic study inasmuch as a Zinfandel has to be made under the same exacting conditions that have been used for hundreds of years as measured by a series of articulated variables (body, acidity, essence, aroma). Some wineries are, in fact, run with the technological precision of a large industry and use classic systems-engineering cycle of *analysis-synthesis-evaluation* as a guide to decision-making. The elements of the process are decomposed into components in a framework that emphasizes feedback, adaptive equilibrium, and cost-efficiency measured by established criteria.

The systems monitors performance, and if perturbations are introduced (early warnings of loss of a grape crop) other options are possible and the system allows for goal change by means of new linkages among elements. Other romantically idyllic wineries are intuitively operated and do not fit the systems model at all with its underlying technicist assumptions. In these wineries the winemaster is an artistic director, more a creator than a producer. Instead of responding to perturbations by adaptive changes in goals, the winemaster invents new wines or wine blends. Efficiency of the processes (e.g., grape crushing) are less important than the quality of the processes. Processes are always being reexamined in the most "romantic" ways. For example, out of love for the grapes, in one winery the winemaster refuses to "crush" grapes. He lets the juice gently ooze from them, with no artificial force applied, relying only on the weight of the grapes on top in the vat. Grape juices are moved only by grativy, not to be disturbed by pumps or propellers. The winery is high on a hill and depends on a vertical arrangement of vineyard, winery, bottling area ordered from top to bottom of the hill. These are "discovered" mechanisms that come out of the concrete embodiments of the local process in a particular landscape. It takes a romantic view, to turn this kind of impractical adversity into an advantage. Yet these instances of "romantic" engineering produce award winning yields. When the stakes are high and the judgment criteria as refined as in wine tasting, ordinary systems-engineering will not suffice; enterpreneurs are not willing to be guided by objective analysis without also consulting their dreams.

Peter Hall (1980) notes parallels in a series of large-scale projects he has analyzed. All of them failed in part due to gratuitous uses of systems-theoretic design and development. Among them are the Concord Supersonic plane and the channel tunnel between France and England. The problem with these projects is not the rationality of systems-theory or the orderly procedures for analyzing processes of inordinate complexity it offers. The systems-approach makes it possible to take apart a problem in which everything impacts on everything else. The difficulty with the theory as used is only that it assumes the objectivity of the "problem space." It uses a phenomenological mapping of the world taken as an *object* system and not a subject system. The concepts of systems, linkages, feedback, and equilibrium are taken as processes in an abstract "mathematical" domain that generate actions and objects in accord with human objectives that are taken to be outside that domain. Systems-theorists treat the phenomenal object-world as if they, themselves are outside it, designing its processes in accord with evaluatable objectives of the system. They are not!

For a *developmentalist* there is no way for a system to be monitored or controlled through "objective" methods alone. Each view of a system reveals only a single component of a total mosaic. Developing the space-shuttle has impacts on particle physics that are unknowable, as are its impacts on national defense or international relations. In some ways, we are at best like Plato's philosopher looking at shadows in the cave (the phenomenal object world). The ways in which we define that object world, the limits we set in bounding it are still a function of values of a local culture operating in its cultural context. It is important for a developmentalist to map the process of generating meanings in the culture. I refer to this process as "entification" or the creation of new meaning-units in the world (cf. Dunn, 1971). Entification is a deliberately evasive term that implies that in the process of creating new artifacts we establish with them new ideologies of living, sentiments (or the loss of old sentiments) and areas of consensus and dissensus in the culture. The anthropology of public policy that I am proposing attempts to capture a quality of design processes in which planners or policy makers are reflexively aware of the consequences of choices for the spate of reality in which they work. The developmental approach focuses, however, on the *meanings* they ascribe to events and the choices they make as to what they use as "source" datum for their actions. In this system there are no simple measures of system performance.

The basic outlines of this theory of practice can be made clear by reference to Table 4.1. In this table I draw a contrast between the "core themes" of systems-theory and those of a developmental approach to practice. I will go through a brief portrayal of the differences between the systems-theoretic and developmental approaches.

A developmental approach requires time to register the nature of the problem by a cohort group and to fantasize different hypothesized solutions to the problem in its immediate context rather than choosing among previously tested, ready-made solutions.

Out of these processes a constituency can develop that can become increasingly agile at scanning the environment for problems and opportunities for consensus-based actions. Actions are then taken in relation to *images* of the future (actions that might provoke animated consensus) rather than

TABLE 4.1[a]

Developmental Approach	Technicist Approach
Entification Categories (Anthropology of Public Policy)	Systems Theory Core Themes (Science and Technology)
Settings of Relevance	Concept of Systems
Role Prescriptions	Linkage and Interaction
Distribution of Functions	Cycles and Cycling
Allocation of Consequences	Feedback
Capabilities Available	Equilibrium
Recognized Contingencies	Systems Energy Flow
Habits of Mind	Hierarchy
Hierarchies of Values	Systemic Evolution

[a]These developmental categories were developed jointly with D. Sam Scheele, *Social Engineering* Technology Inc., Westwood, Los Angeles, as part of work on a contract for the U.S. Office of Education.

deficiency-correcting, error-reducing strategies of most technicist approaches based on objective measures of system-performance.

The developmental approach takes the definition of the SETTING to be a critical determinant of the outcome. The way the problem is bounded and characterized shapes the kinds of strategies and outcomes that are seen as cogent. For example, in studying the redesign of an IBM plant, managers and workers were mutually convinced that the major issue at stake was "cleaning up" or beautifying the environment. As the process proceeded both sides began to realize there were problems with the definition and design of the "work itself" and these new issues were at odds with the upgrading of the environment. They then faced the dilemma of advocating a deeper look at the work itself, at the possible expense of immediate improvement of the environment.

The SETTINGS are not permanent. They are defined through discourse, debate, and political processes. The local culture is modified by this process. As they focus on their shared environment new linkages are formed. The objective of design is to incorporate this breathless flow of human realizations into the result—not to freeze the process of social change.

Each entity we work on, be it a building or an organization, can be thought of as having a "core idea" around which its integrity hangs. In companies this is being referred to currently as "corporate culture;" in a family it may be an underlying metaphorical outlook that leads one family to feel comfortable in a house perched on a precipice while another likes a stone battlement in the middle of a forest. Without the "core idea" there can be no system. The negotiation of these meanings is a major role of the designer, planner, and his/her constituents or clients.

ROLES are ways of dividing the environment into components that are at the same time social and physical. The concept of the "public" implied in the Greek Chorus required the differentiation of the stage into a public central area separated from the audience and actors. All physical settings have some degree of social differentiation. The stage analogy is useful as a source of images that ties social roles to environmental boundaries. It also suggests the variety of ways in which the same idea can be expressed. For example, the stage can be on the periphery. In one theatre in Germany, the audience was actually rotated on a "stage" in the center to face performances on a series of stages all around them.

FUNCTIONS are larger ensembles than roles. They include alternative means of organizing themes (settings) and roles (activities) into larger motifs and compositions.

For example, computers are being designed for commercial use. Systems-designers face choices in their design. This is an instrument at the stage in its evolution that automobiles were seventy years ago. Cars required road building, patterns of urbanization and social life to support their use. These were articulated in relation to the styles of use suggested and options suggested by early artifacts.

By analogy, the "electronic cottage" idea proposed by Toffler, and the concept of telecommuting, involve new notions of relationships of people and environment. People will not travel to work unless they have to. New functions are being shaped, then, by the emergent character of the new technology.

ALLOCATION OF CONSEQUENCES or perceived benefits, impacts and responsibilities, risks and rewards need to be examined. Are the people who are bearing the risks and consequences involved in a process, generating and selecting the options? In the case of new computer technology there is a real danger of loss of jobs and other impacts on the world economy including potential redistribution of world wealth. On the other hand, computers can create thousands of new settings and psychological domains, new languages, and cultural forces.

If they objectify the process of design, systems approaches can result in restrictive technological and electronic versions of the past rather than intuitively transmuted inquiries into the future. There is need to imagine new settings, roles, and functions in addition to rational testing of options based on current settings and roles.

RECOGNIZED CONTINGENCIES and AVAILABLE CAPABILITIES need to be examined in relationship to other demands and priorities. New interest in strategic planning exists as business confront the new turbulence and high uncertainty of the future business environment. Survival depends on a combination of "broken field running" and social intervention. All planning processes need to consider ways of keeping options open, anticipating disrupting events. The success potential of a plan depends on a combination of available capabilities and recognized opportunities. The issue now is not whether an action is worth taking, but how worth it, for whom, and at the expense of what other potential actions.

HABITS OF MIND include the presuppositions, ideas, notions, and folk-theories that a group uses to explain *to themselves* their own activities and motives.

HIERARCHIES OF VALUES are abstract dimensions that underlie choices. They can be examined using multi-dimensional scaling techniques. Diverse groups involved in a design or planning process can be made aware of their own intrinsic criteria in making design choices, providing feedback on their subjective criteria as a basis for planning rather than relying on objective measures of systems-performance.

All these steps in an anthropological approach to systems suggest a high degree of interaction and self-definition of people in relation to technical systems and to PLANNING PROCESSES themselves.

The results of planning are produced by interaction. They can be thought of as a reality construct by the groups involved in the process; not a means of producing a decision among known alternatives to achieve prescribed goals and objectives. As an individual or group enters the planning discourse, the zone of planning issues opens up. More and more of the structure and character of the ordinary world become revealed as products of human interaction as opposed to being seen as the "natural" by-products of social and cultural evolution. In fact, the role of an anthropologically inclined planner is often to slow the process down. Because processes of successive refinement strongly tend to induce convergence, a planner might purposely introduce ambiguities, even disruptions, in order to avoid premature closure on a solution.

The underlying idea is that reality is a negotiable construct. This construct cannot be generated by induction, by simple attempts to gather data, or by rationally defining variables. Information gathering is only a means of defining new options. Using these design intuitions, the environment under consideration is seen as indeterminate, arbitrary, even a "convenient" fiction.

Unlike the Cartesian universe, the "developmentalists" environment will not sit still long enough to be described and analyzed. Imaginative "work" is part of the delimitation of the problem and not merely a mechanism used to create a new situation to an old problem. For example, "synectics" is a problem-solving tool invented by systems-theorists to use imagination (analogizing skills). A biological sphincter mechanism will be "borrowed" to design the automatic top of a new thermos-jug.

In a developmental approach to planning, the problem is not confined to a technical gap that needs to be filled by imaginative discovery; for example, a gate mechanism for a parking garage. Based on the same analogy, no matter how much these approaches value "art" or "intuition," they produce negative effects for their beneficiaries by not involving them in the process. Developmental approaches to planning are based on the building of collective consensus; stimulating and liberating collective imagination.

Very little is known about these kinds of processes.[14] Not all participatory planning and design activities result in positive, structural understanding of the problem, a grasp of its complexity, arbitrariness, and shaping by unpredictable contextual forces. Many "naive" planning groups have waded into a problem of designing for themselves only to emerge with a plan to build a commercial hotel to maximize personal profits.[15]

We do know that complex concepts and images are transpersonal. They can be equilibrial or disequilibrial. They can resist environmental perturbations or yield to them, depending on the power of the "core idea" or myth that serves as their center. Core ideas tend to have a lifespan (or at least a "half-life") that leads to their dissolution and rebirth. Faced with collective images that serve as the "core" of a plan, the professional must adopt the outlook of co-learner trying to stay a step ahead of the growing consensus.

Consensus is not produced by having voting majorities built up around options or choices defined in a political process that is separated from technical analysis. In most planning processes dominated by a technical perspective there is a strict separation of ends and means. Goals are decided by a political procedure, and means of defining actions to achieve these goals in the most efficient manner are the sole responsibility of the technical analyst. In a developmental approach ends and means are intertwined. There are no technical means of solving a problem that are objective or "bias free." In the course of executing actions new goals are discovered. The developmental planner has to be open to an ongoing learning process that involves a reorientation of action and ongoing modifications of project goals. Ultimately, the whole complex of means and ends is a political process in which there is an ongoing negotiation of the meaning of the events by

---

[14]Chris Argyris and Donald Schön (1978) offer suggestions as to how to make people aware of their operating assumptions in organizations. It is difficult to communicate about the power of liberated consciousness in organizations when most people have not had the electrifying experience of the rewards of group consciousness: Therefore, the success of organizations like *EST*, which provide a brief insight into these new processes.

[15]This merely suggests the need for a social learning process. In Holland, for example, great cost and effort is expended in working with communities and sub-communities in a deeply participatory fashion. This is done by having large displays of all plans, encouraging community response to them, negotiating compromises, etc. There are many examples of this work in the U.S. and Canada as well in which architects have stimulated compromise between factions by generating proposals that transcended the historical constraints faced by the divided parties.

groups involved. Tradesmen working on an edifice are not "mere" machine parts executing a project for compensation; they are advocates of a way of building. An open society would not reduce the choice between competing strategies (say industrialized building system vs. hand-made houses) to a simple cost-equation, i.e., selecting the option with the lowest costs and greatest benefits measured in dollars. In this sphere the planners role may be to generate "extra-historical" realities, or scenarios about the future that exist in no time or place, and that can be used to reveal something about the present.[16] These imagined worlds can produce a release from the "zero-sum" character of the present in which one or another group stands to lose. Typically there is a feeling of bad faith about allocation decisions because we view the future as an inevitable extension of the present in which one advocate group will lose. Alternatively, we can see it as a means of utilizing collective experience to initiate new directions of design and development that expand benefits for all groups.

Taken in this way, plans are by no means strictly rational ways of achieving well understood, politically defined goals. Rather, they more or less resemble architecture. There are "core themes" which provide for a project a general direction of development subject to cycles of revision and redefinition. The process is one of mutual learning and discovery as the embedded character of the activity becomes clear. In an imaginative process, obstacles become opportunities rather than being seen as impediments to purified execution of the plan. Finally, the way in which consensus emerges almost always is a surprise and a mystery. In an architectural design process there is a point where the designer surrenders to the building. It now has a life of its own and it appears to "design itself." The lines on the page have become real.

These processes may be translatable some day into algorithmic statements, augmenting, if not replacing current processes with computer planning paradigms that can include the vagaries of emotion and rhapsodic discovery that are familiar to professional planning practice. For the present, impoverished and childlike as our tools of design and participatory planning may be, it is important to keep alive their blend of the rational and the ecstatic.

---

[16]In my own work, I organize debates about projects into "issues" and document them individually. Usually, there is great misunderstanding between factions about the basis for disagreement. If large areas of consensus can be defined, issues can usually be resolved one at a time. Ideological splits usually keep factions from negotiating at the level of individual issues. Hence, the problem set is frozen in rational debate and not allowed to reconfigure itself with new areas of emphasis and urgency constantly coming up, old areas reducing temporarily into the background. Architectural design offers a significant metaphorical ground for this kind of engagement. Like all artistic activities it cannot proceed linearly. At the same time, it has to close on a workable solution. Always it is a risky process that is capable of failure, and cannot succeed without blessing and inspiration.

REFERENCES

Argyris, C., & Schön, D. *Organizational learning*. Reading: Addison-Wesley, 1978.

Arnheim, R. *Dynamics of architectural form*. Berkeley: University of California Press, 1977.

Brown, R. H. *A poetic for sociology*. New York: Cambridge University Press, 1977.

Chodak, S. *Societal development*. New York: Oxford University Press, 1973.

Dunn, E. *Economic and social development*. Baltimore: Johns Hopkins Press, 1971.

Durkheim, E. *Division of labor in society*. New York: Free Press, 1947.

Garfinkel, H. *Ethnomethodology*. Englewood Cliffs, N.J.: Prentice-Hall, 1967.

Gropius, W. *Scope of total architecture*. New York: Macmillan, 1970.

Hall, P. *Great planning disasters*. London: Weidenfeld and Nicholson, 1980.

Jantsch, E. *Design for evolution*. New York: G. Braziller, 1975.

Jencks, C. (Ed.) *Architectural design*. London: St. Martins Press, 1982.

Jenneret, C. E. *Le Modulor*. Cambridge: M.I.T. Press, 1971 (original in French, 1948).

Newman, O. *Community of interest*. Garden City: Doubleday, 1980.

Norberg-Schulz, C. *Existence, space and architecture*. New York: Praeger Paperbacks, 1971.

Palladio, A. *I Quattro Libri Dell'Architectura*. Venice: Appresso Domenico de Franceschi, 1570.

Pevsner, N. *An outline of European architecture*. Baltimore: Penguin, 1974.

Rand, A. *The fountainhead*. Indianapolis: Bobbs Merrill, 1975.

Rykwert, J. *The first moderns*. Cambridge: M.I.T. Press, 1980.

Serlio, S. *Architetura: Regole Generali di Architetura sopra le cinque maniere de gli edifici (Book IV)*. Venitia: 1537.

Steadman, P. *The evolution of designs*. New York: Cambridge University Press, 1979.

Stokes, A. *Greek culture and the ego: A psychoanalytic survey of an aspect of Greek civilization and of art*. London: Tavistock Publications, 1958.

Toffler, A. *The third wave*. New York: Morrow, 1980.

Werner, H. *Comparative psychology of mental development*. New York: Harper, 1940 (Second Ed., Chicago: Follett, 1948; Third Ed., New York: International Universities Press, 1957).

Werner, H. The concept of development from a comparative and organismic point of view. In D. Harris (Ed.), *The concept of development*. Minneapolis, MN: University of Minnesota Press, 1957.

Wittkower, R. *Architectural principles in the age of humanism*. London: A. Tiranti, 1952.

Wittkower, R. *Palladio and English Palladianism*. London: Thames and Hutsen, 1974.

Wolfe, T. *From Bauhaus to our house*. New York: Farrar Straus Giroux, 1981.

Wright, F. L. *A testament*. New York: Horizon Press, 1957.

5 Reflections on Culture and Personality from the Perspective of Genetic-Dramatism

Bernard Kaplan
Clark University and Heinz Werner Institute for Developmental Psychology

INTRODUCTION

Nations fighting over essentially contested territories are likely to deride and ridicule the claims of their opponents to legitimate control of those territories. Even if the nations enter into negotiations, there are likely to be charges of "obstructionism" and "obscurantism" by one or the other when things do not go their way. Each is ready to get on with the solution to the problem, as long as the other yields precedence in determining what shall be done. The same may be said for psychologists or social scientists fighting over essentially contested concepts or terms.[1] Those who are proceeding as if they own the concept or term find those who question that ownership to be "deluded," "counterproductive," "obstructionist," and the bearer of a host of other negative properties. To support their claim to the concept, they may invoke "tradition," "ordinary usage," "divine inspiration," the consensus of their friends and colleagues ("experts"), and so on.

One might think that struggles over the ownership of a term could be more easily resolved than struggles over the control of a physical territory.

---

[1]Some, for theoretical reasons or because of ontological commitments, do not distinguish or wish to distinguish between "terms" and "concepts" (or "sentences" and "propositions"). We shall. Why those who refuse to make, or who collapse, the distinction between terms and concepts fight over possession of the word is more or less easy to understand. Why others, like ourselves, should be concerned with who possesses the "word" is more obscure. It may have something to do with whom one will hire if one is looking, for example, for a *developmental psychologist*. Who controls the "term" has a greater likelihood of having control over the choice.

One of the contestants might yield the "term" to the other, and adopt a different term to represent his/her conception, much as Peirce introduced "pragmaticism" to distinguish himself and his views from James' "pragmatism." It is obvious, however, that such resolutions do not often occur. Social scientists often fight over the possession of the Word, seeking to fill it with their "stuff" rather than allowing others to take it over with their "crap."[2]

Elsewhere (Kaplan, this volume), I have tried to persuade the reader to a certain conception of *development,* arguing, like the Israelis, for legitimate rights to the "territory" on the basis of history, tradition, rationality, etc. Here, we will suppose, even if counter-factually, that we have been granted the rights, and consider how human development-in-culture, a perennial trouble spot, looks from the heights.[3] What should our diplomatic relations be with the overlapping territories of Personality and Culture?

Now, "personality" and its satellites "person," "individual," etc. have always been linked to us. "Culture," on the other hand, has been taken over by a variety of disciplines, and now seems to belong to the "anthropologists." Even among them, it is scarcely an uncontested concept: There are almost as many meanings attributed to "culture" as there are, and have been, anthropologists (see Kroeber & Kluckhohn, 1963). Some have seen "culture" as *sui generis* and have tried to free it from any intrinsic connection with individuals (e.g., L. White, 1949). Others have argued that it had intrinsic connections with "personality": culture influences personality; personality is shaped through culture; personality interacts with culture; and so on.

More recently, some anthropologists have asserted that personality rightly belongs to culture; that one could not understand the formation of the person outside of a socio-cultural context. And, indeed, a few anthropologists have also suggested that "development" belongs to them: It makes no sense, they maintain, to speak of personality, development, or personality development outside of cultural contexts (Geertz, 1966; LeVine, 1980). And one or two have diplomatically asked whether the territory of "psychology" itself is not an artificially established one, one that really belongs, in one part, to biology, and another, to anthropology.[4] A number

---

[2]Hear George Carlin, Monologue. *Johnny Carson Show,* May 19, 1981. Carson Productions, Burbank, CA. Doubtless on tape. Date of permanent recording unknown.

[3]Or the desert depths, if you like.

[4]The rationale underlying this query seems to be somewhat complex. If the formation of the person (and personality) cannot be understood outside of a cultural complex, this must be *a fortiori* true for the functions or activities of a person, for example, remembering, thinking, perceiving, imagining, believing. Indeed, these "functions" themselves are culturally defined, and it is only someone blind to this fact who assumes that these "functions" or "acts" are universal and independent of culture. Thus, one anthropologist (Needham, 1972) has questioned whether the distinctions among activities drawn by one (a limited) group of

of psychologists, ourselves among them, are cautiously sympathetic to these claims, although we also have serious reservations. Some of our sympathies and reservations come out in the following discussion of a number of issues.

DEVELOPMENT AS NORMATIVE:
IMMANENCE AND TRANSCENDENCE

Any universal normative idea of *development* of the kind hinted at in Werner's writings (Werner, 1948/57; see also Werner & Kaplan, 1956), and explicitly advanced by Kaplan (1966, 1983, this volume) is, in this day and age, inevitably subject to challenge or dismissal by historicists, cultural relativists, and others, who reject any claims to the pertinence or validity of normative judgments transcending those indwelling norms obtaining in specific societies in time and space. With the "death of God," the radical decline of beliefs in natural law or natural right (see Strauss, 1953), and widespread rejection of an orthogenetic trend in cultural "evolution" (see Boyd, 1962), transcendent ideals of the good, the true and the beautiful were taken as ethnocentric fantasies, and more or less self-contained socio-cultural entities were proclaimed "absolute monarchs" (Kaplan, 1983).

Although early exponents of the autonomy and sovereignty of cultural entities were often "conservatives," reacting against the denigratory judgments and evaluations of the intellectuals of the "shallow French Enlightenment" concerning the medieval period, the banner of "cultural relativism" in our time has been carried chiefly by "liberal" and "radical" anthropologists, reacting against the racist use of certain standards in evaluating "primitive cultures" (cf. F. Boas, 1911/1963). Such anthropologists challenged attempts to order the beliefs and practices of social orders in some kind of developmental or evolutionary scheme on several different grounds.

First, they challenged the use of the norms and values of one society or one civilization to assess the practices of another society; this procedure was analogous to the practice of using the rules of Latin to evaluate all other languages in terms of excess or defect. Thus, even if it were accepted that

---

psychologists in one cultural tradition for purposes of their study have any pertinence to members of other cultures. It is presumably as ethnocentric to believe that one's psychological categories are universal as to believe that one's values have a universal application. Yet, without this belief, Western psychologists seeking the universal laws and "mechanisms" of abstracted functions of the person are chasing a will of the wisp, or making general claims about human beings on the basis of their own cultural prejudices. Another line of argument questions the justification of separating acts from the objects with which they are involved, that is, talking about "learning," "perceiving," "remembering" as if these could be detached from the objects, learned, perceived, or remembered—objects that are necessarily cultural (see White, 1949).

the practices and instructions characteristic of a society were the objective manifestations of mental functioning,[5] all one could legitimately argue was that mental functioning was *different* in social orders. One could not argue the superiority or higher status of one set of practices and beliefs over another.

The second argument, somewhat at odds with the first, was to the effect that mental processes were everywhere the same; cultural phenomena were merely the variable products of universal mental operations carried out on different material. Thus, everyone learned, or remembered, their beliefs in the same way; people of different societies just learned or remembered different beliefs.

There was also a third argument, somewhat underplayed. If a belief or a practice in another society was assessed as "primitive," an anthropologist could argue (cf. Boas, 1955) that the same kind of practice or belief also was manifested among individuals in so-called advanced societies. This *tu quoque* argument, which conceded that cultural beliefs could be evaluated in terms of transcendent standards, while demanding recognition for the fact that "primitive" or "advanced" mentality was not the peculiar prerogative of any single society or set of societies, was, as noted, generally played down by anthropologists.[6] Only recently has it begun to emerge from the closet.[7]

Despite this occasional concession as to the heterogeneity or stratification of human mentation—a point of course stressed by psychoanalytically-oriented anthropologists (Roheim, Devereux)—the general temper of anthropological thought was in the direction of a high valuation of cultural autonomy and cultural relativism. Although the rise of Hitler, and the prob-

---

[5]This view goes back at least as far as Vico, and was elaborated by Herder and the German idealist tradition. This view accepted by Werner (1957), as well as Dewey, Cassirer, and others allows one to consider cultural institutions—religions, legal systems, languages, etc. as manifestations of mind and locates "mind" first and foremost in culture (see Kaplan, 1967).

[6]Paul Radin (1957), had early argued for advanced forms of mentation in so-called "primitive societies."

[7]Bunzel (1966), a student of Boas had initially rejected Levy-Bruhl's work on "prelogical mentality," but subsequently accepted it with the proviso that the mental processes discussed by Levy-Bruhl also occurred in members of Western societies, and even among scientists. Hallpike (1976) discusses "primitive mentality" in various societies on the basis of Piaget's formulations. With regard to the negative evaluation of Levy-Bruhl, see Kaplan (1966). Once one recognizes that "the fundamental unity of mankind" does not conflict with the heterogeneity of the human mind, wherever it occurs, much of the animus against Levy-Bruhl may dissolve. This is not to suggest that Levy-Bruhl's formulations should be adopted without reservations.

lems of coping with the sovereignty of the Nazi state with respect to norms of justice and truth, was to shake up some relativists among the anthropological fraternity (cf. Redfield, 1953), the interventions of Western nations in third-world societies, under slogans of "developing" these societies, rewakened the doctrine of cultural autonomy and the exaltation of cultural relativism.[8] One had no business assessing others as to their developmental status on the basis of norms or values extrinsic to the sociocultural order itself.[9]

Arguments against transcendent "norms" and "values" seem to have an intrinsic appeal to many of us. We have come to believe that the values of the "good" or "right" and the "beautiful" are "subjective" or "relative." And, although some of us hold on to norms and values of the "true" and "the logical" as transcendent, there seems no good reason to exempt these from the dung-heap of the immanent if one tosses the others on to it. Thus, one may argue that no one from an alien culture can legitimately assess as higher or lower, more advanced or less advanced, any practices, beliefs or conceptions of members of another society. All those cross-cultural studies, so beloved by some Western developmental psychologists, applying concepts, method and elaborate scales to determine the "stages" or "levels" that the aborigines attain, are merely ethnocentric impositions that seek to squeeze others into the Procrustean bed of one's parochial categories. So goes the argument of those who would reject the attempts by psychoanalysts, Piagetians, Wernerians, and others to apply putative culture-transcendent norms and standards to socio-cultural orders other than their own. One has no justification for speaking of the level of cognitive development, moral development, development of concepts of justice, self, or anything else with respect to the practices and beliefs of a

---

[8]"Cultural relativism" as a fact, noted at least as far back as Herodotus, is merely the observation that beliefs, practices, etc. vary from society to society. "Cultural relativism," exalted as a value, leads easily to the normative notion of "cultural sovereignty"—the charge that no one has the right to impose extrinsic standards of the "good," "beautiful," and "true" on an alien social order. It is this latter thesis that leads ineluctably to the normative doctrine of "the absolute sovereignty of the individual" (see footnote 9).

[9]One will note that the same argument has been directed against those who would apply the norms and values of a dominant segment of a society to other groups within the society, for example assessing from a developmental point of view the practices and beliefs of sub-groups or ethnic minorities within a society. The ultimate logic of this position leads to the rejection of the application of cultural norms or sub-cultural norms to individuals in the society. The ultimate upshot of cultural relativism or cultural sovereignty (culture as God) is individual relativism or individual sovereignty (individual as God).

sovereign socio-cultural order other than the one to which one belongs.[10]

If, following this purgative thesis to its sour-tasting end, we decide to abjure the imposition of all value judgments on denizens of another social-order, and even on ourselves incarnating other "roles" from time to time—the only unbiased way open to us, seems to be provided by *met hodos* of positivism. Putting to one side, now, any attempt at rebuttal of the advocates of "cultural sovereignty" and its clone, "individual sovereignty," let us examine this *hodos,* this Way.

DEVELOPMENT AS DESCRIPTIVE (D–D): WHO SHALL DESCRIBE?

Let us take as "positivism" that metaphysical posture which stipulates undistorted Fact as the only transcendent Value.[11] Condemning us for visiting our value judgments on others, those prone to this posture hold that the only permissible activity we should stand for is that of "describing the facts."[12] With respect to the "development" of human beings in societies, this would seem to entail characterizing the changes that occur in some *naturally* given entity, or some "natural" aspect or part of that entity in the course of time. The "natural entity," naturally taken as the object of description, is the human being: sometimes from birth to senescence;

---

[10]Roheim (1973) as a psychoanalytically-oriented anthropologist (or an anthropologically-oriented psychoanalyst) dismissed these rebuffs categorically, insisting on the legitimacy of applying psychoanalytic categories and concepts to archaic societies, but he presents no arguments for the dismissal. In our terms, he appears merely to assert the universality and diaphaneity of the psychoanalytic "terministic screen," as if he and other analysts were discovering the way things are, and not upon "a blue guitar." Whether this dogmatic attitude has been dropped or at least recognized by contemporary analytically-oriented anthropologists remains to be seen. It would involve the realization that psychoanalysis is an hermeneutic system with no privileged position in interpreting what there is. See Burke (1966), Ricoeur (1970), Fingarette (1963), Casey (1971/72). Many Western academic developmental psychologists, intent on applying their developmental tests and scales to children and adults in other societies, have ignored the issue, nonchalantly going ahead with their cross-cultural studies as if there were no fundamental questions about their techniques, procedures, and scoring systems. Others, more flexible in their procedures and less rigidly wedded to any kinds of fixed scales, have questioned assessments of mental levels of individuals in "primitive societies" based on problems and tasks of alien provenance. It is not clear to us whether the latter group has rejected transcendent norms or urged that they be more clearly articulated and grounded, and also more adequately applied.

[11]The transformation of "fact" into a transcedent value is discussed by S. Langer (1942, p. 23 ff), also by H. Margenau, (1961). For an illuminating discussion of the confusion over "fact" by logicians and "philosophers of science," see Dewey and Bentley, 1949, Chapter 1.

[12]It has been observed that proponents of positivism have not been beyond voicing ethical and moral imperatives, despite their charge that such imperatives have no cognitive or factual status and are merely expressions of attitude. See Joad, 1950.

sometimes from conception to the omega point. The selected aspects of the human being—e.g., breathing, remembering, fantasizing, reasoning—are arbitrary only in their selection. They are otherwise given as natural aspects of the natural entity.[13]

The job of the developmental psychologist, on the Way, is to describe, without prejudice, the ways in which given human beings (as natural wholes) or their aspects or parts (as natural parts) change "as a function of" changes taking place either in the parts, or in the naturally given environments that surround the human being. Through various "operations" on their observations of these patterns of change, the developmentalist, as describer of the facts, is able to offer a factual, value-free representation of the nature of human development.[14]

Now, some D–Ds, in our society or civilization, observing that changes in human form and behavior correlate variable with selected aspects of human beings and varying features of the "environment," have sought to go beyond the descriptions of individual human beings changing as a function of x, y and z. Through a range of conceptual, methodological, and statistical operations,[15] presumed to be innocent of any charges of child-molesting, these D–Ds have presented us with a description of *the development of the child* or, more recently, *the development of the human being over the life span*. Through these descriptions, we have ostensibly learned about *the* moral development of the child, *the* language development of the child, *the*—fill it in—development of the child; soon to be heard from, doubtless, are those who will give us pure factual descriptions of *the*—fill it

---

[13]On the changing nature of "the natural," see Lovejoy (1948/52) Lovejoy and G. Boas (1935/65); also M. H. Abrams (1955, 1971); Collingwood (1945). The assumption of natural, unmediated, givens (as wholes or parts) to be the objects of factual description already entails the imposition of a perspective in the apparently neutral descriptive enterprise. See Whitehead, 1938, Chapter 1; Polanyi, 1962, pp. 16, 33f. Those who assert that some object is naturally given characteristically take their terministic screen as "literal" (see Cirillo & Kaplan, this volume).

[14]Some will maintain that we are here characterizing and belaboring a "straw man." No investigator—developmental psychologist or anthropologist believes today that this is what he/she is doing. This may be the case with respect to proclaimed beliefs, but we question whether it is so with regard to the tacit presuppositions. Surely, there are some today, raising the straw man charge, who consider the "human being" as a "natural object" and the actions, aspects of action and characteristics of the environments observed and correlated by the investigator as given to the "innocent eye" (as data). Indeed, they may even deny that the objects of their investigations are the objects of their construction, while concurrently maintaining the "constructivist nature of all human cognitive activity."

[15]One might suggest that theoretical or descriptive concepts are "instruments" and "terministic screens" (Burke) and, so too, are methods. These are likely to disturb and perturb the "facts," giving rise to new "facts" or "facts" that would never come to light without their interventions. This fact, although sometimes acknowledged, is, in fact, often repressed by adulators of the "facts."

in—development of the individual over the life span, demonstrating the relationships of all "variables" to all other "variables."

It is partly against the *definite article* that many D–D anthropologists and an increasingly large number of de-centered psychologists have launched their attack. One cannot talk about *the* development—in a factual, descriptive sense, of anything unless one has examined, comparatively and cross-culturally, human beings who are members of other cultures than one's own. Through such examination, executed *without the importation of ethnocentric* categories,[16] one might find—indeed, one is likely to find—different patterns of human development, in general, and child development, in particular.[17] As long as one follows Spinoza, and shuns ridicule or condemnation, seeking only to understand, one has the opportunity, through cross-cultural study, to determine whether there is one *the* development of the child, or several *the* developments of the child; likely, the latter, since there is considerable evidence of several different developments of the child in one's native society. Propelled far enough by this "latitudinarianism" one might even discover, with omniscient observers doing the descriptions, that there are almost as many developments as there are human beings. Some D–Ds might even conclude that individual longitudinal studies— impartial biographies of everyone—is the only way to go if one really wants to respect cultural and, finally, individual differences in human development.[18]

One might think such a proposal is a figment of a fevered imagination and a jaundiced eye: an attempt at satire, caricature, and ridicule.[19] But are there not D–Ds today, especially among the burgeoning life-span movement,[20] who suggest that "human development" can only be dealt with ade-

---

[16]To anticipate briefly what is to come later, the very conceptual categories of an observer, taken as if they were universal rather than parochial, constitute an "ethnocentric" if not "egocentric" importation. Strangely enough, this seems to be recognized more clearly when academics apply their conceptual categories to members of sub-cultures within their own society. All description is theory—and hence, perspective—laden (see Goethe, "All fact is already theory.").

[17]One might even find that the definition of the human being, taken as a "natural object" to be studied, turns out to be culturally-symbolically constituted. The anthropologist or cross-cultural psychologist who presupposes the naturalness of the human being and the human life span as the objects of investigation may, in the process of trying to overcome ethnocentrism, be ethnocentric in spite of himself/herself.

[18]Recall William Blake's admonition: "To generalize is to be an idiot; individuality is the alone distinction of merit."

[19]As Art Buchwald has observed and demonstrated time and again, the possibilities of satire are sharply limited by the actualities of life.

[20]It should be emphasized that a "movement" is not a theory or even a perspective. It is doubtless salutary to observe that human life may not terminate with, or remain static after, infancy, childhood, or even adolescence. But that insight surely does not constitute a perspective, although it may derive from a point of view.

quately if one employs a multiperspectival, multivariate approach? (See Kaplan, in press b.) Who propose that we find out about the nature of human development by examining the functional relationships of everything to everything else from a multiplicity of (professionally respectable) perspectives?[21] Ostensibly, through such a procedure, we will be enabled to construct a Tower up to the sky, and thereby reach the Empyrean, where the Omniperspectival dwells; or compile an infinitely expandable collection of facts that the Omniperspectival can encompass in a unified theory.[22] Without pretending ourselves, as human beings, to come to any conclusions about the nature of human development, we can at least provide all the pieces from our different jig-saw puzzles so that an eventual Master Builder may fit them all together in one magnificent structure. By enjoining that each investigator stick to the facts, we can insure that the final picture will be uncontaminated by values, having no place in the world of facts (see Köhler, 1938).

The major problem with this attempt to achieve a non-normative, nonethnocentric characterization of human development is, it seems to us, the failure on the part of those pursuing the facts to realize that *facts* are not

---

[21]A careful or even cursory critic might observe that in our *dramatistic* garb, we suggest going even further than those we have just "caricatured," and yet not so far. We have suggested that every situation, small or large, may, in everyday life, be differently defined by different participants. These actor-participants struggle with other actor-participants over what is taking place. Such a struggle, often muted due to asymmetrical power relations or indifference, is also likely to occur between the subjects of psychological or anthropological investigation and the investigators themselves, who construe themselves not as participants but merely as objective spectators. The struggle over the definition of what has been observed and represented by erstwhile "spectators" usually occurs with members of their own peer or professional group who often operate as "presences" on the scene of "field work" even though they are bodily elsewhere. In advocating that one must be sensitive to different points of view applied to situations of whatever scale, we as genetic-dramatists do not suggest that we limit ourselves to the perspectives of professionals or experts *qua* "spectators." Pushing to perfection the principle of positivism, *dramatism* maintains that the subject's perspective be taken into account equally with the investigator's. To justify which of several perspectives be given greater weight, if any, pertains to the "genetic" aspect of genetic-dramatism (see Kaplan, this volume). Such a justification cannot be based on the "facts," but involve normative principles to be arrived at dialectically or through the acceptance of a mythos (see Cirillo & Kaplan, this volume).

[22]We do realize that such "carrying things to extremes" may evoke irritation and provoke the charge that this kind of attitude might lead to scepticism concerning the claims of psychological and anthropological experts. Let us not ignore that possibility. Yet, as Cassirer observes (1944, p. 1), a healthy scepticism is often the forerunner of a resolute humanism. One may also entertain the possibility that some will acknowledge that one *should* take the facts from all perspectives, and should individualize human development, but that one *cannot* because of pragmatic limitations, etc. Agreed. But one should not transform a vice into a virtue. If we acknowledge that the "objects" we *construct* with our concepts, methods, and so on are our constructions, our makings, our "facts" (note the common etymology of fact and fiction), and avoid claims about this is the way things are, we shall at least have acknowledged our sins and limitations.

data. As already noted, facts are not *given* but *made,* and their making involves categories and methods that are of parochial provenance, and thereby inherently ethnocentric.[23] Ingredient in the very language of the outsiders who do the investigating, no matter how much they seek to be insiders, are value distinctions (cf. Louch, 1960), alien to the scenes in which the insiders live. This is even more the case when the outsiders (cross-cultural psychologists, anthropologists) go beyond "description" to "explanation," invoking "metaphors" and "terministic screens" derived from their own scenes of participant-action, their own schemas of making sense, which they take to have some universal warrant and transcendent value.

There are many other *cul-de-sacs* in the Positivist Land of Fact, and the accumulation of more facts through the intrepid adventures of traveling men and women will not lead us out of the blind alleys. Perhaps there is another route.

OUTSIDERS AND INSIDERS:
VOX POPULI, VOX DEI

Once one takes into account the possibility that the facts and explanations of "human development" presented to us by social scientists of whatever discipline are laundered through parochial methods and metaphors of self-selected groups of individuals, contesting for the social roles of men and women of knowledge (cf. Znaniecki, 1968), the question may arise why anyone should accept their parochial representations of the how and why of what takes place. This is likely to occur especially when their representations have nothing to do with our experience.

What gives their constructions any precedence over ours? Any higher value? Especially when, in their constructions, they have sought to eliminate all notions of transcendent values or norms, ultimately locating the sovereignty in all matters in the culture or in the individual person. Why should one accept an alien anthropologist's representation of human development in one's own culture?[24] A D–D psychologist's representation

---

[23]Alas, it may also be that "data" are not data—that is, "givens." See "Myth of the Given." Data are rather "facta" or "danda" treated as if they were given and unproblematic. See Pepper (1942).

[24]Let us try to make the dilemma somewhat more apparent. If "facts" are acknowledged as *made* by agents, and not given to the pristine eye, then they are made according to certain rules, standards, norms, criteria. These rules are not derived from the facts, but are employed by those who accept them to determine what the facts are (and correspondingly, what and where the non-facts are). If such rules, norms, etc. are not assumed to have a transcendent status beyond the inclinations of individuals or groups, but are merely parochial or "idiotic" in a literal sense, then they have no binding force on the makings (facts) of those who opt for

of child development or life span development especially when it may be sharply at variance with what another D–D psychologist says? And even more so when neither of the representations reflect what one experiences oneself?[25] Why accept their facts or makings as any more valuable or better than ours? Enough of that elitism which imports parochial and egocentric value judgments to make the constructions of one group more valid and more relevant than the constructions of another!

The full practice of the principle of *noli me tangere,* entailed by the realization that even the putative "factual description" of the other involves assimilating the other to one's "terministic screen," is rarely, if ever, manifested by descriptive developmentalists. Caught between the Scylla of *distortion* and the Charybdis of *silence,* D–Ds, here and abroad, have moved in two directions, in order to get the insider's story: empathy and autobiography. Instead of trying to represent what takes place in the Other over the course of time through alembicated operations, serving to distill the Other into a set of data for testing one's models, a broad-minded D–D seeks to empathize with the other: to find out how it feels from the inside to live one's life in the strange and varied settings in which the other has lived and lives. One tries to bracket one's own experience, to suspend one's own categories, to erase one's own prejudices, in order to get closer to the near-experience of the other. One strains to attain the status of the native.

But the thought may arise that this *ecstasis,* when represented to one's colleagues back home for purposes of formulating psychological or anthropological generalizations, dissolves into the parochial categories of one's professional discourse. What to do? Let the native speak for himself/herself! Autobiography! In this way one will get the facts of an individual's development (change over time, and his/her beliefs about the reasons and motives for change over time) from the native's mouth.

Now doubtless, autobiographies are interesting. And perhaps the more of them the better. At least they yield the perspectives of the actors in their native habitat, and not the reports of tourists from an alien land. They are clearly more experience-near than any reconstruction or reinterpretation

---

other rules, criteria, etc.; on those engaged in other games. For the D–D then, there are no grounds for stating what the facts are *per se,* but only what the "facts" are as constructed by the particular D–D and those who share his/her sport. Perhaps even more painful for those who like to travel and see the world, the D–D's report of "facts" about the "facts constructed by others" are mediated through the outsider's rules and may easily be at variance with the insider's conception of his/her facts. Should this shock of recognition hit the D–D, inoculated against ethnocentrism, a Protagorean reaction may ensue. Each boy and girl, each man and woman, is the measure of all things. Since there is no ground for invidious distinctions as to quality or validity of descriptions, there is an easy glide to consensus or the Gallup poll. Vox populi, Vox Dei. (See Boas, 1969.)

[25]There is, of course, an enormous advantage in describing the actions and reactions of those who have no instrumentalities (as yet) for describing themselves and their own experience.

that may be placed upon them by anthropological or psychoanalytic "experts."[26] But why would one want to record them, except for one's delectation? And why any particular one rather than another?

MEDITATIONS ON GENETIC-DRAMATISM, CULTURE, AND PERSONALITY

Bracketing the genetic-dramatism perspective, which takes *development* as a *concept by postulation,* a normative concept (cf. Kaplan, this volume) transcending specific societies, we have followed the primrose path, the road paved with good intentions, to see where it would lead. We have seen that an immanent concept of development, albeit still normative, precludes the developmental evaluation of different socio-cultural orders, since that notion of development makes each order a God unto itself. With such a concept, one cannot assess whether one social order is more advanced or more primitive than another, higher or lower, with respect to its promotion or hindering of human perfection.[27] We have also seen that immanence has no natural stopping point: If a socio-cultural order is beyond assessment by a transcendent standard of good and evil, truth and falsehood, rationality and irrationality, why then not any individual in any social order? Development as a movement toward perfection or human liberation (Kaplan, in press, b) then becomes "idiotic"[28] or otiose.

We then followed the vagaries of those for whom the concept of development was ostensibly a *concept by intuition* (Northrop, 1947) something arrived at by impartially examining and recording the facts of change and the conditions under which change takes place over time. We tried to show how those engaged in this presumptively "value-free" and "objective" enterprise imposed ontological presuppositions (*préjuges du monde* of Merleau-Ponty) and parochial "terministic screens" (Burke) on the "data" to secure their "facts," and to indicate that their ostensibly impartial descriptions were inherently partial and perspectival. Their "facts" were characteristically accepted or considered by those who shared their commitments, concepts, and methods, and rejected or ignored by those who espoused an alternative mythos or dogma.

In dealing with these issues, we have alluded only tangentially to the

---

[26]And even autobiographies are likely to be "misrepresented" or "reconstructed" by an agent living in different scenes in later life than he/she lived in an earlier phase in life.

[27]For the contortions of the American anthropologists who adopted this view, when they were faced by the socio-cultural order of Nazi Germany, see Redfield, 1953.

[28]In the original sense of "private, peculiar, one's own."

ostensible themes or content-matter referred to in our title. That is not completely, or even in the main, an oversight. "Culture" and "personality" are not stable "things" or "entities" that subsist outside of the physical, animal and human-symbolic actions and transactions of human beings.[29] They are themselves socially constituted "entities," whose meanings have clearly varied from time to time and group to group (see again, Kroeber & Kluckhohn, 1963; also Kluckhohn, Murray, & Schneider, 1956). They have been formed, deformed, and reformed by human beings cooperating and conflicting with each other in the pursuit of goals and values which themselves have been taken as products of "culture" and "personality." Before we try to deal with these conceptions from our own perspective, or perhaps in dealing with them from our own perspective, it is necessary to get some idea (surely limited, given our human finitude) as to how, why, and in what symbolically constituted scenes, these ideas which are actions have been constructed and deconstructed by different groups. Such critical reflection is a prolegomenon to any attempt to understand "culture" and "personality" not as reified "entities" but as changing acts and processes in human life.[30]

We realize that such an activity implicates us as agents in the pursuit of ends: Ends that include becoming increasingly aware of the historical and social contexts in which we live; the way in which the cultural objects with which we engage in transactions are established, maintained and overturned; the way in which we use symbolic instrumentalities to locate and orient ourselves (as well as dislocate and disorient ourselves) in the process of trying to live, live well, and live better.[31] If these kinds of self-critical awarenesses do not insure a movement toward self-perfection and self-liberation, at least they do not spread dis-ease. And like hospitals, one thing that human beings—aspiring to be men and women of knowledge, both theoretical and practical—should not do, is spread disease.[32]

---

[29]This we take to be true for most if not all "content." The assumption that there is a fixed content that can be examined from different perspectives, as though a content were theory free, is for us a "literalist" illusion, involving a fantasy of "misplaced concreteness" (Whitehead, 1925). The assumption of such "content" is closely linked to the assumption that "facts" are "data."

[30]See the writings of various "critical theorists," e.g., Horkheimer (1974a,b) and Horkheimer and Adorno (1944/72).

[31]The value of freeing ourselves from "the bewitchment or our language" (Wittgenstein) or the tyranny of our "terministic screens" (Burke, 1966)—i.e., literality—is discussed in Cirillo & Kaplan (this volume).

[32]The maxim, "one thing hospitals should not do is spread disease" comes from Florence Nightingale.

ACKNOWLEDGMENT

I would like to thank Angel Pacheco for discussion of some of the issues, and for alerting me to a number of sources. Due to an illness, Dr. Pacheco was unable to collaborate with me—our original intention—in writing this chapter.

REFERENCES

Abrams, M. H. *The mirror and the lamp.* New York: Oxford, 1955.

Abrams, M. H. *Natural supernaturalism.* New York: W. W. Norton, 1971.

Boas, F. *Primitive art* (1927). Dover Publications, 1955.

Boas, F. *The mind of primitive man* (1911). New York: Collier Books, 1963.

Boas, G. *Vox populi: The history of an idea.* Baltimore: The Johns Hopkins University Press, 1969.

Boyd, W. The contributions of genetics to anthropology. In S. Tax (Ed.), *Anthropology today.* Chicago: Phoenix Books, 1962.

Bunzel, R. Introduction to L. Levy-Bruhl. *How natives think.* New York: Washington Square Press, 1966.

Burke, K. *Language as symbolic action.* Berkeley: University of California Press, 1966.

Carlin, G. Monologue. The Johnny Carson Show, May 19, 1981.

Casey, E. Freud's theory of reality: A critical account. *Review of metaphysics,* 1971/72, *25,* 659-690.

Cassirer, E. *An essay on man.* New Haven: Yale University Press, 1944.

Collingwood, R. G. *The idea of nature.* New York: Oxford University Press, 1945.

Dewey, J., & Bentley, A. F. *Knowing and the known.* Boston: Beacon Press, 1949.

Fingarette, H. *The self in transformation.* New York: Basic Books, 1963.

Geertz, C. The impact of the concept of culture on the concept of man. *Bulletin of the Atomic Scientists,* 1966, *22,* 2-8.

Hallpike, C. R. Is there a primitive mentality? *Man* (New Series), 1976, *11,* 253-270.

Horkheimer, M. *Eclipse of reason.* New York: Seabury Press, 1974. (a)

Horkheimer, M. *Critique of instrumental reason.* New York: The Seabury Press, 1974. (b)

Horkheimer, M., & Adorno, T. *Dialectic of enlightenment.* New York: The Seabury Press, 1944.

Joad, C. E. M. *Critique of logical positivism.* Chicago: University of Chicago Press, 1950.

Kaplan, B. The study of language in psychiatry: The comparative developmental approach and its application to symbolization and language in psychopathology. In S. Arieti (Ed.), *American handbook of psychiatry,* Vol. 3. New York: Basic Books, 1966.

Kaplan, B. Meditations on genesis. *Human Development,* 1967, *10,* 65-87.

Kaplan, B. Strife of systems. *Rationality and irrationality in development.* Worcester: Clark University Press, 1983.

Kaplan, B. The past as prologue, prelude, and pretext. In R. Lerner (Ed.), *Developmental psychology: Historical and philosophical perspectives.* Hillsdale, N.J.: Lawrence Erlbaum Associates, in press. (a)

Kaplan, B. Some problems and issues for a theoretically-oriented life-span developmental psychology. In R. Lerner (Ed.), *Developmental psychology: Historical and philosophical perspectives.* Hillsdale, N.J.: Lawrence Erlbaum Associates, in press. (b)

Kluckhohn, C., Murray, H. A., & Schneider, D. (Eds.) *Personality in nature, society and culture.* New York: Knopf, 1956.

Köhler, W. *The place of value in a world of fact*. New York: Liveright, 1938.

Kroeber, A., & Kluckhohn, C. *Culture: A critical review of concepts and definitions*. New York: Random House, 1963.

Langer, S. K. *Philosophy in a new key*. Cambridge: Harvard University Press, 1942.

LeVine, R. Anthropology and child development. *New Directions in Child Development*, 1980, *8*, 71–86.

Louch, A. R. *Explanation and human action*. Berkeley: University of California Press, 1960.

Lovejoy, A. O. *Essays in the history of ideas*. Baltimore: Johns Hopkins Press, 1948/1952.

Lovejoy, A. O., & Boas, G. *Primitivism and related ideas in antiquity*. New York: Octagon Books, 1935/1965.

Margenau, H. *Open vistas*. New Haven: Yale University Press, 1961.

Needham, R. *Belief, language and experience*. Chicago: University of Chicago Press, 1972.

Northrop, F. S. C. *The logic of the sciences and humanities*. New York: Macmillan, 1947.

Pepper, S. C. *World hypotheses*. Berkeley: University of California Press, 1942.

Polanyi, M. *Personal knowledge*. New York: Harper, 1962.

Radin, P. *Primitive man as philosopher*. New York: Dover Publications, 1957.

Redfield, R. *The primitive world and its transformations*. Ithaca: Cornell University Press, 1953.

Ricoeur, P. *Freud and philosophy: An essay on interpretation*. New Haven: Yale University Press, 1970.

Roheim, G. *Psychoanalysis and anthropology*. New York: International Universities Press, 1973.

Strauss, L. *Natural right and history*. Chicago: University of Chicago Press, 1953.

Werner, H. *Comparative psychology of mental development*. New York: International Universities Press, 1948/1957.

Werner, H., & Kaplan, B. The developmental approach to cognition: Its relevance to the psychological interpretation of anthropological and ethnolinguistic data. *American Anthropologist*, 1956, *58*, 866–880.

White, L. *The science of culture*. New York: Grove Press, 1949.

Whitehead, A. N. *Science and the modern world*. New York: Macmillan & Co., 1925.

Whitehead, A. N. *Modes of thought*. New York: Macmillan & Co., 1938.

Znaniecki, F. *The social role of the man of knowledge*. New York: Harper, 1968.

6 An Examination of Studies of Critical Transitions Through the Life Cycle

S. Wapner
Clark University

R. A. Ciottone
*West-Ros-Park CMHC
and Clark University*

G. A. Hornstein
Mount Holyoke College

O. V. McNeil
Holy Cross College

A. M. Pacheco
University of Puerto Rico

INTRODUCTION

In archaic societies, the appropriate way to honor progenitors, mythical or actual, is to repeat their gestures and their sacred words. In "modern societies," the way to show esteem and honor is not to repeat, but to build on; not ritually to invoke, but productively to extend; not to follow in the footsteps but to widen the path. Here, building on Wernerian conceptualization, we extend the organismic-developmental point of view to domains of inquiry Werner did not himself pursue. As shall be seen, in agreement with Werner, we still are oriented toward determining the relations of parts to wholes and of means to ends. We still seek to delineate varying structures for invariant functions in a developmental sequence, a sequence embodying the "orthogenetic principle" (Werner, 1957; Werner & Kaplan, 1956). Moreover, we still do not limit ourselves to "ontogenesis," but consider, from a developmental perspective, variations in adult modes of functioning under different internal or external conditions, modes of functioning manifested in so-called pathological cases, and so on.

We do, however, extend Werner's characteristic focus in at least one respect. Werner was typically concerned with the delineation of the "processes'' or ''modes of functioning'' living entities exercised in coping with their environments, and with the ordering of these processes or modes. He sought to show how these ''developmentally'' different patterns, structures, or means were exemplified by quite different types of living organisms in varying circumstances. One might say that his undertaking was morphogenetic and nomothetic: the development of forms or patterns to realize a function; the emphasis on the general and the common as contrasted with the individual and the specific. In contrast, our interest, still morphogenetic, is idiographic as well: We are concerned with the modes of functioning of specific kinds of socio-historical individuals obliged to deal with the stresses and strains of life in various social settings, under various sociocultural conditions throughout the life cycle.

Moreover, linked with this idiographic, personological interest, we have inclined, more than Werner, to a concern with praxis and intervention. Where specific individuals, in their processes of transaction with sociocultural events, experience demoralization or manifest patterns of action inimical to themselves and/or to others, we have been interested in determining situation-specific and agent-specific ways of assisting such individuals to achieve better, if not optimal, ways of managing their life-situations.

CRITICAL TRANSITIONS

We take it for granted that all human beings, in different times and places, have been obliged to suffer critical or radical transitions. Not only are we all thrown out of a uterine environment into socio-physical settings of a radically different kind, but we are all obliged to move, in the course of our lives, in and through multiple settings or scenes. Consider a typical pattern in middle-class America: from the home environment to nursery school; from family life to adolescent peer-group life; from adolescence to young adulthood; from family-dependence to relative independence in a workforce; from the status of an unmarried person to the status of a married one; from a non-parent to a parent status; perhaps from a status of married to a status of widowed or divorced; from an occupational status to the status of a retiree or an unemployed individual. These, at least, are taken to be critical transitions for the person in the given physico-sociocultural context. And there are many, many others that may intersect with these; forced migration, especially to a setting in which customs and language are unfamiliar; accidents which impair or destroy important instrumentalities for coping with the environment, e.g., loss of a limb, blindness; exposure to natural catastrophes such as earthquakes or floods; being imprisoned or taken hostage (cf., Kaplan, Wapner, & Cohen, 1976; Wapner, 1977, 1978, 1981; Wapner, Kaplan, & Ciottone, 1981; Wapner, Kaplan, & Cohen, 1973).

Now, it cannot be said, unequivocally, that such transitions entail a radical disruption of the person-in-environment system. Much depends on the character of the agent. We expect conduct, feeling, and thought to be disrupted in such circumstances, and we are likely to be surprised and suspicious if they are not. We, therefore, shall assume that these are radical or critical transitions for whomever participates in them, or suffers them, unless the evidence suggests otherwise.

On the other hand, given that the criticality of a transition is, in large part, dependent on the reaction of the agent, we recognize that there are many happenings or events in a life that may occasion a radical transition—a transformation of one's relationships to the environment and one's conception of oneself—without any social or collective expectancy that such an event or happening would typically trigger such a change; for example, a nightmare, a vision, or a strange encounter of any kind. It follows that one can only determine whether a critical transition is taking place on the basis of comparisons among conceptions of the world (including self) by the agent before, during, and after the event.

One need not detail the difficulties in undertaking systematic inquiry with regard to certain radical transitions. Those who are trying to cope with the loss of a loved one, the consequences of a serious injury, the shock of a heart attack are not often inclined to participate in studies until the trauma has passed, if at all. Moreover, even if one could satisfy oneself that no ethical norm were violated, one might still have qualms about decorum or invasion of privacy. This is not to say that such transitions cannot be studied, but the occasions are likely to be unpremeditated and the approaches clinical-therapeutic. There are, however, other transitions, perhaps less traumatic, where one may plan in advance and take on more of a spectator role, at least during initial phases; one is not from the start trapped in the dilemma of being either consoler or voyeur.

In studying such transitions, it is trite to observe that they occur within specific cultural contexts. Yet one must insist on the importance of that fact. Such cultural contexts are not all homogeneous, but are varied in time and place. In such contexts, there are individuals occupying or exemplifying certain culturally established roles with the rights and duties appertaining to these roles; there are socioculturally constituted objects and places whose use and exploitation is enjoined through mores, customs, and laws; there are prescriptions and proscriptions with regard to the appropriate relations individuals occupying certain roles may have with individuals occupying other roles; there are permissible and impermissible ways of acting, expressing thoughts, expressing feelings. It is with these culturally constituted objects, human or otherwise, that one engaged in transactions or manifests reactions to such transactions.

If one is to describe what an individual does or feels, one cannot do so intelligibly without reference to such cultural objects. One cannot speak of a transaction *in vacuo,* indifferent to the objects involved in the transaction. A child does not simply run away; he or she runs away from a home, a school, a parent, a community. A person leaving a job does not merely retire; he or she retires from something and to somewhere. And the specific character of the something and somewhere is significant for characterizing the transaction. Many psychologists in the past have talked of acts as separated from object—as though the acts were psychological while the objects belonged to some other domain. Keeping in mind our tenet of the inseparability of agent and environment, and recognizing the sociocultural-symbolic character of human environments, we hope to avoid this "fallacy of misplaced concreteness." Acts like "running away," "retiring," etc. are cultural acts defined by and within a human community. It is inappropriate to talk about such acts as if they had the same status as physical motions.

We shall present our reflections on our own research pertaining to four such transitions, occurring at different periods in the life-cycle. Some of these, it will be noted, were more than age-related transitions, i.e., they involve the contamination of a transition usually associated with a certain period by other factors that are likely to potentiate the disruption of the person-in-environment system. The transitions are: (1) *from home to nursery school,* in one instance of normal, in another of handicapped children; (2) *from a native habitat to an unfamiliar place (migration)* by young people also subjected to the pressures of emerging adolescence; (3) *from high school to college,* in some instances complicated by the fact that the one in transit enters an ethnically and racially alien milieu; and (4) *from membership in the work force to the status of retiree.* It was our belief that if we could discern developmental transformations in self-world relationships in these situations, *regressions and progressions,* we would have reasonable grounds for expecting even more clear-cut regressions and progressions in those variable and unanticipated traumata that may strike any of us at any time.

Our detailed studies on these four types of transitions during the lifecycle have been discussed in their specificity and distinctiveness elsewhere. (References are indicated in later sections as each study is discussed.) Here, we would like to focus less on the detailed findings we have obtained through the methods and techniques employed in the various inquiries, and more on the problems involved in arriving at a developmentally relevant description of these transitions. Let us make this point clear. In examining the various transitions in separate studies, we have been guided by developmental conceptualization but have deviated occasionally by using other perspectives to characterize the complex nature of the transitions.

The issue is not whether it is invalid to examine transitions from different perspectives. Clearly, one is warranted in using whatever perspective one wishes in the analysis and description of "what there is." The objection is rather to the agglutination of observations and inferences derived from a variety of different and incommensurable perspectives, as if the "facts" thus agglutinated were thereby rendered perspective-free or theory-independent. If one is to examine critical transitions from a Wernerian or neo-Wernerian perspective, one is obliged to formulate one's questions, construct one's methodologies and techniques, and interpret one's findings in terms of the fundamental categories and concepts of that perspective. Insofar as the "findings" and "facts" derived from other points of view are amenable to re-interpretation in terms of the Wernerian framework, they may be used to help answer questions or evaluate the hypotheses formulated in that framework.[1]

In our perspective, development is *defined* in terms of *increased differentiation and hierarchic integration.* One agent is taken to be more developed than another, the more diverse his/her domains of activity, the more internally articulated these various domains, and the more integrated and interdependent these differentiated domains. This holds whether one compares two distinct individuals or the same individual at different time-slices. The more developed the individual, the larger the range of distinguished realms in which the individual is capable of participating and the more these divided and distinguished "worlds" are harmoniously interrelated.

One is taken to be more highly developed the more one has a knowledge of all the modes of being and action of individuals and groups *within the particular social order.* Modes of being and distinctions among them will vary in nature and degree in different social orders. One must be careful not to impose, without reflection and justification, the modes of being of one's own social group upon others. One need not observe that even such a culturally-relative telos is achieved by no one. Its importance lies in the

---

[1]Kenneth Burke, who has devoted considerable attention to the problem of perspectives and "terministic screens," discusses this issue in *Dramatism and Development,* 1972, p. 35–36. Objecting to those who suggest combining insights derived from several different disciplines (analogous to combining insights from several different perspectives), he asks for the *methodological* grounds underlying the choice of such insights. He remarks: "Usually the problem is 'solved' by not even being considered. You pick from different fields items that you like, as though interdisciplinary [or interperspectival] decisions were not much different from shopping at a department store—and that's what it amounts to, so far as the methodology of your choice is concerned." For us, as for Burke, the relevant methodological approach that is justifiable in recruiting insights obtained through other perspectives is one that is formulable in one's own perspective.

regulative principle or standard that it provides and against which members of a community assess the developmental status of individuals, including themselves.

If we now leave this empyrean realm and return to the mundane one, it is reasonably clear that the division of any sociocultural universe into different regions is already partly given as environment to individuals in the processes of ontogenesis in a specific sociocultural world. The differentiation of a school sphere and a home sphere is not in the nature of things, but is socially constituted. Distinctions as to where one eats, sleeps, works, engages in recreation, etc. are socioculturally established, and one is obliged to accommodate or adapt to this environment before one can ever attempt to transcend it. It is obvious that one must be at least partially "socialized" before one can "transcend" one's parochial social order. Thus, if we want fully to understand how a particular individual differentiates and integrates his or her transactions with environments, we must have some idea of what this cultural environment is for the hypothetical ideal observer, or, in G. H. Mead's phase, "the generalized other."

The kinds of problems and issues—both general and specific—with which we were and still are confronted in struggling to attain a relatively adequate *developmental description* of the phenomena inherent in critical transitions are perhaps best clarified through a reconsideration of the four kinds of transitions to which we have referred above.

DEVELOPMENTAL ANALYSIS

As neo-Wernerians, developmentalists in Werner's sense, we pose the question, "What is the telos?"[2] We may sometimes try to suppress this question, but sooner or later, it comes back to haunt us. Unless one has some end in view—ultimate or proximate—either attributed to the subject of investigation or posited by the investigator, one has no grounds for viewing actions or patterns of action as means to an end, and no grounds, therefore, for a developmental analysis. One may see here the radical difference between a Wernerian "developmental psychology" and those developmental psychologies that limit themselves to "causal" or "antecedent-consequent"

---

[2]This kind of question should make it clear that Wernerians take "development" to pertain to form-function or means-ends relations. In the jargon of Jean Piaget, it is a way of ordering variable structures with respect to functions taken as invariant. It is principally concerned with formal and final determinants rather than material and efficient "causes" (see Kaplan, 1966, 1967). For a discussion of the need to disentangle "form" and "causality," see Cassirer, 1961, Chapter 10. Such a disentangling does not mean that Wernerians eschew an examination and analysis of conditions ("causes") facilitating or hampering development progression either in general or in individual cases. It does mean that we distinguish development in itself from the factors occasioning progression or regression in actual human beings.

analysis, or that construe "development" as whatever takes place during the course of earthly existence. One way of summing up the difference is that Wernerians take "development" to be a way of representing phenomena or a mode of analysis, whereas the other "developmental psychologies" restrict development to age differences.

The ultimate telos for Werner was maximum differentiation and hierarchic integration. In *Comparative Psychology of Mental Development,* Werner tended to conflate "development" as an ideal notion with the actual phenomena of ontogenesis, phylogenesis, neurogenesis, etc. That is, he seemed to claim to "read off" development from phenomena, occurring in a temporal sequence. In his joint work with Kaplan (Werner & Kaplan, 1956, 1963) and in his 1957 paper, however, development was logically disentangled from ontogenesis, phylogenesis, etc. and became a "norm" for assessing actual change. This disentanglement led to the formulation of the "orthogenetic principle" (Kaplan, 1967). An "organism"[3] approximated (the never attainable) full development to the extent that the organism distinguished what was conflated or syncretically fused and, concurrently, united these divided and distinguished spheres into an integrated world. Applying this telos to abstracted domains or spheres of functioning (as if the "organism" were collapsed into a cognitive being, an emotional being, a linguistic being, etc.), Werner was able to talk of cognitive development, emotional development, perceptual development, language development. (See Wapner & Werner, 1957; Werner, 1926, 1940; Werner & Kaplan, 1963; Werner & Wapner, 1949, 1952.)

The problem for us was how to interpret or specify the orthogenetic principle with regard to the range of phenomena we have called "critical transitions." If an individual were to undergo a "critical transition" in his or her transactions with the environment, this would entail—we realized only gradually—an arrest or regression, a dedifferentiation and disintegration, relative to the individual's developmental status prior to the transition. But what would constitute developmental progression beyond the individual's status prior to the transition?

This was an especially crucial issue for us because the radical alterations in mode of living with which the various agents were obliged to cope were not in the nature of things, but were imposed on them by forces in their environment, their sociocultural environment. A dislocation from the home for a period of time to participate in a nursery school is not an intrinsic feature of the human condition, but comes about because someone other than the agent decides, for a variety of reasons and motives, that such a transition ought to be made. A migration from one sociocultural domain to another, and especially the kinds we have looked at, is not necessarily

---

[3]The term "organism" is not restricted here to a biological entity, but is also used to pertain to societies, etc., i.e., to any entity, considered as a complex unit.

gleefully entered into by an agent to expand his or her range of experiences and modes of actions, but may be enjoined by socio-political-economic circumstances. There is nothing intrinsic to the nature of human life to necessitate that one must go from a local high-school to a distant and alien college, and especially to one in which one's ethnic group is marginally represented either in the student body or the faculty. To be obliged to retire from one's occupational role at a certain age is not a phenomenon of nature, but a stipulation of a socioculture community.

It is important for us to stress this point because we have found ourselves, on occasion, assuming that an agent who accommodated to or adapted to the culturally imposed state of affairs manifested a higher level of functioning than one who refused to adapt to the externally imposed situation. The ultimate consequence of this unwitting and unwarranted assumption is that adaptation to cultural demands or institutions is taken to be an intrinsic desideratum—a telos. This is a position we would surely not want to maintain. That is not to say that we automatically reject adaptation to cultural institutions as a desirable end. It does mean that we must consider, from the point of view of optimal human development, whether specific cultural institutions conduce to such optimal development or militate against it.[4]

One may, of course, with full recognition of the limitations and reservations surrounding such a step, provisionally consider the culturally imposed conditions as if they were acts of fate, ineluctable alterations in the human environment, with which human beings must cope and come to terms. "Coming to terms" with such "naturalized" conventional situations would then be the telos, and the different ways of coping would then be the variable "means" to the end. In that process, the different modes of coping would be amenable to assessment in terms of the orthogenetic principle and thereby susceptible to a developmental ordering. In the main, this has been the assumption guiding our studies of the four above mentioned transitions. With our new-found recognition of the limitations and reservations involved in making such an assumption, we now turn to these specific inquiries.

FOUR PERSON-IN-ENVIRONMENT TRANSITIONS

As noted earlier, our review of the four transitions is presented as a context for: (1) raising questions about the form developmental analyses might take rather than presenting empirical findings; (2) seeking suggestions about techniques, methods, and conditions that might serve as the occasion for

---

[4]This questioning or rejection of the absolute sovereignty of a culture or sub-culture entails a rejection of "cultural relativism." For elaboration see Kaplan's discussion in Reflections on culture and personality from a Genetic-Dramatistic perspective (Chapter 5, this volume).

developmental change; and (3) formulating ways of intervening that can facilitate progressive development.

In all four transitions—home to nursery school; migration; high school to college; work to retirement—a developmental analysis involves at least three general issues and tasks. The first is assessment of the developmental status of the focal person or agent. Such assessment ideally is made prior to the transition, during the transition, and then again during the later phases of the transition, including adaptation to the new milieu (if that takes place). The second task is to assess contextual conditions or circumstances that might serve as the occasion for change in developmental status. The third task is to describe some reasonable interventions that might help to free transitions from trauma and where there is a trauma to seek interventions that might facilitate higher level transactions, indicative of more optimal person-in-environment relationships.

We shall characterize the particular transition in general terms and address most of these issues and tasks for each of the four transitions.

Home to Nursery School

In trying to understand, from an idiographically oriented developmental perspective, the nature of a child's responses to the hypothetical "obligatory" transition to a nursery school, it is imperative that we realize that one cannot talk about such a transition in general terms: just as one child is not another child is not a third child, so one home is not another home is not a third home; nor is it the case that if you have seen one nursery school you have seen them all.[5] One must know in detail the nature of the home environment prior to the transition and the nature of the nursery school into which the child is placed. Nor is it enough to know the material aspects of the home and school "culture." One must get some sense of the non-material, "spiritual" atmosphere. Indeed, optimally, one would have to undertake something akin to an ethnographic analysis of a singular culture, determining the formal and informal rules and regulations governing the focal child's actions and transactions in the home world. A depth as well as surface analysis is needed to ascertain how the child responds to such rules and regulations. In that "culture," are specific demands, if any, characteristically made upon the child by the mother, the father, the siblings? In that "culture," are there specific rewards and punishments for actions executed by the child? Does that "culture" enjoin different types of

---

[5]One recent study (Quirk, Ciottone, & Wapner, 1980) suggests that, in general, and with the usual caveat of "other things being equal," mothers of handicapped children look to nursery school to help their children gain a greater degree of "social maturity," while mothers of nonhandicapped children seem to send their children to nursery schools to acquire "cognitive skills." Another study (Quirk, 1982) is seeking to uncover relationships between mother's values and mother-child transactions.

action in different places or does it allow different types of action to take place in the "same locale"? In that "culture," is the child sent to nursery school in the hope and expectation that the child will benefit socially and intellectually from the experiences in the new environment? Or is the child sent to nursery school as a means of obtaining "custodial care" for him or her during the day?

These questions, and others like them, are enormously difficult to answer, even if one has skilled social workers, clinicians, and anthropologists present often enough to make a reasonable assessment. In the absence of such experts, we have thus far, been obliged to rely on global judgments concerning the status of the focal child in the pre-transition phase. It is clear that subsequent research with regard to this transition will require the appropriation of techniques from all of these disciplines.

Beyond the determination of the characteristics of the home environment in which the child lives, we also require means for assessing the developmental status of the pre-transition child. Can we make some relatively precise evaluation of the extent of differentiation of the child from his or her parents and siblings? Can we assess the level at which the child characteristically deals with a range of intellectual problems, social conflicts, etc.? It is only with a relatively precise assessment of the levels of performance exemplified by the child in different domains that one can determine whether the transition to nursery school engenders that kind of regression and/or progression that warrants considering the transition as a critical one.

Experience in the new school world may disrupt the child's typical patterns of transactions and induce regressive transactions in both the home and school contexts. Departures from developmental advance may occur since the environmental transition is a perturbation that may impose stress on all system components—for example, mother, siblings, teachers, peers, etc. Since such a stress may be experienced as mild or severe by different individuals, the transition may profile the adaptive potential of the person involved, that is, there may occur a pattern of arrest, of regression or of progression. Ideally, the child must operate effectively in two contexts, each with different demands, and must be able to organize his or her transactions at home and at school into differentiated and integrated spheres of activity (multiple worlds).

What are some possible indicators of developmental status at this ideal level, or at those which fall short of it? When children import behavior as well as objects from one setting to the next indiscriminately, they are exhibiting developmentally less advanced transactions since such behavior implies fusion of the home and school settings. If with further exposure, their transactions are appropriate to the context—for example, the child states, "I am going to *play* school here at home"—then the child is exhibiting transactions indicative of more advanced developmental status. Further, means and ends can be ordered developmentally in the context of environmental transition. For example, to what extent does the child behave in ways that reflect a diffuse sense of the means by which to achieve his or her goals (e.g., acting as if blocks and crayons serve the same purpose) as opposed to a differentiation of means-ends transactions with the environment (e.g., tower building with blocks and coloring with crayons)?

Over and above such inquiry directed to elaborating a developmental description of the construals and transactions of the focal agent during the transition, there is the further question of the *circumstances or conditions* under which developmental transformation is arrested, reversed or advanced. The impact of the environmental transition will vary depending on the characteristics of the agent, the environment, and the interrelation of the two. A mother of a handicapped child who seeks to protect her child rather than challenge him or her maintains a set of demands differing from those of a young, change-oriented teacher who values increasing independence in children. In this way, the child is presented with contradictory demands from both the home and school worlds. Such contradictory demands may make for advancement or retardation, and this may vary depending on the degree of conflict between the demands. Mild conflict may make for advancement, severe conflict for retardation (cf. Wapner, 1976). Considering differences in environment, what is the impact of nursery schools with varying degrees of structure in their programs? Further, considering interaction of agent and environment, does a child who is handicapped construe and transact differently and exhibit more marked developmental advance in a "mainstream" as compared with a "segregated" environment?

Given that for some children the experience of transition to nursery school is conflicted and traumatic, what conditions can help in advancing social and cognitive developmental status of the child undergoing that transition? We know that in the development of a cognitive organization of the spatial features of a new environment the person utilizes an anchor point or home base (Schouela, Steinberg, Leveton, & Wapner, 1980). We know that in exploring a new environment a child will utilize his or her mother as anchor point (Ainsworth & Wittig, 1969; Rheingold & Eckerman, 1969, 1970). Will fostering the child's use of an anchor point (whether an actual or symbolic object) in the new environment help the child move closer to the developmental ideal of integrating the new world of school with the old world of home and in experiencing stability, comfort, and satisfaction in both?[6]

---

[6]In this connection, we have found that adaptation is more effective for residents of nursing homes who are permitted to bring personal objects with them than for those residents not permitted to do so (Schmitt, Redondo, & Wapner, 1977).

Migration of Adolescents

The challenges of facing a new environment are strikingly evident in *migration,* that is, moving from one to another region of the world, a complex act that generally entails adaptation not only to a change in climate but to a radical change in the environment of places, people, and customs. One is obliged to cope with alterations in all aspects of the surrounding environment: Physical, biological, psychological, and sociocultural and often all at the same time. The developmental status of the migrant is of significance. For example, when the focal person is a teenager, as in our own studies of Puerto Rican migration,[7] the transition is made more complex by the emergence of adolescence, which in itself may very well be a critical transition (Lucca-Irizarry, Wapner, & Pacheco, 1981; Pacheco, Wapner, & Lucca-Irizarry, 1979).

A developmental analysis is ingredient in the general goals of migration as indicated by the form of the acculturation adopted by the migrant. For example, there may be assimilation and identification of self with the new culture (e.g., "melting pot"); there may be isolation from and/or conflict with the culture of the host environment (e.g., ethnicity), or there may be flexible maintenance of both values of the culture one leaves as well as the culture one enters (e.g., biculturalism [Ramirez III & Castaneda, 1974]). These alternatives formally parallel the self-world relationships implied in the orthogenetic principle as ranging from lesser to more advanced developmental status, that is, from (1) de-differentiated to (2) differentiated and isolated, or (3) differentiated and in conflict to (4) differentiated and hierarchically integrated.

Assessment of the developmental status of the migrant in the home environment is almost impossible since he or she will, for the most part, not become available as a subject until after entry in the new environment. The assessment of developmental status, the determination of expectations, and of goals for the new environment is largely retrospective. The migrant has come from a different culture, with its correlative features of family, school, mores, and customs, which differ drastically from the environment he or she now enters. His or her expectations are formed in terms of that environment and will vary depending on whether the migration is voluntary or involuntary.[8]

---

[7]This research was supported, in part, by grant MH–32904 from the National Institute of Mental Health. Support to Angel Pacheco from the National Research Council and the National Institute of Mental Health (MARC Program) is gratefully acknowledged.

[8]For one voluntary migrant in a pilot study, the expectations regarding the new life were joyful excitement about entry into school. These highly positive expectations were, however, quickly replaced by misery, loneliness, gloom, and unhappiness because of lack of friends, doing poorly in schoolwork, and feelings that others were prejudiced (Redondo, Pacheco,

What means or instrumentalities does the adolescent migrant (return migrant) use to cope with the demands, stresses, (e.g., prejudice, rejection), expectations of the host environment, as well as to cope with the migrant's lack of "fit" between self and world? Are these means orderable developmentally? Generally, migrants might feel uprooted as they compare their life in the old and new environments. Such a lack of consonance in the person-environment relationship could spread across all environmental features. For instance, the migrants might dislike the climate, find the trees beautiful but feel strongly that almost all other features of the urban environment are ugly. They may feel constrained, lament the lack of recreational facilities and criticize the slow pace of life in the new environment. Migrants may report a sense of diminished personal freedom (Lucca-Irizarry, Wapner, & Pacheco, 1981) insofar as their lives are constantly under surveillance and scrutiny by the members of the host community. In schools and community gatherings the migrants may feel out of place and create islands within the island which serve as pockets of resistance for those who, faced with conflict, attempt to personalize their environment according to their own goals and preferred instrumentalities. Indicators of coping strategies might include: overt criticism of the community; clinging to dating habits, dress codes, styles of communication and social interaction characteristic of the pre-migration community; showing off ability to speak English; speaking in a dialect-wise "Span-Glish" mode that is not easily decoded by the locals, thereby isolating one's self or withdrawing from the new environment; coming together in groups with others like themselves; and being in conflict with authorities in the host environment.

Isolation of self from environment involves differentiation and accordingly represents more advanced developmental status than where the migrant yields to every pressure from the host environment (fusion; dedifferentiation). However, isolating self from and being in conflict with the environment is less advanced developmentally than is the case where there is differentiation and hierarchic integration. Such differentiation and hierarchic integration may be expressed when the migrant is able to withstand the pressure from the host environment when he or she so desires, and, flexibly to shift toward agreement with the host environment on those issues which are in concordance with his or her belief(s).

What conditions or circumstances serve to help the migrant cope with various features of the new environment? Are there key people in the new environment, for example, kin or friends who will become instrumental in the development of the social network of the migrant, and then serve as an-

Cohen, Kaplan, & Wapner, 1982 (in press). Adolescent migrants returning involuntarily to Puerto Rico are often rebellious, openly express frustration over being uprooted, are uncomfortable in the homes of their relatives, and are overtly hostile to them, the community, and the school (Pacheco, Wapner, & Lucca-Irizarry, 1979).

chor points or referents for establishing the migrant's social world? Parents, relatives and/or friends, may be the key persons who guide migrants in their first steps through the intricate web of new environmental features. Those who serve as anchor points for the "newly arrived" may fulfill not only an orienting function (differentiation) in terms of self-world relations but also facilitate hierarchic integration as "anchor people" fostering movement on the part of the migrants toward a more optimal person-environment fit.

To be sure, many migrants may feel comfortable in the new environment. Although they may face the difficulties of learning about the environment, they may report a positive feeling of being in the new environment. Do they learn to share with others and engage in a "give and take" process in which they show others their ways while they also learn from them? Do they appreciate many facets of the new culture and yet maintain some values of their native cultures? Do they come close to adopting the developmentally advanced bicultural stance?

High School to College

Young people enter college with multiple goals. They aim to obtain a general education, to meet friends, to prepare for a career, and to become more aware of themselves as individuals. In other words, the individual looks for opportunities to expand his or her knowledge of the world in which he or she lives, to develop intellectual skills, to acquire specialized knowledge, to prepare for entry into graduate/professional school or the work force, to establish a variety of interpersonal relationships, to enhance self-awareness, and to develop the values by which he or she ought to live and act. For the person entering college, the change in setting represents a shift from the familiar to the unfamiliar, from a setting where living and schooling is separate to a setting where for the most part living and schooling have merged. An array of strangers are present who may have drastically different values. The individual must become self-reliant. Marked changes in status may be experienced. On the positive side, there may be exhilaration from the new feeling of individual freedom, and the shift from being bored to being intellectually challenged. On the negative side, there may be a change from campus leader to an ordinary member of the group, from the decision maker to the follower, from being the top achiever to becoming an average student, etc. Therefore, some young people entering college may experience, to varying degrees, a sense of disappointment, disillusion, and alienation during their college careers. Generally, it is assumed that such feelings and sentiments stem from discrepancies between what the entering and perservering student wants from college life and what the college setting as a whole provides (Buckley, 1971; Gibbs, 1973; Pate, 1970; Reiner & Robinson, 1970; Risch, 1970).

Here, as for the other transitions, it would be ideal to assess[9] the experience and transactions of the person prior to, during, and following entry into the new environment. This is not so easily accomplished. To date, for example, in our own work, we have made only a limited beginning in assessing the experience of sub-freshmen by asking them, prior to college entry, to write a description of their feelings, thoughts and expectations about the impending experience. However, such data are difficult to obtain.

Some features of this transition are different from the transition to nursery school and are similar to the adolescent migrant's transition. Though we shall not elaborate these differences systematically, it is worthy of note that the entering college student, like the migrant and unlike the young child, has a fairly clear notion of and can express immediate and long-term goals and expectations. These expectations relate specifically to academics, to social interrelationships, and to preparation for entering the work force. They may be in conflict with actions that in fact take place in these areas. Given a transactional conflict with actuality falling short of expectation (it could, of course, exceed expectation), it is possible to describe means of handling the discrepancy in terms which are orderable developmentally. One such set of developmentally ordered means of coping was described by Apter (1976) in a retrospective study with undergraduates who recalled incidents making for such transactional conflict and the ways in which they themselves had handled those conflicts. She described the following means of handling conflict as representing respectively lesser to greater developmental progression: (1) *accommodation* (going along with or accepting status quo); (2) *nonconstructive ventilation* (exhibiting an aggressive act toward source of conflict, without suggesting constructive ways of remedying the situation); (3) *disengagement* (distancing self from the situation by laughing, becoming cynical, etc.); and (4) *constructive assertion* (recommending planned action and different, creative alternatives for achieving a

---

[9]Again, in the studies of this transition, the technique we have used so far is a comprehensive in-depth interview covering cognitive, affective, and valuative experience of the physical, interpersonal, and sociocultural aspects of the environment. In addition, we have employed: descriptions and drawings of the environment (cf. Wofsey, Rierdan, & Wapner, 1979; Edelman, Rierdan, & Wapner, 1977); topographic sketch maps (Schouela, Steinberg, Leveton, & Wapner, 1980); psychological distance maps, in which participants are asked to represent their feelings of psychological closeness to places, people, and sociocultural rules that constitute their psychological environment (cf. Wapner, 1977); and intensive interviews regarding the construction of the maps and items placed on it.

goal). We might anticipate that means of coping similar to these might occur in terms of academic goals.[10]

The feelings of transactional conflict and ways of handling it may vary with any entering student but may be more salient for women and blacks, especially when such conflict occurs in a particular college context that was until recently restricted completely to white men. In a larger sense, such feelings of conflict may derive from the nature of the material taught in college classes, which is based on the experience, history, and ideas of white men; it is often difficult for women or minority men to identify with this material or see its relevance to them.

Because the college context involves a period of rapid expansion of the academic and social-interpersonal worlds, there is special opportunity in this transition to learn about the developing relationship between these two worlds. Dedifferentiation or fusion of the two worlds would be exhibited if the straight A student's academic performance shifts to failure when there is trouble with his or her affective life. The compartmentalization of each world through isolation involves differentiation and represents a somewhat more developmentally advanced status, but is less advanced than obtains for the student who can flexibly subordinate one or the other world depending on his or her long term goals and the demands of the situation.

Finally, another opportunity for developmental analysis is linked to the significance of the transition as an occasion for the development of, for definition of, and for the structuring of one's work world. How such a definition becomes articulated and then becomes structured involves assessing one's abilities, skills, potential, and their relation to the demands of different occupations and professions.

What are some of the conditions of developmental change? Consider what happens to the student when his or her personal, academic, and social expectations, values, and goals for self and for the relations of self to college are increasingly discrepant with actuality. How does the student who does not have the intellectual skill necessary to achieve a long-term goal handle such a discrepancy? Does he or she persist in pursuing the goal and continuing to suffer a loss of self-esteem from questioning his or her intellectual capacities? Does this experience, albeit negative, also serve the positive function of fostering greater self insight and providing the formal

---

[10]There is some evidence along these lines in a study (McNeil & Wapner, 1981) currently being conducted, which is concerned in part with conflict in the academic sphere. These means include: (1) accepting self and academic world without attempting to change either; (2) withdrawing; (3) attempting to change self to meet the demands of the situation by changing study habits, shifting schedules, etc.; and (4) attempting to change the situation to better match one's self-interest and ability (e.g., by asking the instructor to switch from essay to objective examinations or vice versa, by moving to another section of the course, or by selecting a different subject area).

condition of "dissolution of a prior organization of self" thereby permitting a creative reorganization of self and relation of self to academic goals? This reorganization may serve as a means for developmental advance by instituting other forms of self-integrity and self-esteem. Do these, in turn, make possible some movement toward actualization of optimal self-world relationships? Does the principle of "reculer pour mieux sauter (draw back to leap)" operate as a condition for creative developmental advance?

Work to Retirement

In a culture such as ours, in which social status and self-identity are defined to a significant extent in terms of occupation, and where the value of a person depends largely on his or her ability to remain employed, the shift from *full time work to retirement* has come to be one of the most critical transitions in the life cycle. It has the potential to change basic elements of an individual's life, e.g., his or her self-identity, sense of importance and value as a person and as a member of society, relationships with family and friends, daily activities, financial status, and living arrangements.[11]

In retirement, there is a change from living in two or more worlds (work, family, friends, recreation, etc.) to leaving the work world and living in the other worlds only. What is the impact of such a perturbation? The ongoing organization of worlds constituting one's universe of experience is disturbed since one part is excised. A reorganization is required. Can one describe the disorganization and the course of reorganization in developmentally relevant terms? Is there regression, arrest or advance in self-world transactions, in construals of self and world? What indicators are there of such change? Given the reality of retirement, the retiree who keeps getting ready for work every day, who "hangs out" at the diner to which his *ex*-fellow workers like to go for lunch surely suggests arrest, let alone regression if such transactions persist. Such rigid adherence to transactions no longer appropriate to the new context formally parallels the irrelevant importations of the nursery school child early in the transition process. A shift from acting out these transactions to internalizing them in reverie or in imagination would seem to represent a developmental advance. Stated more generally, a crucial question is whether the formal structure that existed among the worlds prior to retirement (e.g., whether one's worlds are fused, isolated, conflicted, or integrated) also exists for those worlds that now remain and have been added.

Some clues on the ways in which this transition could be analyzed developmentally, by considering the structure of one's multiple worlds, may

---

[11]The study of this transition was supported, in part, by a grant to Clark University from the NRTA-AARP Andrus Foundation.

be seen in a study in which we had the goals of: (1) describing a retiree's experience just before or at time of versus some months soon after retirement; (2) establishing groupings of retiree's experiences; and (3) seeking links between such experience and the formal ways in which the person's universe of worlds is structured in relation to the work world (Wapner & Hornstein, 1980; Hornstein & Wapner, 1981).

Intensive semi-structured interviews conducted with retirees and members of their support system, and analyzed by phenomenological methods (Giorgi, 1971; Watkins, 1977), revealed four qualitative different types of retirement experience:

In one type of experience, the significance of retirement is that it is felt to be a *transition to the last phase of one's life, old age.* Retirement is a time to wind down, a time in which to order one's life, to put it into perspective, and to prepare psychologically for the process of aging.

For a second group, retirement represents the *welcome beginning* of a new phase of life. It signifies the time in one's life that one can live in accordance with one's own needs, desires, and goals, free of the requirements and demands of others. It is a time to embark on new projects, to energetically pursue long-awaited goals, and to live and enjoy life to its fullest.

For a third group, retirement is *not experienced as an event of major personal importance.* There is a basic continuity to the pattern of these individuals' lives pre- and post-retirement and retirement per se does not really constitute a critical transition in a psychological sense.

Finally, for a fourth group, the significance of retirement is that it constitutes the *loss of a highly valued sphere of activity.* It is as if a part of the self has also been removed. These individuals often adjust to this loss after some time, but an underlying feeling of disquiet remains, reflecting their sense that they have made the best out of a situation that was neither sought nor really desired.

The common themes and similarities in the four groups were: coming to terms with the issue of aging and death; a slow process of separation from one's company or organization; the development of an internal organization to replace the external structure provided by work; and the development of a new sense of identity through support of the social network of family and friends.

One of the dimensions identified, sense of self, reveals interesting differences among the four groupings of retirement experience, which may have significance for a developmental analysis. Change in self identity is most evident in the fourth group, where retirement is experienced as the loss of a highly valued sphere of activity. This loss is tantamount to the experience that a part of the self, identified with work, has been removed. These individuals seem to reorganize their worlds after some time, but the issue remains problematic. For the first and third groups, there seems to be continuity in the experience of self. For the second group, retirement allows reorganization in a sense for the "birth" of a new part of the self.

The developmental status of the structure of the retiree's worlds of experience (work isolated from, versus integrated with, other worlds) prior to and following retirement, and its relation to the retirement experience is worthy of exploration. There is some limited evidence that the first group (retirement is indicative of aging) and the second group (retirement is a beginning) shows greater integration between the work world and other spheres of activity prior to retirement, and that the fourth group (retirement is the loss of a highly valued activity) shows greater isolation. (The first two groups also appear to have a more successful adaptation than the latter groups.) If such relationships hold, and if further investigation shows that the formal features of structuring one's worlds of experience are highly correlated with or change systematically compared to structuring at later stages in retirement, then this may have bearing on the manner in which intervention can be introduced.[12]

Relevant to intervention is the question of the conditions or circumstances that might make for more optimal experiences during retirement. Since retirement means different things to different people, such conditions must take into account individual differences in the ways in which retirement is experienced. But to develop pre-retirement counseling programs, the difficult problem remains of knowing some five or more years ahead of time what the person's retirement experience will be like. If people can accurately identify themselves in relation to a given experiential profile, then the task will be much easier. Should it turn out that the structure of the person's worlds prior to retirement is linked to the retirement experiences in a specific way, then the general issue of developmental change or constancy of the structure of the person's multiple worlds is relevant. It is entirely possible that for people in the fourth group who experience retirement as a devastating affair, continued contact with one's fellow workers rather than a sudden break with the work world might make it easier to adapt. Such may not be the case with those persons who experience retirement as a "welcome beginning" or a "transition to the last phase of life, old age."

---

[12]Some open questions remain that must be answered before either accepting these findings as definitive or posing further developmental questions. For example, are the four groupings obtained by our methods replicable with other subject samples and data analysts or by other methods? Can some of the dimensions that we have identified in our data—meaning of retirement; style of transition; dominant emotions, attitude toward work; sense of self, orientation toward time; change in pre-retirement life focus; level of activity; nature of goals and activities; and attitude toward aging—be scored in a systematic way, and if so, can they be related to a developmental analysis?

The developmental organizations and reorganizations we seek to understand during, in the course of, and following critical person-in-environment transitions are complex, profound, and pervasive, and require intensive long-term, systematic study. We have only made some small beginnings in stating our questions so that they are amenable to developmental analysis. The empirical road ahead should provide some interesting answers.

ACKNOWLEDGMENT

The authors gratefully acknowledge the suggestions and contributions of Bernard Kaplan whose perspicacious views on the nature of psychological development have added immeasurably to our understanding.

REFERENCES

Ainsworth, M. D., & Wittig, B. A. Attachment and exploratory behavior of one-year-old children in a strange situation. In B. M. Foss (Ed.), *Determinants of infant behavior* (Vol. 4). London: Methuen, 1969.

Apter, D. Modes of coping with conflict in the presently inhabited environment as a function of variation in plans to move to a new environment. Masters thesis, Clark University, 1976.

Buckley, H. D. A comparison of freshman and transfer expectations. *Journal of College Student Personnel,* 1971, *12,* 186–188.

Burke, K. *Dramatism and development.* Barre, MA: Clark University Press with Barre Publishers, 1972.

Cassirer, E. *The logic of the humanities.* New Haven, CT: Yale University Press, 1961.

Edelman, E., Rierdan, J., & Wapner, S. Linguistic representation of a macroenvironment under three communication conditions. *Environment and Behavior,* 1977, *9,* 417–433.

Gibbs, J. T. Black students/white university: Different expectations. *Personnel and Guidance Journal,* 1973, *51,* 463–469.

Giorgi, A. Phenomenology and experimental psychology: I and II. *Duquesne studies in phenomenological psychology, Volume 1.* Pittsburgh, Duquesne University Press, 1971.

Hornstein, G. A., & Wapner, S. *Modes of adaptation during the transition from full-time work to retirement.* Presented at Eastern Psychological Association Meetings, New York, April, 1981.

Kaplan, B. The comparative developmental approach and its application to symbolization and language in psychopathology. In S. Arieti (Ed.), *American handbook of psychiatry, Vol. III.* New York: Basic Books, 1966.

Kaplan, B. Mediations on genesis. *Human Development,* 1967, *10,* 65–87.

Kaplan, B., Wapner, S., & Cohen, S. B. Exploratory applications of the organismic-developmental approach to man-in-environment transactions. In S. Wapner, S. B. Cohen, & B. Kaplan (Eds.), *Experiencing the environment.* New York: Plenum Press, 1976.

Lucca-Irizarry, N., Wapner, S., & Pacheco, A. M. Adolescent return migration to Puerto Rico: Self-identity and bilingualism. *Agenda,* 1981, *11,* 15–17, 33

McNeil, O. V., & Wapner, S. Developmental analysis of means of coping with conflict induced by transition from high school to college. Working Notes, 1981.

Pacheco, A. M., Wapner, S., & Lucca-Irizarry, N. Migration as a critical person-in-environment transition: An organismic-developmental interpretation. *Revista de Ciencias Sociales (Social Sciences Journal),* 1979, *21,* 123–157.

Pate, R. H. Student expectations and later expectations of a university enrollment. *Journal of College Student Personnel,* 1970, *11,* 458–562.

Quirk, M. *Values, beliefs and transactions of mothers of handicapped and mothers of non-handicapped pre-schoolers.* Doctoral dissertation, Clark University, 1982.

Quirk, M., Ciottone, R., & Wapner, S. Similarities and differences in the values held by mothers of handicapped children and mothers of non-handicapped children for their pre-schoolers. In symposium on "Parenting: A constructivist perspective." Presented at Eastern Psychological Association Meetings, Hartford, Connecticut, April, 1980.

Ramirez, M., III, & Castaneda, A. *Cultural democracy, bicognitive development and education.* New York: Academic Press, 1974.

Redondo, J. P., Pacheco, A. M., Cohen, S. B., Kaplan, B., & Wapner, S. Issues and methods in environmental transition: Exemplars from Puerto Rican migration. *Interamerican Review,* 1982 (in press).

Reiner, J. R., & Robinson, D. W. Perceptions of college environment and contiguity with college environment. *Journal of Higher Education,* 1970, *41,* 130–139.

Rheingold, H. L., & Eckerman, C. O. The infant's free entry into a new environment. *Journal of Experimental Child Psychology,* 1969, *8,* 271–283.

Rheingold, H. L., & Eckerman, C. O. The infant separates himself from the mother. *Science,* 1970, *168,* 78–83.

Risch, T. J. Expectations for the college environment. *Journal of College Student Personnel,* 1970, *11,* 463–466.

Schmitt, V., Redondo, J. P., & Wapner, S. *The role of transitional objects in adult adaptation.* Unpublished Report, Clark University, 1977.

Schouela, D. A., Steinberg, L. M., Leveton, L. B., & Wapner, S. Development of the cognitive organization of an environment. *Canadian Journal of Behavioral Science,* 1980, *12,* 1–16.

Wapner, S. Process and context in the conception of cognitive style. In S. Messick (Ed.), *Individuality in learning: Implications of cognitive styles and creativity for human development.* San Francisco: Jossey Bass, 1976.

Wapner, S. Environmental transition: A research paradigm deriving from the organismic-developmental systems approach. In L. van Ryzin (Ed.), *Proceedings of the Wisconsin Conference on research methods in behavior-environment studies.* Madison: University of Wisconsin, 1977.

Wapner, S. Some critical person-environment transitions. *Hiroshima Forum for Psychology,* 1978, *5,* 3–20.

Wapner, S. Transactions of persons-in-environments: Some critical transitions. *Journal of Environmental Psychology,* 1981, *1,* 223–239.

Wapner, S., & Hornstein, G. A. *Transition to retirement.* Final Report to NRTA-AARP Andrus Foundation, December 31, 1980.

Wapner, S., Kaplan, B., & Ciottone, R. Self-world relationships in critical environment transitions: Childhood and beyond. In L. Liben, A. Patterson, & N. Newcombe (Eds.), *Spatial representation and behavior across the life span.* New York: Academic Press, 1981.

Wapner, S., Kaplan, B., & Cohen, S. B. An organismic-developmental perspective for understanding transactions of men in environments. *Environment and Behavior,* 1973, *5,* 255–289.

Wapner, S., & Werner, H. *Perceptual development.* Worcester, MA: Clark University Press, 1957.

Watkins, M. *A phenomenological approach to organismic-developmental research.* Unpublished manuscript, Clark University, 1977.

Werner, H. *Einführung in die Entwicklungspsychologie.* Leipzig: Barth, 1926. (2nd ed., 1933; 3rd ed., 1953; 4th ed., 1959).

Werner, H. *Comparative psychology of mental development.* New York: Harper, 1940 (2nd ed., Chicago: Follett, 1948; 3rd ed., New York: International Universities Press, 1957).

Werner, H. The concept of development from a comparative and organismic point of view. In D. B. Harris (Ed.), *The concept of development.* Minneapolis: University of Minnesota Press, 1957.

Werner, H., & Kaplan, B. The developmental approach to cognition: Its relevance to the psychological interpretation of anthropological and ethnolinguistic data. *American Anthropologist,* 1956, *58,* 866–880.

Werner, H., & Kaplan, B. *Symbol formation.* New York: Wiley, 1963.

Werner, H., & Wapner, S. Sensory-tonic field theory of perception. *Journal of Personality,* 1949, *18,* 88–107.

Werner, H., & Wapner, S. Toward a general theory of perception. *Psychological Review,* 1952, *59,* 324–338.

Wofsey, E., Rierdan, J., & Wapner, S. Planning to move: Effects on representing the currently inhabited environment. *Environment and Behavior,* 1979, *11,* 3–32.

7 Regression Revisited: Perceptuo-Cognitive Performance in the Aged

Robert H. Pollack
University of Georgia

It has been traditional to look upon the aging process as a continuous inexorable deterioration of both physiological and psychological functions. Theories of regression, either historic or formal, have been applied to cognitive processes especially. The general assumption is that cognitive or more specifically intellectual functioning reaches its peak in early adulthood, remains on a gently downward sloping plateau until late middle age and then declines in accelerating fashion until death. It has been argued that these functions can be divided into those underlain by crystallized intelligence (such as long-term memory, comprehension of information, etc.) and decline more slowly than those functions underlain by fluid intelligence (including acquisition of new knowledge, problem solving, etc.). Nevertheless, the overall pattern of aging remains one of deterioration and decline. There are enough individual and group exceptions to the expected patterns of behavior, however, to make a congenital skeptic question both the assumptions and the data and to argue for a radically different view of adult development and aging.

There are a number of more or less complementary theoretical frameworks for accounting for physiological aging and death including genetically programmed limits on the number of cell divisions that must eventually lead to organ death (Hayflick, 1965; Lesher, Fry, & Kohn, 1961; McDonald, 1961; Rubner, 1908; Saunders, Gasseling, & Saunders, 1962; van Scott & Ekel, 1963; Sohal, 1976), programmed changes in endocrine production, which bring about metabolic dysfunction (Freeman, 1959; Shock, 1962), breakdown of the immunity functions, which lays the organism open to disease (Shock, 1976), and a breakdown of the oxygen transport system, which leads to a chronically acclerating hypoxia especially in brain tissue that never rejuvenates or replaces itself (Heinrich, 1959; Himwich & Himwich, 1956; Thompson & Marsh, 1973; Wolff, 1959). Recent discoveries concerning body chemistry (Orgel, 1963; Sun & Sun, 1979), nutrition (Eklund & Bradford, 1977; McCay, Crowell, & Maynard, 1935; Silberberg & Silberberg, 1955), and the possible replacement of certain vital substances offer some hope of slowing down physiological aging in the future (Aune, 1976; Linn, Kairis, & Holliday, 1976; Mindus, Cronholm, Levander, & Schalling, 1979; Pines, 1978; and Reisberg, Ferris, & Gershon, 1979). What we are not at all clear about is the temporal ordering of events in the physiological aging process as it impinges on cognitive functioning. It has always been assumed that performance decrements in cognitive tasks reflect, primarily, aging of those brain centers responsible for either the most complex or the most hierarchically superior mental operations (depending on one's theoretical preference) and furthermore, that in general, Hughlings Jackson was correct in assuming that regression continued from higher to lower or simpler functions with the passage of time. It is precisely here that I wish to say NO! to the system.

Much of the impetus for a notion of formal regression as the reverse of progressive development comes from the work of Goldstein (1939) and Werner (1957). The argument is that regression proceeds from higher to lower levels of functioning and involves dedifferentiation and the loss of the hierarchization of function. Elements of the higher levels are retained, however, but are set in a more concrete lower level of organization. This theoretical model is based largely upon the effects of disease and damage to the nervous system—that is, upon trauma to those structures underlying the very organization of behavior. If one examines the data gathered from diseased and damaged patients, the evidence for the regression model seems overwhelming. There are, nevertheless, data from the normal healthy course of aging that do not fit this picture.

Werner (1937) provided perhaps the most important caveat of all when he clarified the distinction between process and achievement. He argued most cogently against inferences concerning developmental levels and processes based solely on the appearances of performance. He pointed out that one level of development (genotype) could produce many kinds of behavioral performance (phenotypes) and that any given performance (phenotype) could result from more than one developmental level (genotype). The coincidence of phenotype and genotype, while it does occur with some regularity, is not guaranteed and may not always be inferred from the observation of behavior, especially in naturalistic settings. I submit that Werner himself, and many of the current workers in the field of aging, have ignored the process-achievement distinction with referent to aging.

The basic reason for the failure to apply the process-achievement distinction is the typically western assumption that optimal physical performance is somehow linked to optimal cognitive functioning and that maximal speed of performance somehow reflects top level, top quality intellectual activity. People slow down as they grow older, both in terms of physical movement and in the speed with which they make decisions (Birren, 1970; Birren & Riegel, 1962). Does the latter reflect the physical deteroiration that produces the former? Other societies venerate the aged, looking upon them as mature in judgment and rich in wisdom. They are shielded from their physical infirmities and appreciated for their wisdom in decisions that affect the running of their societies. Senility and retirement are largely western concepts. It is interesting, however, that we tend not to choose Presidents under the age of 50, nor are corporate chiefs and board chairmen noted for their youth. In our hypocrisy, we avoid contradictions by declaring such older persons as exceptions or as well-preserved or, frequently, as canny, yet burned out, tyrants holding on to power that should be passed to younger men!

I could use analogies from machines, but I will stick to human beings to keep the examples as cogent as possible. One over-riding methodological principle must be stated as a preamble to meaningful discussion. The older people we study must resemble as closely as possible the healthy, well-nourished, educated autonomous children, adolescents, and young adults who produce the data base for our theories of progressive development in the early part of the life span. If we study the middle aged and elderly people who are sick, senile, malnourished, and institutionalized, we will make inferences based on physical and social pathology qualitatively different from the normal aging process. The norms must come from the healthy, the vigorous, and the independent in the older population. Regardless of their numbers, they set the standard against which we measure the ravages of pathology. The fact that the statistical norm in youth is health as compared to a culture stereotype of infirmity in old age is no reason to alter the data base upon which we build developmental theory anywhere in the lifespan.

Given this caution, we can proceed to examine just what psychophysiological functions age in what order, at what developmental level and what their effects are on various aspects of general cognitive operation. Is it necessarily the case that the aging process causes deterioration in those brain centers that underlie the conceptual level of intellectual activity? Is it possible that subordinated perceptual or even sensorimotor functions deteriorate that preclude the manifestation of conceptual functions whose underlying structures are still intact? Could the installation of hard- and soft-ware sensorimotor and perceptual prosthetic devices produce the reappearance of high level behavior?

Let us choose one obvious, even banal, example from the experience of each of us before I go on to research-based examplars. Presbyopia is universal in the human animal. The lens of the eye from shortly after birth progressively becomes more yellow, dense and stiff (Leopold, 1971). The last phenomonen makes accommodation progressively more difficult so that comfortable near focusing is possible at three inches in middle infancy, 15 inches in early adolescence, and exceeds arm's length in the mid-to-late forties. If our society had no artificial lens technology or had not discovered that a small artificial pupil gives unlimited depth of focus, middle-aged people would give the appearance of having lost their capacity to read the sort of abstract material that appears in books with small print, but they would still read the concrete things that are written large on posters and road signs. What an obvious indication of intellectual deterioration we would have! Of course, the symptoms disappear when our population wears corrective lenses. Let us not pass off the obvious too lightly.

In our first study (Lee & Pollack, 1978), we attempted to extract some likely variables that would influence task performance at the perceptuo-cognitive border. Many investigators consider the embedded figures test (EFT) to be primarily a problem solving task representing the outcome of various cognitive strategies and even a reflection of cognitive style. It could be looked upon, as well, as reflecting the sensitivity of the visual system to camouflaged figure-ground segregation. All previous investigators agreed that performance time should increase in old age and the number of correct solutions should decline. If performance were to be tied to age-related changes in perceptual searching, the classical regression notion would retain support. If not, other possibilities would suggest themselves and further work would be worthwhile. In short, we followed the Wernerian strategy of the *experimentum crucis* at the outset, or as I have called it, the outrageous experiment.

We selected our subjects (all female due to scarcity of healthy elderly males) so that they were healthy, free living, middle class individuals all of whom had no visual resolution problems with our stimuli. The standard EFT Procedure was followed with one exception. No time limit was imposed so as to avoid test anxiety and overcautiousness. Time scores were obtained and scored raw or in EFT fashion (3 min limit). The scoring method had no effect on the data analysis. As expected, the time taken to find the figures increased with age and the number actually found declined. What was surprising was the shape of the curve. All of the decline in performance took place between the decade of the forties and the decade of the sixties with most of it between the forties and fifties. The expected acceleration of deterioration with increasing age did not occur. The sixties and seventies were almost alike. At the other end of the curve, the twenties, thirties, and forties were similar. Each subject was questioned after the fact on how she went about the task. The tape recorded protocols were classified in Wernerian terms as global or analytic at two levels within each category. Some people were classified at a third higher level as analytic-synthetic.

There were no differences in searching strategies across ages nor were there relationships between strategies and successes. The results, therefore, indicated not cognitive regression, but either a deterioration in figure-ground segregation or a change in overall cognitive style in the direction of field dependence.

By the way, there was no relation between task performance and such general personality variables as neuroticism or introversion-extraversion.

Our second study (Lee & Pollack, 1980) attempted to replicate the findings using other tasks related to the field dependence-independence continuum. The tasks involved were the portable rod & frame test and two versions of an ambiguous figure series that depicted a change from one figure to another (tree to house and dog to cat). Using the same sort of subjects in the critical decades, we were unable to find reliable age differences. If anything, our older subjects were more flexible in the ambiguous figures test and the apparent decline in rod-frame performance fell far short of significance. We suggested that general cognitive style is not a factor in determining EFT performance, and that the source of the performance drop in middle age lies in the operation of the visual system as it underlies figure-ground segregation.

In order to confirm and strengthen the notion of aging of the mechanism of figure-ground segregation, a third study has been carried out (Schwartz & Pollack, 1981). Essentially, it replicates the original EFT study and adds a new embeddedness task. This new task, taken from the comic strip section of a local newspaper involves two full color cartoons identical except for six changes that involve the elimination of details, the alteration of details in terms of extent, or the alteration of details in terms of orientation. Thus, the task is similar to EFT in that figure-ground segregation is involved, but there is no camouflage either geometric or by color. Embeddedness is achieved by location within the content context of the cartoons. In short, the task is more concrete than the EFT, but it still requires that the subject alter figure and ground voluntarily.

The quantitative results of the EFT resemble the findings of the original study. The time needed to identify each embedded figure increased sharply after the fourth decade and leveled off after the seventh. The overall trend, however, was linear, with significant paired comparisons largely between 20-30 and 60-70. The number of items solved showed no age effect at this time. In contrast, the cartoon task exhibited no significant time effect. The number of changes identified appeared to increase from the third through the fifth decades but decreased thereafter. There was, however, no significant age effect. The shape of this curve resembles somewhat that obtained by Heyn, Barry, and Pollack (1978) in a study of problem solving performance in young, middle aged, and older subjects. In that investigation, middle aged and older subjects took longer to solve reasoning, spatial, and numerical problems than young subjects, but the middle aged subjects solved significantly more problems than either of the other groups.

These results show, therefore, that perceptual embeddedness is a descriptive concept that includes a multiplicity of phenomena produced apparently by a number of non-equivalent underlying processes. The ability to segregate figures embedded in concrete pictorial content appears to be similar to that required for cognitive problem solutions. The difficulties encountered by subjects in their 40s, 50s, 60s, and 70s with the EFT seem to be quite different and to be independent of their problem solving abilities and strategies. This finding gives added support to the earlier conclusion (Lee & Pollack, 1980) that the source of those age differences lies in the operation of the visual system and not in cognitive functioning.

The qualitative data from the retrospective interviews concerning the strategies employed for finding the embedded figures show no age related differences for either task. Older and younger women do not do as well as middle aged women on the "Hocus Focus" problem. Further detailed analysis of the exact errors made may yield some clues setting off the youngest from the oldest subjects. Heyn, Barry, and Pollack (1978) found, for example, that while younger subjects made more errors of commission in problem solving, older subjects made more errors of omission. In the EFT, the hidden figures have either become much more difficult to separate and hold in view or the ground of camouflaging lines and colors has become more difficult to suppress. At any rate, the shapes of the age functions for solution time are different and the net loss from young to old age is much less for "Hocus Focus" than for EFT.

The "Hocus Focus" task has provided another interesting finding. Items that are different by virtue of being absent in the second picture are easier to detect at all age levels than items whose extent or orientation has changed. This difference is smallest in the 40–49 year old group whose performance is superior to all other groups with both item types. We see, therefore, a relatively flat age function for items correctly identified, except perhaps, for some improvement in extent and orientation items by the 40–49 year olds.

Where do we go from here? Despite the intrinsic interest generated by the "Hocus Focus" data, further investigation of that task will be delayed temporarily. The variables underlying EFT performance are of considerably more theoretical and empirical interest right now. Two lines of research need to be pursued. The first involves parametric studies of the camouflaging factors in the EFT itself. Jo Ann Lee is planning, as a first step, a series of studies on the effects of the colors used in the EFT. Particular dimensions are the presence or absence of color, the effects of short versus long wavelengths and the effects of particular color pairings. We know from our previous work with the block design subtest of the WISC and WAIS that the yellow-blue version of the test is more difficult than the red-white or a red-green version for darkly pigmented subjects (Mitchell & Pollack, 1974; Mitchell, Pollack, & McGrew, 1977). We also know that putting a neutral density filter in front of lightly pigmented eyes stimulates the effect of dark fundus pigmentation (Mitchell, Pollack, & McGrew, 1977). Other data indicate that yellow tends to bleed across borders (Skoff & Pollack, 1969). We are not, therefore, wading into unknown waters. Later studies will probably vary chroma and value as well. The next logical step after that would be the variation of the number and orientation of the camouflaging lines.

The second line of research will be concerned with configuration, and here the search is for other tasks whose age courses will mimic the EFT results. David Schwartz and I will work with the configuration problems involved in tests of color defect.

It has long been a part of the unpublished folk lore of color deficiency testers that tests of the Ishi-Hara type (Ichikawa et al., 1978) involving the identification of numbers made up of colored dots could not be used with children six years old and younger. If simple geometric forms (triangle and cross) and used (Hardy, Rand, & Rittler, 1957) and perhaps Pflügertridents (Velhagen, 1980) the problem disappears. When the American Optical Company abandoned geometric forms in favor of numbers several years ago, there was a wave of futile protest from the testers. It remains to be seen whether Velhagen has provided an equivalent alternative.

It is our intention to investigate possibly differential declines in color vision performance comparing Ishi-Hara type items with the HRR-American optical plates and the new Velhagen designs. We will also vary the order of the tests systematically in search of transfer effects. We may, of course, find a universal drop in color configuration performance in the 40- to 60 year-olds, which would go a long way toward solving our problem of identifying the visual process underlying the performance drop in the EFT. If we get differential results, we shall have to look at shape and lightness factors as well.

In summary, the main points to be made, using the above research with the EFT as an illustrative example, are that we cannot look at age differences through adulthood as reflecting an overall decline in performance underlain by regression characterized as a mirror reversal of progressive development, nor can we ignore the possibility that the loss of relatively low level performances can mask the appearance of undiminished higher level activities under certain definable circumstances. In other words, the process-achievement separation must be maintained and carefully investigated before we apply genetic principles either ortho or anti-ortho to data in gerontological research.

I will conclude by suggesting some practical applications for the theoretical modifications suggested and the laboratory results obtained. It appears that unlike the problems of acuity due to eyeball shape or accommodation or lens occlusion in vision or various hearing loss difficulties, individual hardware prostheses (spectacles and hearing aids) cannot solve the figure-ground segregation problems encountered above. In order to provide an effective visual environment for the aged with respect to the domains of signals, signs, and symbols, certain relatively simple rules need to be followed. First, all such stimuli should have high figure-ground lightness or brightness contrast ratios. Second, backgrounds should have matte rather than glossy finishes. Third, illumination should be strong with a peak of intensity in the orange-yellow region of the spectrum; short wave light should be avoided. Fourth, backgrounds should be plain—not noisy. Fifth, color coding, if used, should employ high saturations and emphasize longer wave hues. Clear verbal substitutes for diagramatic representations need to be developed. This list is far from exhaustive, but I did not want to stray too far from the situations discussed in this chapter.

I believe that cognitive prostheses can be developed for older people that will allow them to continue indefinitely at their previous high levels of performance. The work place in particular can be modified to get around sensory, perceptual, and speed constraints in order to make use of the experience, judgment, and wisdom of the elderly. The consequence of such an investment could mean an enormous profit in terms of quality control. It would also mean an end to wasting the older half of the labor pool in a population whose average age is rising inexorably. More important perhaps, such a policy would promote feelings of confidence and self worth in a part of the population now coming to be viewed as an increasing social burden to the young and productive. Given the appropriate application of science to relatively simple technology, it *can* be demonstrated that orthogenesis continues well beyond the third decade.

REFERENCES

Aune, J. Ultrastructural changes with age. In R. G. Cutler (Ed.), *Interdisciplinary Topics in Gerontology,* 1976, *10,* 44–61.

Birren, J. E. Toward an experimental psychology of aging. *American Psychologist,* 1970, *25,* 124–135.

Birren, J. E., & Riegel, K. F. Age differences in response speed as a function of controlled variations of stimulus conditions: Lights, numbers, letters, colors, syllables, words, and word relationships. In C. Tibbitts, & W. Donnahue (Eds.), *Social and psychological aspects of aging.* New York: Columbia University Press, 1962.

Eklund, J., & Bradford, G. E. Longevity and lifetime body weight in mice selected for rapid growth. *Nature* (London), 1977, *265,* 48–49.

Freeman, J. T. The mechanisms of stress and the forces of senescence. *Journal of the American Geriatrics Society,* 1959, *7,* 71–78.

Hardy, L. H., Rand, G., & Rittler, M. C. *AO—HRR pseudoisochromatic plates.* American Optical Company, 1957.

Hayflick, L. The limited in vitro lifetime of human diploid cell strains. *Expl. Cell Research,* 1965, *37,* 614–637.

Heinrich, A. Beitraege zur physiology des alterns. In K. Wolff (Ed.), *The biological, sociological and psychological aspects of aging.* Springfield: Charles Thomas, 1959.

Heyn, J. E., Barry, J. R., & Pollack, R. H. Problem-solving as a function of age, sex and the role appropriateness of the problem content. *Experimental Aging Research,* 1978, *4,* 505–519.

Himwich, H. E., & Himwich, W. A. Brain metabolism in relation to aging. In *The neurologic and psychiatric aspects of the disorders of aging.* Baltimore: Williams & Wilkins, 1956.

Goldstein, K. *The organism.* New York: American Book Company, 1939.

Ichikawa, H., Hukami, K., Tanabe, S., & Kawakami, G. *Standard pseudoisochromatic plates.* New York: Igaku-Shoin Medical Publishers, 1978.

Lee, J. A., & Pollack, R. H. The effects of age on perceptual problem-solving strategies. *Experimental Aging Research,* 1978, *4,* 37–54.

Lee, J. A., & Pollack, R. H. The effects of age on perceptual field dependence. *Bulletin of The Psychonomic Society,* 1980, *15,* 239–241.

Leopold, I. H. The eye. In J. F. Corso, Sensory processes and age effects in normal adults. *Journal of Gerontology,* 1971, *26,* 90–105.

Lesher, S., Fry, R. J. M., & Kohn, H. I. Influence of age on transit time of cells of mouse intestinal epithelium. *Lab. Invest.,* 1961, *10,* 291–300.

Linn, S., Kairis, M., & Holliday, R. Decreased fidelity of DNA polymerase in aging human fibroblasts. *Processes of the National Academy of Science, USA,* 1976, *73,* 2818–2822.

McCay, C. M., Crowell, M. F., & Maynard, L. A. The effect of retarded growth upon the length of the life span and upon the ultimate body size. *Journal of Nutrition,* 1935, *10,* 63–79.

McDonald, R. A. Life span of liver cells. *Archives of Internal Medicine,* 1961, *107,* 335–343.

Mindus, P., Cronholm, B., Levander, S. E., & Schalling, D. Piracetam-induced improvement of mental performance: A controlled study on normally aging individuals. In B. Reisberg, S. H. Ferris, & S. Gershon, Psychopharmacologic aspects of cognitive research in the elderly: Some current perspectives. *Interdisciplinary Topics in Gerontology,* 1979, *15,* 132–152.

Mitchell, N. B., & Pollack, R. H. Block design performance as a function of hue and race. *Journal of Experimental Child Psychology,* 1974, *17,* 377–382.

Mitchell, N. B., Pollack, R. H., & McGrew, J. F. The relations of form perception to hue and fundus pigmentation. *Bulletin of Psychonomic Society,* 1977, *9,* 97–99.

Orgel, L. E. The maintenance of the accuracy of protein synthesis and its relevance to aging. *Processes of the National Academy of Science, USA,* 1963, *49,* 517–521.

Pines, M. The riddle of recall and forgetfulness. In C. Kennedy, *Human development: The adult years and aging.* New York: MacMillan, 1978.

Reisberg, B., Ferris, S. H., & Gershon, S. Psychopharmacologic aspects of cognitive research in the elderly: Some current perspectives. *Interdisciplinary Topics in Gerontology,* 1979, *15,* 132–152.

Rubner, M. *Das problem der lebensdauer.* Berlin, 1908.

Saunders, J. W., Jr., Gasseling, M. T., & Saunders, L. C. Cellular death in morphogenesis of the avian wing. *Developmental Biology,* 1962, *5,* 147–178.

Schwartz, D., & Pollack, R. H. *Hocus Focus and the EFT: Effects of age on perceptual problem-solving strategies.* Presented at the annual UGA Convention for the Behavioral Sciences, April 1981.

Shock, N. W. Systems integration. In C. E. Finch, & L. Hayflick (Eds.), *Handbook of the biology of aging.* New York: Van Nostrand Reinhold Co., 1976.

Shock, N. W. The physiology of aging. *Scientific American,* 1962, *206,* 100–110.

Silberberg, M., & Silberberg, R. Diet and life span. *Physiological Review,* 1955, *35,* 347–362.

Skoff, E., & Pollack, R. H. Visual acuity in children as a function of hue. *Perception and Psychophysics*, 1969, *6*, 244–246.

Sohal, R. S. Metabolic rate and life span. In R. G. Cutler (Ed.), *Interdisciplinary Topics in Gerontology*, 1976, *9*, 25–40.

Sun, A. Y., & Sun, G. Y. Neurochemical aspects of the membrane hypothesis of aging. *Interdisciplinary Topics in Gerontology*, 1979, *15*, 34–53.

Thompson, L. W., & Marsh, G. R. Psychophysiological studies of aging. In C. Eisdorfer, & M. P. Lawton (Eds.), *The psychology of adult development and aging.* Washington: *American Psychological Association*, 1973, 112–148.

van Scott, E. J., & Ekel, T. M. Kinetoics of hyperplasia in psoriasis. *Archives of Dermatology*, 1963, *88*, 373–381.

Velhagen, K. *Pflügertrident-Plates for Testing the Sense of Colour.* German Democratic Republic: VEB George Thieme Leipzig, 1980.

Werner, H. Process and achievment. *Harvard Educational Review*, 1937, *7*, 353–368.

Werner, H. The concept of development from a comparative and organismic view. In D. B. Harris (Ed), *The concept of development: An issue in the study of human behavior.* Minneapolis, Minn.: University of Minnesota Press, 1957.

Wolff, K. Sul problema dei tumori. In Wolff, K. *The biological, sociological and psychological aspects of aging.* Springfield: Charles Thomas, 1959.

8 Process and Achievement Revisited

Edith Kaplan

Boston Veterans Administration Medical Center and Department of Neurology, Boston University School of Medicine

INTRODUCTION

In a classical paper entitled "Process and Achievement: A Basic Problem of Education and Developmental Psychology," Heinz Werner (1937) argued that it is erroneous to assume that any achievement, that is, the final solution to any problem, is an objective measure either of a developmental stage or of some unitary underlying mechanism. Borrowing the concept of analogous function from Biology and Anatomy, that is, that a given function may be accomplished by organs distinctly different in structure, Werner suggested that the final solution to a problem may be arrived at via diverse processes which themselves may reflect the activity of various structures in the Central Nervous System (CNS). To provide evidence for his observations, Werner presented illustrative material drawn from research in perception, memory, and concept formation, both in normal development and in pathology following brain damage. Werner's observations provide a foundation for a perspective in the assessment of intellectual and cognitive activities that more accurately delineates an individual's abilities and deficits. In fact, the application of this approach in the newly evolving field of clinical neuropsychology has proven to be particularly fruitful in describing brain-behavior relationships for: clinical diagnosis; rehabilitation; and an orientation to data collection for theoretical research. In order to illustrate the impact of Werner's process orientation on neuropsychology, in this chapter, I present material drawn from the observations of patients with verified focal lesions, normal children, and normal and pathological elderly individuals.

Underlying Werner's organismic-developmental approach to the analysis of behavior is the assumption that any cognitive act involves an "unfolding process" over time or "microgenesis" (Werner, 1956). Thus, the close observation and monitoring of behavior en route to a solution (process) provides more useful information than can be obtained from a correct/incorrect scoring of the final response only (achievement). This orientation fosters a patient-centered clinical approach, which is sensitive to a variety of "individual" variables such as age, sex, handedness, familial history of handedness, educational background, pre-morbid talents, etiology of CNS dysfunction, lateralization and locus of lesion. Obviously these variables contribute to the current neuropsychological status of the patient, and together with the nature of the task and the stimulus parameters, determine both the expression of spared and impaired functioning as well as the strategies the individual will employ to compensate for his/her impairment(s). A process-oriented, patient-centered neuropsychological assessment more effectively speaks to prescriptive rehabilitation efforts than an achievement-oriented, "fixed-battery" approach. Though the focus of this chapter is not rehabilitation, it should be noted, nonetheless, that the recovery course in rehabilitation underscores a microgenetic development that is best monitored and evaluated by a process-oriented approach.

VISUO-SPATIAL EXEMPLARS

Block design.   The distinction that can be drawn between the "process" and "achievement" approaches is clearly illustrated by performance on the Block Design subtest of the Wechsler Adult Intelligence Scales (WAIS, WAIS-R [Wechsler, 1955, 1981]). Figure 8.1 demonstrates three identical final solutions that are correct within the allotted time (60 seconds), and are given the sum score of four points. However, by keeping a running record (a flow chart) of the successive moves en route to the same final solution, three *different* strategies become apparent. The young, unimpaired adult (Young Control in Fig. 8.1) begins, as normal right-handers typically do, in the upper left corner and works from left to right systematically, without error. The other two examples (right frontal and left frontal) are characteristic of patients with lateralized focal frontal lesions. The patient with the frontal right hemisphere lesion, using his non-hemiparetic preferred right hand, begins in the lower right quadrant of the design (i.e., in the hemi-attentional field contralateral to his non-compromised cerebral hemisphere) and proceeds to work from right to left. This patient makes no errors while working toward his final correct solution. If he had made a self-corrected

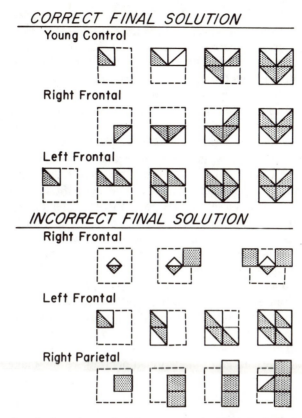

FIG. 8.1   Sample flow charts of performance on the Block Design subtest of the Wechsler Adult Intelligence Scale (Adapted from Albert & Kaplan, 1980, p. 425).

error, it would typically have occurred on the left side of the design, i.e., in the hemi-attentional field contralateral to his lesioned hemisphere. On the other hand, the patient with the left hemisphere frontal lesion (third row from top in Fig. 8.1), typically hemiparetic on the right side of his body, and using his left, non-preferred hand, begins to work on the left side of space, or the hemi-attentional field contralateral to his non-lesioned right hemisphere and the hemisphere controlling the motor output of his left hand. Though the position of the initial block placement is identical to that of the normal young control who had used his right hand to execute the design, the underlying mechanism may in fact be quite different. It should be noted further that the patient with the left hemisphere lesion makes a perseverative error on the right side of the design, which he self-corrects within the allotted time.

The three incorrect final solutions in the lower half of Fig. 8.1 are typical of errors made by patients with different focal lesions. The two patients with right hemisphere lesions (first and third solutions) do not maintain the 2 × 2 configuration matrix (broken configuration). Note that the patient with the frontal lesion lateralized to his left hemisphere (incorrect solution 2) typically does not violate the 2 × 2 matrix. Furthermore, whereas the left side of the design is intact, the two blocks in the right hemi-attentional field (contralateral to his lesion) are in error. Although broken configurations are more characteristic of right-hemisphere lesioned patients, the patient with the more anterior lesion preserves the physiognomic "V-ness" of the chevron-like figure. Thus, in this Right Frontal patient's construction the saliency of the lower point of the stimulus model is reflected by his selection of a single block to characterize it, which he places first. The construction of the Right Parietal patient (more posterior, right hemisphere parietal lesion) bears no relation to any aspect of the stimulus model. Within the framework of an "achievement" approach, the errors, either en route to, or in the final solution are not distinguished. The significant information provided by starting position, side of error, and qualitative differences between the final products—all scored zero—is irretrievably lost.

The importance of this type of neuropsychological analysis has recently been confirmed in a study of patients with focal lesions verified by CAT scan (Kaplan, Palmer, Weinstein, & Baker, 1981). Patients with lateralized lesions significantly more often start their constructions in the hemi-attentional field ipsilateral to the lesioned hemisphere and make significantly more errors (of the types exemplified above) in the hemi-attentional field contralateral to the lesioned hemisphere.

Object assembly.   We turn now to an analysis of differential stimulus parameters and their relevance for the understanding of brain-behavior relationships. The Object Assembly subtest of the Wechsler Intelligence Scales (WISC and WISC-R for children [Wechsler, 1949, 1974] and WAIS and WAIS-R for adults) contains assemblies that differ with regard to the presence or absence of internal details. The puzzles, that are rich in internal detail (e.g., WISC, WISC-R Automobile containing door, windows, and wheel lines), demand a capacity for a feature analytic approach. The puzzles that are devoid of internal features required a sensitivity to external contours (e.g., WISC, WISC-R Horse and WAIS, WAIS-R Hand). Patients with lesions confined to the left hemisphere have greater success with puzzles that load heavily on the dimension of contour, and relying on an edge alignment strategy, are frustrated by puzzles that require internal feature analysis for adequate solution. Patients with right hemisphere lesions, on the other hand, tend to fail the puzzles that require an appreciation of the saliency of contour and meet with greater success on those puzzles that feature internal details. Success may be precluded for both the left and right hemisphere lesion patients on those puzzles which simultaneously demand internal feature and external contour apprehension (e.g., WAIS, WAIS-R Profile). It is of interest that the two easier puzzles on the WISC, WISC-R (the Horse and the Apple) provide contour information and that as the child matures and there is increasing focalization in the language zone of the left hemisphere, the more difficult puzzles, which require feature analytic strategies are more readily solved. In contrast, the two easier puzzles on the WAIS, WAIS-R, the Mannikin and the Profile, are much richer in internal detail than the Hand and the Elephant, which lack internal detail and which become increasingly more difficult with advancing age. It is obvious that an achievement approach could result in the same score for two patients, one with a lesion lateralized to the left hemisphere and one with a lesion lateralized to the right, for successes on quite different stimulus items.

These findings make it abundantly clear that the visuo-spatial functions involved in constructional tasks such as Block Design and Object Assembly require the integrity of both cerebral hemispheres, and that lacking such integrity because of a lesion in either hemisphere, visuo-spatial functioning will be compromised in very particular ways. By manipulating the stimulus parameters described above, differences may be induced in the quality of performance of a patient with a given lesion or in the very young or very old.

Hooper visual organization test.   This task (Hooper, 1958), which requires the subject mentally to integrate component parts of line drawings, provides a further opportunity to examine stimulus parameters (see Fig. 8.2). Unlike the Object Assembly test, which does not require a verbal identification of the object assembled, and unlike the Object Assembly pieces, which do not lend themselves to being mislabeled as integral objects in isolation from the other pieces, the Hooper test is remarkable for the role the verbal task requirements play. Thus, patients with lesions involving the right hemisphere and an over-reliance on relatively preserved left hemisphere functions, have greater difficulty integrating the elements of particular items in which one or more of the component parts can readily be labeled in isolation. For example, in Fig. 8.2, the tail segment of the rat is frequently seen as a pipe, the key is often mislabeled as a utility knife or the profile of a person (e.g., Benjamin Franklin), and the cup identified as bookends or a handbag. Each of the separate components of the cat, on the other hand, lacks a compelling and "labelable" structural form; however, on a feature analytic basis, the detail of the eye permits the correct inference (cat) without necessitating a mental object assembly. Those patients with right hemisphere lesions, who, as on the Block Design subtest, focus on bits of information provided in the right hemiattentional field, may erroneously

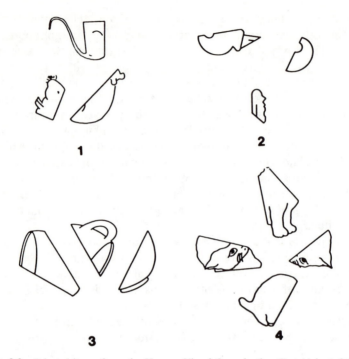

FIG. 8.2 Selected items from the Hooper Visual Organization Test (Adapted from Albert & Kaplan, 1980, p. 421).

identify the ear of the cat, on the right side, as the beak of a bird. Item 1 of the Hooper test (Fig. 8.3) is characteristically misidentified as a flying duck because of the critical feature on the right side of space.

The test requirement to name the items on the Hooper test probably, by virtue of engaging the language zone and thereby activating the left hemisphere (Kinsbourne, 1972, 1973), exacerbates the propensity towards a feature analytic mode of processing found in patients with right hemisphere lesions. Patients with left hemisphere lesions, including patients with word finding difficulties, secondary to a lesion in the language zone (aphasics), do not demonstrate these difficulties and are able to communicate their knowledge of the object in one way or another (e.g., by circumlocution).

NAMING

The ability to name the line drawing of an object (confrontation naming) is significantly impaired as a result of a lesion anywhere in the language zone. Further, a given score reflecting the absolute number of errors made on the 60 item revised Boston Naming Test (Kaplan, Goodglass, & Weintraub,

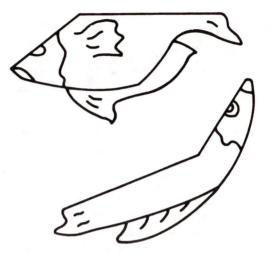

FIG. 8.3 "Fish" from Hooper
Visual Organization Test.

1982) may be obtained by non-aphasic patients with right hemisphere lesions, by the elderly, as well as by aphasics with classical syndromes
(Broca's, Wernicke's, Conductions and Anomics). These groups are dif-
ferentiable only with regard to the nature of the errors that are made
(Goodglass, 1980; Goodglass & Kaplan, 1972). Aphasics typically make the
following types of error:
      Literal paraphasias—phonologically based errors involving the substitu-
tion, deletion, addition or misordering of sound elements (Broca's and
Conductions);
      Verbal paraphasias—substitution of a word that may be semantically
related, that is, a word in the same category, or contextually associated, or
words that are remotely related (Wernicke's);
      Circumlocution—describing the object or indicating its function (Wer-
nicke's and Anomics).
      The above errors in accessing the lexicon, with the exception of cir-
cumlocutions in the elderly, are not evidenced by non-aphasic patients.
Rather, misidentification is based on highly significant perceptual features
of a stimulus or prominence of features on the basis of color and/or redun-
dancy (e.g., the harmonica [Fig. 8.4] is frequently misidentified as a double
decker bus or factory because of the "windows"). Misidentification is
characteristically observed in right hemisphere lesion patients and in the
elderly, but not in aphasics. The features of the stimulus that give rise to the
misidentification are virtually in all cases readily identifiable. This non-
aphasic misnaming is a result of an inability to organize the percept, and to
integrate the multiple aspects of the stimulus, but does not reflect an inability to access the lexicon as is the case in aphasic naming problems.

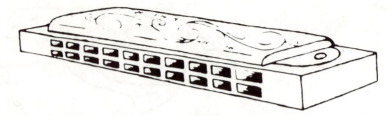

FIG. 8.4   "Harmonica" from Boston Naming Test.

IMMEDIATE MEMORY

The misidentification of a stimulus object that is a consequence of either partial or incomplete perceptual analysis, or stimulus boundedness (i.e., the inability to resist a pull to the sensory-perceptual aspects of the stimulus) severely limits veridical reproduction. Obviously, such superficial encoding strategies may be mistaken for a memory or retrieval problem in patients with CNS dysfunction and in the elderly. This is shown in the characteristic errors patients with lateralized lesions make in the immediate reproduction (lower half of Fig. 8.5), following a 10 second exposure of the stimulus shown in the upper half of Fig. 8.5. The left hemisphere lesion patients again are noted to process the major configurational component, that is, the "X," making only rotational errors with regard to the "flag" features. The patients with lesions in the right hemisphere typically lack the X configuration. Though each feature, viz., the two lines and four flags may be present, the integration of these components is wanting. Figure 8.6 presents the characteristic error patterns of a large sample of men and women between the ages of 55 and 89 to the same stimulus shown in the upper half of Fig. 8.5). Based upon performance on a brief neuropsychological screening test they were divided into high, middle, and low scorers. A flow chart capturing the sequence and direction of the lines drawn permitted the analysis of the process underlying both correct and incorrect drawings. Taking only correct final reproductions, it was possible with the help of the flow charts to identify by far the most common strategy (drawing the X first and adding the flags second) employed by between 80% and 90% of the high cognitive scorers at age 55 to 64. Figure 8.7 reveals a sex difference favoring women 65 years and older. The high cognitive scoring women appear to maintain the typical strategy even after age 75, whereas the high cognitive scoring men show a significant decline relative to the women as early as age 65. This sex difference would not have emerged from a dichotomous scoring system (viz., correct vs. incorrect), since all the reproductions were correct. Though it is tempting to assume that this finding indicates some sort of superiority or resistance to aging effects in women, until the analysis of the varieties of

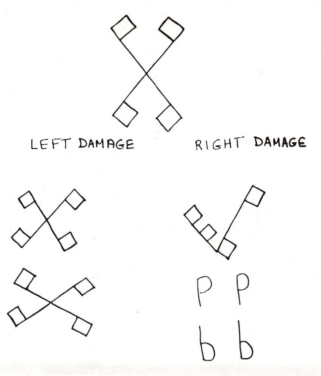

LEFT DAMAGE   RIGHT DAMAGE

FIG. 8.5   Visual Reproduction Errors in patients with lateralized lesions (Adapted from E. Kaplan, 1980).

alternative strategies employed by both the high and low scorers has been conducted, such as conclusion would be premature.

The similarity between the segmented, poorly integrated reproductions of the low cognitive functioning elderly subjects (Fig. 8.6) and right hemisphere lesion patients (Fig. 8.5) is striking and raises the possibility that the functions subserved by the right hemisphere are more vulnerable to the effects of aging than are those subserved by the left hemisphere (Albert & Kaplan, 1980; Kaplan, 1980).

GESTURAL REPRESENTATION

The ability to represent gesturally an absent implement to verbal command (praxis) for example, "Show me how you would brush your teeth with a toothbrush" has been studied in ontogenesis (Kaplan, 1968), in pathology (Goodglass & Kaplan, 1963) and in the elderly (Kaplan, 1978).

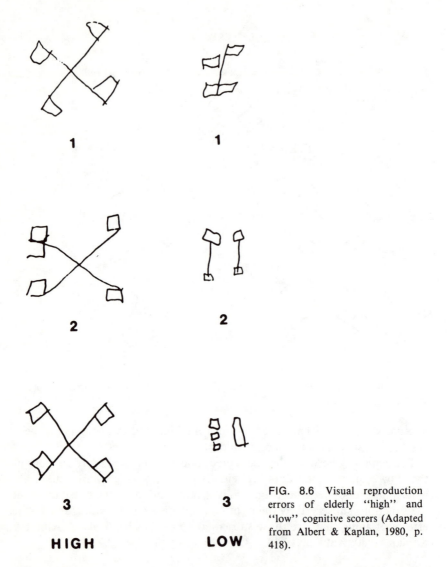

1   1

2   2

3   3

FIG. 8.6 Visual reproduction errors of elderly "high" and "low" cognitive scorers (Adapted from Albert & Kaplan, 1980, p. 418).

HIGH   **LOW**

Development of praxis.   In accord with the orthogenetic principle of development (Werner & Kaplan, 1963), as a normal child increases in age, gestural representation of the utilization of an absent implement, for example, toothbrush, reflects an increase in the degree of differentiation and hierarchic integration of the components of the referent, that is, the agent (you), the action (brush), the object of the action (teeth), the implement (toothbrush). An analysis of the modes of response reveals a distinct developmental progression as follows:

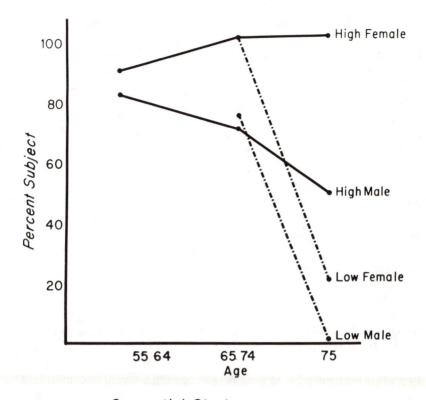

Sequential Strategy

FIG. 8.7 Percentage of correct responses with sequential strategy in the elderly (Adapted from Albert & Kaplan, 1980, p. 417).

Level 1—Deictic behavior.   Pointing to the locus of the action, for example, index finger pointing into mouth. *Manipulation of the object of the action.* For example, rubbing teeth with fingertips. These responses focus entirely on the object of the action. The implement is in no way depicted.

Level 2—Body-part-as-object (BPO).   The index finger, positioned as if it were the toothbrush, vigorously rubs teeth in brushing motion. Here the implement and the characteristic action of the implement are represented by a part of the body. At this level of representation there is a lack of differentiation between the agent and the implement.

Level 3—Holding without extent.   The hand is positioned to hold the absent toothbrush but the positioned hand is too close to the teeth. The implement itself is not fully articulated.

Level 4—Holding with extent.   The hand is positioned to hold the toothbrush and the hand is held at a sufficient distance from the mouth, i.e, empty space is used to represent the extent of the absent implement. At this level the agent, action, object of the action and implement are all fully differentiated.

Normal children below the age of 4 gesture at level 1, at age 4 level 2 predominates, at age 8 level 3 has been attained, and by age 12 children are primarily gesturing at level 4. The developmental status of the child is reflected in his characteristic mode of gestural representation.

Apraxia.   The inability of some aphasic patients to use pantomime to circumvent their language impairment was at first thought to be a symbolic, or central communication disorder. Since the turn of the century, however, gestural impairment has been ascribed to a movement disorder (Geschwind, 1965; Goodglass & Kaplan, 1963; Liepmann, 1905). Apraxia is defined as an inability to perform movements to verbal command (with the disability not attributable to an auditory comprehension problem, a motor or sensory loss). When a brain damaged apractic patient is verbally required gesturally to represent absent implement usage, he may produce a body-part-as-object response (BPO), which is formally similar to the BPO response of the young child. However the initiation of the response is distinctly different. The apractic adult may make groping movements and appear to be attempting to posture his hand prior to what may be for him a way of circumventing his disorder. In contrast, the young child hesitates not at all. In fact, he produces a BPO immediately and with certitude. It is clear that the process underlying the BPO of the adult is distinctly different from the process underlying the BPO response of the child. For the developmentally immature child the lack of differentiation between components of the symbol situation accounts for the response. For the apractic adult the locus of the anatomical lesion causes a disconnection between the idea and the motor execution of it.

BPO representation in the elderly.   BPO responses are encountered in elderly individuals performing at a lowered cognitive level. Again, though these responses are formally similar to those of the child and those of the apractic adult with brain damage, the underlying defect is different. In the low cognitive scoring older person, BPO responses are probably secondary to a dedifferentiation at the symbolic level. Such individuals respond at a more concrete level, interpreting the command to perform some movement as a mandate to, e.g., really brush his teeth. This behavior may be likened to concrete responses on other symbolic tasks (e.g., Gorham's proverbs).

SUMMARY

The survey of exemplars demonstrated the power of a patient-centered, process-oriented approach to the neuropsychological assessment of patients who have sustained insult to the central nervous system. The exemplars illustrate the variety of ways in which a process-oriented approach, as opposed to an achievement-oriented approach, deepens our understanding of the functioning of a given individual by closely examining the course of problem solving behaviors. The process approach informs us of the compensatory strategies, both adaptive and maladaptive, that an individual has developed to cope with his or her deficit(s). In addition, the process analysis provides information concerning the individual's differential response to varying task demands as well as stimulus parameters that may induce a more or less effective response. This body of information is critical for the formulation of interventions that immediately address the profile of spared and impaired functions. At the same time a process analysis permits sensitive, dynamic monitoring of the efficacy of these interventions and the ongoing reformulations during the developmental course of rehabilitation.

ACKNOWLEDGMENT

The author wishes to express gratitude to Dr. Elisabeth Moes for her help in the preparation of this chapter.

REFERENCES

Albert, M. S., & Kaplan, E. Organic implications of neuropsychological deficits in the elderly. In L. W. Poon, J. L. Fozard, L. S. Cermak, D. Arenberg, & L. W. Thompson (Eds.), *New directions in memory and aging*. Hillsdale, N.J.: Lawrence Erlbaum Associates, 1980.

Geschwind, N. Disconnexion syndromes in animals and man. *Brain,* 1965, *88,* 585–644.

Goodglass, H. Naming disorders in aphasia and aging. In L. K. Obler, & M. L. Albert (Eds.), *Language and communication in the elderly*. Lexington, Mass.: Heath, 1980.

Goodglass, H., & Kaplan, E. Disturbance of gesture and pantomime in aphasia. *Brain,* 1963, 703–720.

Goodglass, H., & Kaplan E. *The assessment of aphasia and related disorders*. Philadelphia: Lea and Febiger, 1972.

Hooper, H. E. *The Hooper Visual Organization Test. Manual*. Los Angeles: Western Psychological Services, 1958.

Kaplan, E. *Gestural representation of implement usage: An organismic-developmental study*. Unpublished doctoral dissertation, Clark University, 1968.

Kaplan, E. *Symbolic, motor and spatial components of praxis: Lifespan overview*. Paper presented at International Neuropsychology Symposium, Oxford, England, 1978.

Kaplan, E. Changes in cognitive style with aging. In L. K. Obler, & M. L. Albert (Eds.), *Language and communication in the elderly.* Lexington, Mass.: Heath, 1980.

Kaplan, E., Goodglass, H., & Weintraub, S. *The Boston Naming Test (Experimental edition-revised)* Boston, 1982.

Kaplan, E., Palmer, E. P., Weinstein, C., & Baker, E. *Block design: A brain-behavior based analysis.* Paper presented at the International Neuropsychological Society, Bergen, Norway, June, 1981.

Kinsbourne, M. Head and eye turning indicate cerebral lateralization. *Science,* 1972, *176,* 539–541.

Kinsbourne, M. The control of attention by interaction between the cerebral hemispheres. In S. Kornblum (Ed.), *Attention and performance IV.* New York: Academic Press, 1973.

Liepmann, H. Der weitere Krankheitsverlauf bei dem einseipig Apraktischen und der Gehirn-befund auf Grund von Serienschnitten. *Monatschrift Psychiatrie und Neurologie,* 1905, *17,* 289–311.

Wechsler, D. *Wechsler intelligence scale for children.* New York: Psychological Corporation, 1949.

Wechsler, D. *Wechsler adult intelligence scale.* New York: Psychological Corporation, 1955.

Wechsler, D. *Wechsler intelligence scale for children-revised.* New York: Psychological Corporation, 1974.

Wechsler, D. *Wechsler adult intelligence scale-revised.* New York: Psychological Corporation, 1981.

Werner, H. Microgenesis and aphasia. *Journal of Abnormal and Social Psychology,* 1956, *52,* 347–353.

Werner, H. Process and achievement: A basic problem of education and developmental psychology. *Harvard Educational Review,* 1937, *7,* 353–368.

Werner, H., & Kaplan, B. *Symbol formation.* New York: Wiley, 1963.

9 Some Aspects of a Developmental Analysis of Perception

Ricardo B. Morant
Brandeis University

INTRODUCTION

In this chapter I indicate some ways to use developmental theory to study perceptual processes. My point of departure is Heinz Werner's holistic, organismic view of development and I relate it to a series of experimental studies under current investigation in my laboratory. Although I begin by noting Werner's influence on the investigation of the microgenesis of form perception, most of the discussion refers to problems of orientation and the perception of visual and haptic space. The first set of experiments deals with the effect of prismatic rearrangement on the perception of the vertical, the second has to do with auditory and visual localization under conditions of labyrinthian stimulation, and the third studies the development of visual-haptic organization in young infants. The results of the first two sets of experiments are seen to fit the main theoretical formulations of sensory-tonic theory and to underscore the importance of analyzing the temporal course of development of perceptual experiernce. They indicate that perception is best understood as a continuously transforming relationship between sensory-motor subsystems and the proximal stimulation provided by the environment. Some suggestions are made for future research on the microgenesis of perceptual adaptation and some implications of the results of the experiments for image and spatio-temporal flow theories of perception are noted. In the penultimate section, I discuss the development of the experience of intersensory unity in relation to the results of the third experiment in which infants reach for virtual objects. The essay concludes with a brief discussion of the orthogenetic principle as a definition of an ideal movement towards perfection.

WERNER'S IMPACT ON PERCEPTION

Werner's conceptualization of perceptual development was meant to encompass all instances of sensory interaction with the environment as it occurs over time. The basic principle, that perception proceeds from global, unanalyzed units to forms of organization where the whole is differentiated into articulated parts clearly related to the whole and to one another, was seen to apply not only to the ontogenetic development of the organism but also to the changes in organizational patterning occurring from the time a sensory subsystem is stimulated to the emergence of a final perceptual structure. This conceptualization and the experimental strategies that Werner formulated to demonstrate it anticipated much of contemporary thinking and research in diverse areas of sensory-perceptual functioning. For example, his investigations of the way in which visual contours are formed under conditions of tachistoscopic exposure laid the foundation for much of the recent work on contour interaction. His studies on the microgenesis of visual form showing that contours develop over time and can influence one another (Werner, 1935, 1940) was the direct precursor of the whole body of work on metacontrast and visual masking. A third paper in this series of "Studies on contour" (Solomon & Werner, 1952) anticipated the current interest, re-introduced by Kanizsa's work on contours without gradients (Kanizsa, 1976), in interrelating attention, apparent brightness, and contour processes (for example, Kennedy, 1976).

Werner's application of what he and Kaplan came to call the orthogenetic principle (Werner & Kaplan, 1963) to problems of perceptual functioning in psychopathology, "primitive" cultures, and lower animals did not fare as well. Aside from occasional references to physiognomic perception, synaesthesia, and the difference between objects as perceived in static terms or as perceived as things of action, little has been made of Werner's brilliant speculations regarding the formal similarities among all primordial forms of perception.

Perhaps Werner's greatest influence on perceptual theory has come from the series of investigations applying the principles of the sensory-tonic theory, which he developed during the last 15 years of his life in conjunction with Seymour Wapner and a group of young collaborators at Clark University. These studies continue to have broad implications for current workers in such areas of investigation as body imagery, sensory-motor coordination, figural and adaptation aftereffects, visual space integration, vestibular functioning, prism adaptation, event perception, and geographic orientation.

A DEVELOPMENTAL APPROACH TO
SENSORY-TONIC THEORY

The basic thrust of sensory-tonic theory for the study of developmental processes was that perception should be conceived as an ongoing transaction
between sensory and intra-organismic factors which change over time. The
development of any perceptual act was viewed as a continuously transforming relationship between intra-organismic state and the proximal stimulation provided by the environment (Werner & Wapner, 1956; Wapner &
Werner, 1965). The application of the theory to ontogenetic perceptual
development has been formally delineated in a theoretical paper by
Wapner, Cirillo, and Baker (1969). They argue that the characteristic structure of the system that underlies the changing environment-organism transaction as the child grows up conforms precisely to the orthogenetic principle of development. The hierarchical relationship between the organism and
the environment is conceptualized in their scheme as the interaction of three
levels of organization with distinct equilibrial tendencies whose relative
precedence change as the child matures. The three levels, sensory-motor action, objectification, and experienced relations between percepts, are meant
to characterize the increasing emergence of cognitive processes, particularly
intentionality, as organism-environment transactions occur over time. The
two poles of the system, the organism and the environment, are seen to be
increasingly differentiated from a primitive state of immediate motoric
responsivity to environmental signals, to a distancing between the organism
and the environment through a process of objectifying the world and, finally, to a hierarchic integration of different object percepts including the
perception of the body itself.

The differentiation between object and self is conceived as a dynamic
process wherein earlier forms of organization become subsystems of the
emergent higher-forms so that disturbances of any one subsystem influences
the performance of the others in the mature organism. This rich developmental schema is then used to re-interpret many of the findings of early sensory-tonic research including the studies on the effects of body tilts, prismatic
adaptation, tactual-kinaesthetic interactions and child/adult differences in
the perception of spatial localization. One illustration of this reinterpretation refers to earlier studies on the perception of straight-ahead. Wapner
and Werner (1957) had originally shown that the effect of exposure to
background asymmetrical light stimulation was to induce a torsion of the
head away from the light. Wapner et al. (1969) now note that whether or
not this actually occurs depends on the task set by the perceiver. The asymmetrical stimulation will have different effects depending on whether the
perceiver adjusts by yielding to the imbalance or by counteracting it. The
immediate sensory-motor response to the asymmetry runs free or is subordinated to a higher system depending upon the overall goal of the organism.

But there is an even more direct response possible to resolve such an organism-environment disequilibrium. The perceiver can change the environment directly so as to rectify the imbalance and provide more symmetry. Indeed under natural conditions, after an initial change in body posture, the preferred mode of resolving the conflict induced by an unbalanced visual field is for the organism to change the properties of the field directly. One such instance can be observed by hanging a picture askew on the living room wall and observing the response of newly arrived guests. The initial resolution of the disequilibrium between object tilt and upright posture is to incline the head so as to bring the observer in line with the main organization of the picture space. The invariable second response is to reach out and straighten the picture and so also straighten the head. The point is that adjustment to symmetry depends not only on the perceiver's goals but also on the constraints to response imposed by the environment. If the environment can be manipulated directly, then it is. If it cannot be manipulated, then other sensory-motor subsystems, functioning vicariously, come into play to resolve the imbalance.

ADAPTATION TO PRISM REARRANGEMENT

How is body-environment disequilibrium resolved when experimental circumstances allow neither an adequate change in body posture nor a change in the environmental field? The following set of studies were designed to investigate what occurs when constraints disallow direct resolution of asymmetrical conflict. The results indicate that under such circumstances a set of adaptation processes come into play that highlight the hierarchic relationship between vision and posture in the organization of visual space.

Asymmetry was induced by having subjects wear a binocular prism device that tilts the visual world clockwise (CW) or counterclockwise (CCW) in the fronto-parallel plane. The subject wore the device while walking about in a normally lit environment, in this case the halls of a university laboratory. Let us jump to the end result first. The aftereffect of wearing prisms that tilt the visual world, say CW, is that after removal of the prisms a vertically oriented line, viewed in a dark room, appears tilted CCW. It is the mechanism underlying this change in the line's apparent orientation, or to put it another way, the mechanism responsible for the change in the position of visual space which is considered vertical, which we want to determine.

We begin with the observation that as soon as a subject puts on the prisms and begins to walk about, he inclines his head in the direction of visual tilt induced by the prisms. If the prisms tilt the visual field CW, the head is inclined towards the right shoulder, if the prisms tilt the visual field CCW, the head is inclined towards the left shoulder. When queried, subjects seem unaware of their head tilt. This laboratory situation, however, is critically different from our tilted picture in the living room demonstration. Here the head inclination rather than resolving the visual-body posture asymmetry tends, if anything, to exacerbate it, for as the head rotates in space, so do the prisms. Each attempt to resolve asymmetry by rotating the head in the direction of visual displacement induces a comparable tilt of the visual field. Our first question was to determine whether the head inclination during exposure was related to the change in the apparent vertical after exposure when the head was reoriented to the normal upright position. The second was to analyze the time course of head tilt during exposure and relate it to the visual aftereffect.

The initial study was done some years ago with two of my students, David Lotto and Allen Kern. It tested the following four assumptions: (1) During prism exposure the head inclines in the direction of prismatic tilt; (2) The subject tends to accept this tilted head position as vertical and consequently, after prism exposure when the head is placed at true vertical, it feels tilted in the opposite direction; (3) For a line to appear vertical it should be in the same position as the apparent vertical position of the head; and (4) Since the felt head position is changed after prism exposure, there should be a concurrent change in the position of the apparent visual vertical.

What we did was to compare the results of conditions in which the subject walked freely about while wearing tilting prisms with conditions when the head was physically restrained at varying degrees of lateral inclination. Briefly, we found directionally equivalent head posture and visual vertical aftereffects in both types of conditions. The magnitude of the effects could not, however, be compared since the subjects were mobile in one condition and stationary in the other and, more importantly, the actual degree of head rotation involvement in the prism conditions was unknown.

A second study, conducted in collaboration with Steven Shulman, was designed to monitor the head tilt occurring during prism exposure so as to compare the magnitude of both visual and felt head position aftereffects after prism-induced and equivalent non-prism-induced head tilts. This experiment consisted of two main parts. Part one involved a 30 minute exposure to 40° CW or CCW tilting prisms. During this inspection period the subject walked up and down the hallway in a specially designed "walker" that restricted trunk movements by means of arm rests, shoulder straps, and hip pads. While walking about, the subject bit firmly onto a biteplate mounted on the walker. The biteplate was free to rotate CW or CCW and therefore could be used to monitor the subject's head position (see Figs. 9.1 and 9.2). Thirty measures of head position were recorded, one after each minute of prism exposure. The mean reading of each subject's actual head

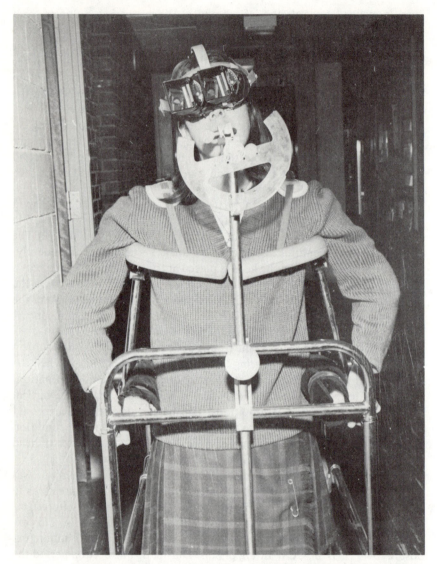

FIG. 9.1   "Walker" with head tilt measuring device: Front view.

position during the first, second, and third 10 minute segments of prism exposure were calculated for use in the second part of the experiment.

The procedure during the second part was identical to that of the first with one exception. Instead of wearing the prisms during the inspection period, subject's head was locked by means of the biteplate at head tilts equivalent to those registered when prisms had been worn. The head was locked at the average positions observed during the three 10-minute seg-

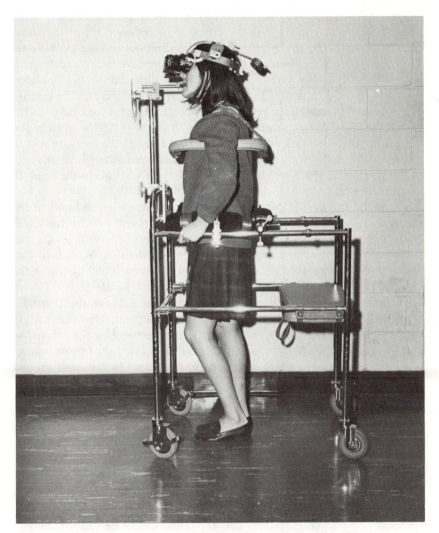

FIG. 9.2 "Walker" with head tilt measuring device: Side view.

ments of the original inspection period. During inspection in this second part then, the subject walked up and down the corridor in the walker with his eyes open, without prisms, but with his head position fixed in the manner described. Total body posture therefore mimicked that of the first part of the experiment although, since the prisms were not worn, the retinal flow pattern of visual stimulation was substantially different. Again, we found that equivalent head and visual aftereffects are obtained when the head is held without prisms in the same position as that to which it spontaneously tilts while wearing prisms.

The results can be summarized as follows. When prisms were worn, the head spontaneously inclined in the direction of apparent tilt of the visual field. With 40° tilting prisms, the head inclined on the average slightly over 11° towards the right shoulder if the prisms were CW tilting and towards the left shoulder if they were CCW tilting. Visual tilt and head tilt aftereffects were also in the direction of the original prism tilt and were on the average 2.2° and 2.6° in magnitude respectively. These measures were taken at the end of the 30 minute exposure condition with the head held at upright and the prisms off. The task of the subject in the visual tilt measure was to rotate an objectively vertical field of lines viewed in an otherwise dark room to the position in space which he considered to be vertical. In the head tilt measure, the task was to incline the head until it felt to be straight up and down on the trunk. Comparable measures taken in the second part of the experiment, without any prism exposure whatever, were 1.8° for the visual aftereffect and 3.5° for the head aftereffect. Each of the four results was statistically significant at a probability level of less than .01. What is of particular interest is that the findings obtained in the second condition, with the head inclined but without wearing prisms, were not significantly different from those obtained after wearing prisms. For these studies then, we conclude that the visual tilt aftereffect is not directly attributable to adaptation to the changing visual stimulus flow pattern introduced by the prisms, so much as it is to the aftereffects of head inclination that the prisms induce. More recent studies in which only one eye is exposed to prismatic tilt and then either that eye or the other is tested tend to confirm these findings. Results of conditions where head-trunk exercises are introduced between prism exposure and testing, and conditions where the head is forcibly inclined towards one shoulder while opposite tilting prisms are worn, are a bit more complex but essentially congruent with our other results. They demonstrate that change in the visual perception of the vertical is integrally related to change in the apparent felt position of the head.

These results underscore Wapner's and Werner's insistence that "a perceptual property (in this case verticality) is an experience which corresponds to a particular relation between organismic state and stimuli issuing from an object" (1957, p. 1). We should add that the experience changes as the stimulus modifies both the sensory and motor systems over time. Lashley in his seminal paper on the integrative action of the nervous system reminds us that all sensory systems have diffuse rather than specific projections (Lashley, 1951). The determination of the temporal course of the effects of sensory stimulation as they modify the motor systems and postural tonus and are then consequently modified in turn is a critical problem for future research on the genesis of short term perceptual experience. A few such studies related to perceptual adaptation and aftereffects are suggested in the following section.

SUGGESTED STUDIES ON PERCEPTUAL
ADAPTATION AND AFTEREFFECTS

The developmental change in perceptual processing due to restructuring of salient stimulation over exposure time has commanded little attention in space perception research thus far. A microgenetic approach to how perceptual adaptation changes in the course of stimulus exposure might clarify the interrelationships among various of the supposedly different adaptation and perceptual aftereffects reported in the literature. For example, the following longitudinal study of a set of perceptual experiences might allow the results of prismatic tilt aftereffects to be related both to the Witkin and Asch tilted room, and rod and frame effects (1948) and the Werner and Wapner starting position effects (1952a, b). The essence of the study is to plot both adaptation and aftereffects at various intervals during exposure to prismatic rearrangement and see how they change over time. We begin with the observer first sitting and later walking about. Adaptation is measured by having the subject adjust a rod to vertical against the visual background (a cluttered laboratory room) seen through the tilting prisms. Aftereffect is measured by having the subject remove the prisms in the dark and adjust the now illuminated rod to vertical in the absence of any other comparison visual contours. Preliminary observations indicate the following course of adaptation and aftereffects.

The first few minutes of looking at the optically tilted room is paradigmatic of the Witkin and Asch (1948) tilted room situation. Since the subject is seated with the head stationary, there is no optical transform contingent upon motion and as Witkin and Asch showed, the room tends to be accepted as less tilted than it really is and the rod adjusted accordingly. However, this adaptation does not result in an aftereffect. When the lights are shut off, the adjusted rod, which looked vertical in the light, now appears tilted once again and must be readjusted to just a few degrees off true vertical in order to appear straight up and down.

This last observation is congruous with results obtained in the rod and frame task showing large immediate adaptation effects but small aftereffects (Morant & Aronoff, 1966). The point is that the subject when first confronted with the prismatically tilted world tends to accept its main directions as defining upright and minimizes cues coming from his own body. When the rich visual field is removed in the dark-room condition, the visually given directional characteristics are eliminated, and only the equivalent of a "starting-position" aftereffect is left.

As the subject now gets up and walks about while wearing the prisms, something new occurs. The very act of moving forces the subject into an immediate awareness of the discrepancy between his body posture and the visual environment. Adaptation, as measured by the adjustment of the rod,

drops off and again there is no aftereffect in the dark. However, with pro-
longed walking about the sensed body position begins to change. Body cues
now are now no longer ignored but are reinterpreted. The result of this
reinterpretation—a sensory-motor relearning—is reflected in large aftereffects. It should be noted that at both times, at the beginning and at the end
of inspection, subjects report that the visual field normalizes. It is only at
the latter time, however, that this prismatic adaptation is reflected in the
dark room aftereffect tests. It is apparent, then, that the dominance of the
various subsystems that determine both the adaptation and aftereffect processes change during the course of the observations. To understand these
changing interactions and how they are hierarchically integrated requires
longitudinal determination of the ongoing perceptual experience.

More systematic studies are needed to specify which sensory and motor
subsystems are most directly influenced by which stimulus conditions in
order to determine how they are hierarchically integrated. For example, we
should know whether the visually determined position in space regarded as
vertical is more influenced by apparent eye scan, or by head inclination or
by trunk tilt and how the relative influences change as the systems are
systematically disarranged. Suppose the vertical is determined haptically
rather than visually, do the same relationships hold? Are the relationships
equivalent for the horizontal? That is, do the vertical and horizontal constitute a unitary Cartesian coordinate system such that postural and/or
visual adaptation to one is equivalent to adaptation to the other?

Or, to take another example, in a conflict situation between visual and
haptic or auditory localization, is visual capture the rule or does sensory
dominance depend upon the task at hand? We certainly localize the ven-
triloquist's voice in the dummy's mouth, but we hear what is said and not
what might be phonetically mimicked by the wooden lips. If we turn to the
problem of stimulus integration directly, are touch and audition dominant
in the perception of temporal patterns and vision dominant in perceiving
spatial patterns? Clearly, there is scattered information in the literature on
some of these relationships, but unfortunately it is often contradictory.
More specific study of each of these questions is required in order to better
understand the ground rules of how sensory-motor systems are interrelated
and how they change over stimulus exposure.

One general formulation for future research is that more attention be
paid to having laboratory testing conditions more nearly correspond to
those encountered in the normal environment in which the organism
habitually acts. Results from the laboratory too frequently have little to say
to what is happening in the real world. One reason, at least for studies in
space perception, is the artificial quality of stimulus configurations used.
One example should illustrate the point. Stimulus arrays used in laboratory

studies of spatial perception are generally considered solely in terms of their geometric patterns. In studying adaptation to visual spatial reorientation, for example, the observer typically is exposed to fields of tilted lines viewed in isolation. The lines, for example, are exposed in a reduction screen or illuminated in an otherwise dark room. It is well known that adaptation under such conditions occurs so as to minimize the tilt of the lines from the axis from which they deviate least. If the lines are tilted less than 45° from vertical, adaptation is toward the vertical, if more than 45°, it is toward the horizontal (Gibson, 1937). However, as we have noted elsewhere (Morant, 1965, 1968), adaptation to such simple geometric properties of stimulus configurations is a special case of a more general formulation that visual adaptation actually occurs towards the norm from which the observer *believes* the stimulus array deviates. Geometric lines in a dark room have no intrinsic normal orientation and so the observer defines their location only in terms of whether they lie closer to the vertical or to the horizontal. However, if the contours of the visual array represent real objects a different situation prevails. Objects have meaning, a history of preferred positions, which isolated lines do not and it is towards these experientially determined preferred norms that adaptation occurs. Thus if the field viewed is composed of objects or pictures of objects that have a normal orientation, say tables and walls and buildings, then adaptation occurs so as to restraighten the visual configuration irrespective of whether it actually is displaced least from the vertical or the horizontal axis. It appears then that adaptation and displacement effects are determined not by the properties of the projection field created but rather by the properties of the memory traces to which they give rise. It is the memory trace invoked by the sensory process that determines the direction of adaptation and not the sensory process itself. Experiments in which exposure histories of subjects are manipulated or where ongoing changes in the meaning of the stimulus configurations are introduced should help to bridge the results of the laboratory with those reported in studies with natural environments.

Kurt Goldstein was fond of pointing out that laboratory studies are experiments in pathology. The restraints imposed upon the organism in the laboratory are sometimes similar to those imposed by neurological deficiencies. The results of studies both in the laboratory and with the neurologically impaired are important because they enhance understanding of lower level process operations that may be masked under more normal conditions in which higher functions prevail. But it is precisely for this reason, that such studies primitivize conditions by isolating organismic systems from one another, that their results should not be accepted automatically as indicators of how the organism under more normal circumstances actually functions in coming to terms with the environment.

THE RESULTS BRIEFLY RELATED TO
IMAGE AND FLOW THEORIES OF PERCEPTION

The results of the experiments on prismatic rearrangement together with those to be shortly presented on spatial localization and intersensory coordination, are in general accord with Werner's holistic, organismic approach to perceptual development. Furthermore, they point out the essential difficulty of the classical image theory of perception and I think go beyond the spatio-temporal information flow theories postulated in recent years by James Gibson (1979) and Gunnar Johansson (1975).

The classical theory of Wundt and Helmholtz postulated retinal images whose characteristics bridged those of the distal object stimulus and its perception. Elaboration of the retinal image through the interplay of experiential factors was assumed to account for the developing veridical nature of the percept as the organism matured. According to Gibson (1979), however, the relationship between the distal object and its percept can be specified more parsimoniously by considering the primary proximal stimulus to be the spatio-temporal flow of information across the retina rather than a static image. This emphasis on the stimulus energy flux on the eye has the added advantage of emphasizing the active character of perception. The mobile perceiver is conceived as responding to the geometric invariances of the stimulus flow across the retina that have been generated in part through his own locomotion in the environmental field. The development of increasingly veridical perception is attributed to an increasing ability of the infant to abstract out from the environment the invariant structures it contains.

Gibson's view that the primary visual stimulus has more the character of flux than image is undoubtedly correct. However, in essentially restricting his analysis of the perceptual outcome to the invariances of the visual flow, Gibson fails to do justice to the influence of intra-organismic factors, especially the impact of the changing flux of stimuli that may be impinging upon other sense receptors at the time. It is precisely this emphasis, that perception must be seen as a reflection of the interaction between the proximal stimulation and ongoing organismic state, which was the cornerstone of Werner's developmental theory of perception. It should be clear that the information read out from the environment is determined at least as much by how it is processed as it is by the sensory influx. We will return to this issue after presenting the results of the next set of experiments.

THE AUDIO AND OCULOGYRAL ILLUSIONS

The studies reported thus far refer to orientation to a physically defined norm—verticality. Precisely the same hierarchic interaction of sensory-motor subsystems can be demonstrated in the changing orientation to an egocentrically defined norm—the straight ahead. Straight-ahead is objectively defined as the extension of the median sagittal plane of the body. Normally, objective and subjective straight-ahead are identical but under certain conditions they do not coincide. One such condition is obtained when an observer is angularly accelerated around the midbody vertical axis (Z axis). Furthermore, during such labyrinthian stimulation, the position in space considered as straight-ahead appears to be determined by the sensory modality used to judge it. Defined visually, straight-ahead is opposite to the direction of acceleration (an object rotating with the observer and physically straight-ahead of the nose is seen displaced in the direction of acceleration); defined auditorily, it is in the direction of acceleration (the object, as sound source, is heard displaced opposite to the direction of acceleration).

Some years ago, Gene Lester and I demonstrated that the auditory displacement, the so-called audiogyral illusion, is probably based on a vestibularly-induced change in felt head position (Lester & Morant, 1969, 1970). In order to localize a sound relative to the body midline, the observer must consider the position of the head. Sound clues allow the sound to be localized directly in front of the face, but in order to refer the sound to some locations in space, the position of the head must be taken into account. Observations made in our laboratory showed that rotary acceleration changes the apparent position of the head with respect to a fixed reference point—the chair in which the observer is rotating. The head, which is actually fixed straight-ahead through a bite-plate arrangement, feels rotated towards the left shoulder under CW acceleration and towards the right shoulder under CCW acceleration. Since sound cues inform the observer that the sound is directly in front of the face, the sound is mis-localized in agreement to where the head is felt to be directed. It can be shown also that inducing tension on the neck muscles by direct muscle strain augments or diminishes the extent of auditory displacement depending upon whether the tension is complimentary or antagonistic to that induced by the labyrinthian stimulation.

The visual displacement, known as the oculogyral illusion, is somewhat more complex. At least three pieces of information are required to specify a visually determined spatial location. In addition to considering the position of the object relative to the gaze of the eyes and the position of the head relative to the trunk, the position of the eyes relative to the head must also be specified. The oculogyral illusion is probably related both to the felt rotation of the body and to the consequences of the attempt to inhibit nystagmic eye movements induced by the labyrinthian stimulation. The illusion has three components, one to do with movement, another with displacement and a third with acceleration.

A spot of light attached to a rotating chair and viewed in an otherwise dark room appears both to move through space in the direction of acceleration and to lead the observer. Even though the dot does not move physically with respect to the observer and there is no visual background for reference, explanation of the seen motion is straight-forward. Since the observer feels himself to be rotating and the dot remains in front of his eyes, the dot must also be seen to move to keep pace with the sensed body rotation. A comparable effect is found when the observer is suddenly stopped. Deceleration engenders a feeling of counter rotation and therefore an apparent movement of the dot synchronous with the new felt rotation of the body. The quality of motion, then, is wholly determined by the relationship of the stimulus object to felt body changes of the observer.

The displacement of the dot, or what it amounts to, a change in the visually sensed position of straight-ahead, is probably related to the reflexive nystagmic movements of the eyes, which are inhibited by fixating the target dot (Whiteside, Graybiel, & Niven, 1965). Either efferent stimuli induced by the inhibited eye movements or incomplete inhibition of the nystagmus resulting in a displaced nodal point would account for the dot being seen as leading the observer.

The motion and displacement effects, however, are compounded by a third component of the illusion. Curiously, the target dot appears to be moving more rapidly than the observer although it retains its same position in the visual field. The apparent speed of the trajectory gives the impression that the dot will move out of the field of view and yet it remains in the same relative position to the observer.

Richard Teixeira and I have recently begun a series of studies to investigate the interrelationships among these three components of the illusion. In one set of studies we are looking at the interaction between real and illusory motion. Briefly, what we attempt to do is to influence the path of seen motion of a specified visual flow pattern by changing the apparent motion of the observer. Let me give one illustration.

Duncker (1950) long ago noted that in looking at a rolling wheel, we see both the rotary motion of the rim around the hub and the forward translation of the whole wheel. Physically, a single spot on the rim describes a cycloidal motion—a combination of its forward and rotary motions. Perceptually, however, the spot is seen to move in a full circle around the hub with the whole wheel translating forwards. If the spot is now made luminous in a dark room both the forward and rotary motions disappear and the physically defined cycloidal movement is seen. What we have found is that comparable patterns of motion are obtained if real circular motion is imposed on apparent translatory motion.

In one set of observations the wheel with its illuminated spot is fixed directly in front of the observer at eye level in the fronto-parallel plane. In the dark, and with the chair stationary, observers correctly report the circular pattern described by the dot. Under conditions of rotary acceleration of the observer, however, the circular pattern disappears and a cycloidal motion whose loop is related to the apparent lateral motion of the dot is seen. The equivalence of real and subjective lateral motion in generating interactive movement patterns with rotary motion is of basic theoretical significance. It indicates that motion is analyzed at a level in the central nervous system where it can be integrated with body position cues. In a series of elegant demonstrations, Johansson (1975) has argued that what is seen in any complex motion pattern can be understood by assuming a hierarchically integrated series of component motions perceptually analyzed out of the total optical flow pattern. The demonstration reported here, however, would seem to argue against his further assertion that such optical flow patterns over the retina necessarily take precedence over other sensory stimuli present at the same time. Indeed, flow patterns must be interpreted against the background of all other stimuli impinging on the organism. Contextual factors provided by such mechanisms as sensed body posture are as important in determining visual localization, orientation, and pattern perception as are the specific properties of the retinal flux (see for example Cohen, 1981; Lackner, 1978, 1981).

THE PHENOMENOLOGICAL UNITY OF PERCEPTION

We implied earlier that it is difficult to identify criteria to specify which sensory-motor subsystems are most directly influenced by which stimulus conditions. One reason is that it is difficult to relate the performance of the subsystems to the final perceptual act. This problem, it should be noted, is similar to one confronted in contemporary research on feature detector mechanisms. Although it can be demonstrated that single neurons are differentially responsive to isolated specific properties of given visual patterns, it is unclear how other stimulus variations impinging on other feature detectors modify the final neural messages. The problem of understanding how information from perceptual subsystems or from feature detectors is integrated in perception and how the integration develops and is modified through experience and growth is formidable. At its basis is the question of how the functional characteristics of both feature detectors and perceptual subsystems conform to phenomenological experience. There is little reason to suppose that the shape of what we sense or feel or experience has much in common with that of the systems which bring it about. Characteristics of phenomenological experiences and those of the functioning of sensory-motor systems belong to different levels of discourse.

Werner puzzled over this issue and speculated about the development of phenomenological experience as perceptual subsystems change through growth and experience. The philosophical background of his speculations and the influence that his speculations had on psychoanalytic and anthropological thought, in addition to developmental psychology, have recently been traced by Barten and Franklin (1978). The third experiment that I briefly want to present relates to one hypothesis formulated by Werner and Wapner to account for the changes in mechanisms underlying the onto- genetic development of phenomenologically stable perceptual world. The hypothesis is that there exists "an earliest period in the life of the child at which object and self are not separated, where no perceptual organization of space, no frame of reference, exists" (Wapner & Werner, 1957, p. 63). The hypothesis is not unlike James' notion that "the first sensation which an in- fant gets is for him the Universe" and that the elaboration of the plurality of sensations and the separation of outside object from inner state comes about from a "dissociation of unsuspected varieties within the unity" (James, 1890, V. 2, p. 8–9). The experiment in progress is being conducted by David Starkey. It is designed to investigate one aspect of the unity of the perceived world—the integration of visuo-haptic experiences by infants.

Utilizing two 60 inch parabolic mirrors of optical quality, Starkey studies what occurs when infants attempt to grasp an object and do not get cor- responding tactual feedback. The approach is similar to that taken by Bower (1974) and Field (1977) and should help resolve their discrepant find- ings. Unlike Bower, who used polarized goggles that were poorly tolerated by his infants, and Field, whose Fresnel lense provided virtual images less luminous and well defined than their corresponding real objects, the optical mirrors create virtual objects of the greatest realism without infringing on the free movement or comfort of the infants.

In Starkey's procedure, the image is sometimes of an object that the in- fant knows well, a favorite toy, and sometimes of an object that is un- familiar. On half of the trials the actual object is substituted for its image. The infants' hand movements and facial expression are photographed on videotape and the heart rate is monitored. The study is designed to test 3, 5, 7, and 9 month old infants and although the results have not yet been fully analyzed, some preliminary observations can be reported.

The older infants are particularly disturbed by reaching for the virtual ob- jects. After a few encounters, they begin to cry, look around at mother and give every indication of what to an onlooker seem to be overt reactions of surprise, concern, and anxiety. The emotional upset is unrelated simply to seeing a desirable object that cannot be grasped. Plane mirror images or ac- tual objects held beyond reach do not elicit this sort of emotional response. Roughly every other 5-month-old and an occasional 3-month-old tested also show behavioral distress to the virtual objects. However, when heart rate data is considered it appears that most infants at all ages tested respond dif- ferently to the experience of reaching for virtual as opposed to real objects. Preliminary findings also indicate some difference in exploratory hand movements, with more older than younger infants poking at the virtual ob- jects.

It appears then that for infants as young as 3 to 5 months of age, a different reaction is obtained to real ojbects that can be grasped and virtual objects that cannot. Furthermore, although reaching and not touching engages the attention of very young infants, their response to the experience differs at different ages. For example, lack of correspondence between visual and tactual space engages the attention of the very young without, however, always resulting in the overt emotional upset characteristic of older infants. Let me mention without further elaboration that these data fit neither Bushnell's model of the ontogeny of intermodal relations (Bushnell, 1981) nor Kagan's timetable for the development of retrieval memory in infancy (Kagan, Kearsley, & Zelazo, 1978).

What are the implications of these results for the development of visual and haptic space? Bishop Berkeley's position that there are no ideas common across the senses (Berkeley, 1709), that, as Russell stated, "different senses have different spaces [and] . . . it is only by experience in infancy that we learn to correlate them" (Russell, 1914, p. 113), might be interpreted to indicate that very young infants should not manifest surprise when nonconordant visual and haptic stimuli are encountered. But how old is "very young"? Three-month-old children after all have already had substantial experience with eye-hand encounters. On the other hand, Wapner and Werner's (1957) speculation about a primitive phenomenological state leads us to expect an early period in life where sensory experiences are not differentiated, but "early" is also not well enough specified. Clearly, this study is not an *experimentum crucis* nor is it obvious that one can be readily designed in this area.

Problems abound. For example, the very concept of a primordial sensory unity is unclear. Is it suggested that the new organism does not experience a stimulation as having the discrete quality of touch or of sight or of hearing but rather that it experiences another more primitive feeling from which these sensations later differentiate? Or is what is proposed the belief that the senses have their neurologically defined specificity from the outset, that is that they are differentiated, and it is the integration between the senses which is what is already laid down at birth? Is there a common sensory register that differentiates in development or a differentiated sensory register whose connections have been prefixed? Or is the problem not one of neurological specificity at all but rather one of the infant's growing conceptual awareness of discriminative possibilities in the stimulating environment?

These questions are difficult to formulate operationally. What is possible is to ask specific questions that will more adequately describe the ontogenetic timetable of such things as sensory-motor coordination in reaching and postural adjustment, or the intermodal equivalences in the perception of texture or shape, etc. Studies of this type in which intersensory sensations are studied, in which the environment is manipulated so that information does not covary across the senses, should lead to better understanding of how and when the organism extracts which kinds of qualities from the flux of stimulation impinging on the end organs, the extent to which these qualities have common characteristics, and the ways in which they are coded, stored, and integrated. The beginning of precisely this sort of research has been well documented in an excellent recent survey edited by Walk and Pick (1981).

Adult perception is unitary, we see the texture that we feel and feel the form that we see. Stimulation to one receptor is integrated with other stimuli impinging on the organism and although in the adult each receptor gives rise to a unique sensory experience, we sense only one world. How it got that way and the nature of the integrative mechanisms responsible continue to be, as they were for Werner, the critical problems of developmental perceptual theory.

THE ORTHOGENETIC PRINCIPLE: DEVELOPMENT VERSUS CHANGE

There is one further aspect of Werner's thinking about perceptual development that I should like briefly to discuss. In his classic book, *Comparative Psychology of Mental Development,* Werner (1948) with obvious approbation, refers to a passage from Goethe's *Morphologie* in which development is equated with perfection (p. 40). Goethe is quoted to indicate that perfection and development go hand in hand; that the more perfect the creature, the higher the development as specified by the extent of differentiation of morphological parts to one another and their subordination to the functioning of the organism as a whole. Furthermore, according to Kaplan (1981), it appears that both Goethe and Werner assumed that "time was the mother of perfection" and therefore that development, in the sense of a change towards perfection, could be read off from what occurs over time.

But, and this at least in part is the thrust of the Genetic-Dramatist approach espoused by Kaplan in this volume, development and change should not be confounded. The concept of development is reserved for those changes which not only follow the orthogenetic principle of organization but also have a directional valence. Change is simply alteration. Development implies a goal or ideal; a movement towards perfection. Experimental psychologists as well as historians or biologists, to the extent that they fail to formulate an ideal towards which change is directed, address only questions of variation. Only those variations which are valued can be considered developments. Judgments of better-worse, higher-lower, advanced-primitive require a benchmark of value against which the direction of change can be plotted.

Can we provide such a benchmark for the ontogenesis of perception to determine whether or not it follows the orthogenetic principle? The task of doing so is fraught with difficulties. Perfection does not come labeled in nature and therefore cannot be identified empirically. Perfection, or the tendency thereto, is a consensual judgment susceptible to changing standards and theories and experimental psychologists are notorious for their insistence on going it alone. Let me phrase the question in terms of an issue that I have already touched on. Should we consider as a more perfect perception one that more nearly resembles what is painted on the eye or one that more closely represents the distal stimulus configuration? One difficulty, as I indicated earlier, is that many regard what is painted on the eye to have little in common with what is perceived. The problem of the correspondence between the painted image on the retina and phenomenological awareness is not unlike that confronted in the history of representational art (Gombrich, 1960). How do we distinguish between what is "seen" and what is inferred to be seen, what is detected and what is construed, between what is sensed and what is known?

The specification of the distal stimulus is a particularly hoary problem. As I have noted elsewhere (Morant, 1975), the notion that we can distinguish between illusions that do not reflect reality and perceptions that do reflect reality is particularly unproductive in the study of perception. For reality, like a modest maiden, hides her true appearance from prying eyes behind a facade of relative images.

Though we might eventually agree on a characterization of how some of the mechanisms involved in perception evolve over time, I feel less hopeful about reaching agreement on what constitutes perfect perception. And it is questionable in the absence of such agreement whether the pertinent perceptual subsystems can be identified to determine the extent to which their development follows the Werner-Kaplan orthogenetic principle.

ACKNOWLEDGMENTS

The experiments on prism adaptation and labyrinthian stimulation were supported by Grant M-3658 from the National Institutes of Health. The developmental study was supported by a grant from the Spencer Foundation.

REFERENCES

Barten, S. S., & Franklin, H. B. (Eds.) *Developmental processes.* New York: International Universities Press, 1978.
Berkeley, G. *A new theory of vision.* London: Dent, 1963 (Published originally in 1709).
Bower, T. G. R. *Development in infancy.* San Francisco: Freeman, 1974.
Bushnell, E. W. The ontogeny of intermodal relations: Vision and touch in infancy. In R. D.

Walk, & H. L. Pick (Eds.), *Intersensory perception and sensory integration*. New York: Plenum Press, 1981.

Cohen, M. M. Visual-proprioceptive interactions. In R. D. Walk, & H. L. Pick (Eds.), *Intersensory perception and sensory integration*. New York: Plenum Press, 1981.

Duncker, K. Induced motion. In W. D. Ellis (Ed.), *A source book of Gestalt psychology*. New York: The Humanities Press, 1950.

Field, J. Coordination of vision and prehension in young infants. *Child Development*, 1977, *48*, 97–103.

Gibson, J. J. Adaptation, after-effect and contrast in the perception of tilted lines. II. Simultaneous contrast and the areal restriction of the after-effect. *Journal of Experimental Psychology*, 1937, *20*, 553–569.

Gibson, J. J. *The ecological approach to visual perception*. Boston: Houghton Mifflin, 1979.

Gombrich, E. H. *Art and illusion: A study in the psychology of pictorial representation*. Princeton: Princeton University Press, 1960.

James, W. *The principles of psychology*. Vol. II. New York: Henry Holt, 1890.

Johansson, G. Visual motion perception. *Scientific American*, 1975, *232*, 76–88.

Kagan, J., Kearsley, R. B., & Zelazo, P. R. *Infancy: Its place in human development*. Cambridge: Harvard University Press, 1978.

Kanizsa, G. Subjective contours. *Scientific American*, 1976, *234*, 48–52.

Kaplan, B. Personal communication, August, 1981.

Kennedy, J. M. Attention, brightness and the constructive eye. In M. Henle (Ed.), *Vision and Artifact*. New York: Springer Publishing, 1976.

Lackner, J. R. Some mechanisms underlying sensory and postural stability in man. In R. Held, H. Leibowitz, & H. L. Teuber (Eds.), *Handbook of sensory physiology. Vol. 8: Perception*. Berlin: Springer Verlag, 1978.

Lackner, J. R. Some aspects of sensory-motor control and adaptation in man. In R. D. Walk, & H. L. Pick (Eds.), *Intersensory perception and sensory integration*. New York: Plenum Press, 1981.

Lashley, K. S. The problem of serial order in behavior. In L. A. Jeffress (Ed.), *Cerebral mechanisms in behavior: The Hixon symposium*. New York: Wiley, 1951.

Lester, G., & Morant, R. B. The role of the felt position of the head in the audiogyral illusion. *Acta Psychologica*, 1969, *31*, 375–384.

Lester, G., & Morant, R. B. Apparent sound displacement during vestibular stimulation. *The American Journal of Psychology*, 1970, *83*, 554–566.

Morant, R. B. Adaptation to prismatically rotated visual fields. *Science*, 1965, *148*, 530–531.

Morant, R. B. Factors influencing adaptation to rotated fields: The role of meaning. In M. L. Simmel (Ed.), *The reach of mind: Essays in memory of Kurt Goldstein*. New York: Springer, 1968.

Morant, R. B. Review of *Illusion in nature and art*, R. A. Gregory & E. H. Gombrich (Eds.), *Art Bulletin*, 1975, *57*, 601–604.

Morant, R. B., & Aronoff, J. Starting position, adaptation, and visual framework as influencing the perception of verticality: *Journal of Experimental Psychology*, 1966, *71*, 684–686.

Russell, B. *Our knowledge of the external world*. Chicago: Open Court, 1914.

Solomon, P., & Werner, H. Studies on contour: III. Negative after-images. *The American Journal of Psychology*, 1952, *65*, 67–74.

Walk, R. D., & Pick, H. L. (Eds.) *Intersensory perception and sensory integration*. New York: Plenum Press, 1981.

Wapner, S., & Werner, H. *Perceptual Development*. Worcester: Clark University Press, 1957.

Wapner, S., & Werner, H. (Eds.) *The body percept*. New York: Random House, 1965.

Wapner, S., Cirillo, L., & Baker, A. H. Sensory-tonic theory: Toward a reformulation. *Archivio di psicologia, Neurologia e Psichiatria*, 1969, *30*, 493–512.

Werner, H. Studies on contour: I. Qualitative analyses. *The American Journal of Psychology,* 1935, *47,* 40–64.

Werner, H. Studies on contour: II. Strobostereoscopic phenomena. *The American Journal of Psychology,* 1940, *53,* 418–422.

Werner, H. *Comparative psychology of mental development.* New York: International Universities Press, 1948.

Werner, H., & Kaplan, B. *Symbol formation.* New York: Wiley, 1963.

Werner, H., & Wapner, S. Experiments on sensory-tonic field theory of perception: IV. Effect of initial position of a rod on apparent verticality. *Journal of Experimental Psychology,* 1952, 43, 68–74.

Werner, H., & Wapner, S. Toward a general theory of perception. *Psychological Review,* 1952, *59,* 324–338.

Werner, H., & Wapner, S. Sensory-tonic field theory of perception: Basic concepts and experiments. *Rivista Di Psicologia,* 1956, *50,* 315–337.

Whiteside, T. C. D., Graybiel, A., & Niven, J. I. Visual illusions of movement. *Brain,* 1965, *88,* 193–210.

Witkin, H. A., & Asch, S. E. Studies in space orientation: IV. Further experiments on perception of the upright with displaced visual fields. *Journal of Experimental Psychology,* 1948, *38,* 762–782.

10 The Aesthetic Mode of Consciousness

Sybil S. Barten
*State University of New York,
College at Purchase*

INTRODUCTION

More than fifty years ago, Cassirer (1927/1978) argued that a given sensuous form (e.g., a line pattern) may have either an expressive, a representative, or purely significative function, each rooted in a distinct orientation or "form of consideration." Cassirer (1957) felt that an orientation toward expression was inherent in the transformation of a spatial image into an aesthetic image, and he describes this orientation in detail as follows:

> Let us, for example, consider an experience from the optical sphere. Such an experience is never composed of mere sensory data, of the optical qualities of brightness and color . . . . We can consider an optical structure, a simple line, for example, according to its purely expressive meaning. As we immerse ourselves in the design and construct it for ourselves, we become aware of a distinct physiognomic character in it. A peculiar mood is expressed in the purely spatial determination; the up and down of the lines in space embraces an inner mobility, a dynamic rise and fall, a psychic life and being . . . . the form gives itself to us in an animated totality, an independent manifestation of life. It may glide along or break off suddenly; it may be rounded and self-contained or jagged and jerky; it may be hard or soft: all this lies in the line itself as a determination of its own reality, its objective nature [p. 200].

Several elements of this account, such as the degree of subject-object interpenetration, the heightened awareness of affective and gestural qualities, have been described in similar terms by writers on art (Langer, 1957; Milner, 1973; Moncrieff, 1978) and artists (Kandinsky, 1964; Klee, 1961). For example, in the words of Paul Klee (1961):

> And every figure, every combination, will have its particular constructive expression, every form its face, its physiognomy. The pictures of objects look out at us, serene or severe, tense or relaxed, comforting or forbidding, suffering or smiling. They look out at us in all the contrasts of the physical-physiognomic dimension; . . . The forms . . . also have their own postures, which result from the way in which the selected groups have been put in motion [p. 91].

These descriptions from several sources suggest that the understanding of the aesthetic should be rooted in a consideration of the agent's intentionality or orientation, rather than from an examination of properties of art objects alone. In this chapter I argue that the aesthetic mode of consciousness constitutes a distinct orientation toward the world. Aesthetic consciousness, in this account, is not to be identified with the manner of viewing works of art, nor operationalized as the manner in which artists experience the world. Rather, I assume that description of the aesthetic mode of consciousness logically precedes inquiry into its manifestation in certain individuals (e.g. artists) or its embodiment in certain objects of experience (e.g. works of art). In investigating this mode of experience, however, observation and description are intertwined, and it is reasonable to arrive at a clear conception of the aesthetic mode of experience by observing it in its purest form, namely in the ways in which artists perceive their world. Adopting this strategy, I hope to be able to distinguish aesthetic consciousness from other intentionalities, particularly the mundane orientation towards the world. This is not to suggest that artists exclusively possess an aesthetic orientation, that artists' entire experience reflects an aesthetic orientation, nor that such an orientation alone distinguishes artist from non-artist.

The aims of this chapter then are threefold: (1) to delineate characteristics of aesthetic consciousness by distinguishing it from other modes, particularly the mundane; (2) to present evidence that artists do habitually experience the world in a manner distinct from non-artists; and (3) to suggest certain conditions for aesthetic consciousness. The studies to be presented here were inspired by Heinz Werner's interest in and conceptualization of the aesthetic, and I shall present the outlines of Werner's views, after a brief account of the distinction between an aesthetic and a "mundane" orientation toward objects, a distinction that is only implicit in Werner's formulation.

AESTHETIC VERSUS MUNDANE MODES OF CONSCIOUSNESS

The distinction between the aesthetic and the mundane mode of experience assumes that the same *physical* object may constitute one of two kinds of "things" or objects of consciousness, determined by what Cassirer has termed its specific "form of consideration." As a mundane or everyday thing, an object (e.g. a shoe[1]) has a consensually fixed or determinate identity, given to it by virtue of its class membership. In contrast, identification and classification are frequently (if not always) of secondary importance when an object is aesthetically viewed. Thus, it is reported that Matisse, when asked whether a tomato appeared the same to him when he ate it as when he painted it, replied "No, when I eat it I see it like everybody else." (cited in Arnheim, 1954, p. 134).

Second, mundane objects are embedded in a context of action, are physically manipulable, while the relation of person and aesthetic object is one of interaction at a distance: An aesthetically apprehended object or event is a *contemplative* object. Third, the mundane object, belonging to the pragmatic-causal world, is not viewed in and for itself, but in relation to other objects and in relation to the agent's pragmatic aims. As such, the mundane object may become mere instrumentality. In contrast, an aesthetic object cannot function as means to an extrinsic goal without losing its status as aesthetic. Thus, if we climb upon a sculpture or use a painting as a tray, in the act they are no longer experienced as aesthetic objects. To summarize, an aesthetic object is not consensually identified in its meaning, is not acted upon but viewed at a distance, and does not form a link in a pragmatic-causal nexus.

The above distinctions refer to external relations of the object viewed as a whole. Aesthetic and mundane objects also differ in terms of their internal properties. Here Werner's distinction between geometric-technical properties and physiognomic properties is germane. Whereas mundane objects tend to be constituted by "physical" properties such as size, color, weight, and shape, aesthetic objects are experienced in terms of pervasive dynamic or expressive qualities. As early as 1931, Werner stated, "Expressive lines, colors, and forms are the primary building material of the artist" (Werner, 1931, p. 250).[2]

A related distinction between mundane and aesthetic experience lies in the degree of subject-object polarization. In the everyday mode of apprehending, certain ("objective") properties tend to inhere in external objects while other ("subjective") properties such as intentions, feelings, and thoughts belong to persons. Within aesthetic experience, this relatively clear demarcation of the perceptual and the motor-affective is diminished. Ar-

---

[1]As MacLeod (1970) pointed out in an illuminating essay, our language confounds phenomenological analysis. Thus, terms such as "object" are taken to refer both to the physical object and to the object as construed within a particular intentionality. Even assigning a name ("shoe") to a physical object implies that the object *is* a shoe independent of an agent's orientation.

[2]"Innerhalb der aesthetischen Welt sind Farbe, Linien, Formen 'ausdruckend': ausdruckshafte Linien, Farben, Formen sind erst der Stoff mit dem der Kunstler baut."

tists and philosophers have described such loss of subject-object separateness in various terms. Thus, Merleau-Ponty (1964) writes, "Indeed we cannot imagine how a *mind* could paint. It is by lending his body to the world that the artist changes the world into painting" (p. 162), and, expanding on this theme, he states, "Things have an internal equivalent in me; they arouse in me a carnal formula of their presence" (p. 164). Milner (1973) speaks of "spreading the imaginative body to take the form of what one looked at" (p. 55); and Langer (1957) states "The arts objectify subjective reality, and subjectify outward experience of nature" (p. 74). Moncrieff (1978) provides a vivid illustration of the experience of "one-ness" that he believes to be an essential ingredient of aesthetic consciousness:

> I was immediately caught up in the music. I didn't know what was happening to me. I found myself crying. My body felt like it would sink into the chair. I personally was gone, into the radio, into the music. I don't know where. I was one with the music [p. 363].

Two essential constituents of aesthetic awareness are highlighted: (1) the expressivity of objects aesthetically apprehended, an awareness of gestures, intentions, feelings, vitality in objects; and (2) the lessened distance between self and object, the way in which the self imaginatively enters the object apprehended.

All of the specific characteristics of aesthetic consciousness noted above may be seen as emerging out of a particular aim or intentionality of consciousness. What uniquely describes aesthetic consciousness is its aim: experiencing and enjoying the harmony and unity of form, whatever the medium in which that form is presented or embodied. This orientation toward experiencing the wholeness of aesthetic objects, of grasping their structure, rhythm, and textures is the fundamental directive and integrative aim from which all other characteristics spring.

In this connection—in relation to the aim of aesthetic consciousness—it would be well to mention another mode of consciousness that also involves a departure from the mundane or everyday mode of experience, namely the so-called altered modes of consciousness. The notion of an "altered" state suggests a contrasting "normal" state, and, as such carries an unfortunate connotation of deviation comparable to the distinction between illusory and veridical perception. Characteristics of drug states, hypnotically induced "regression" and meditative phenomena (see Deikman, 1963), like aesthetic experience, involve a departure from mundane modes of appreciation, a more diffuse boundary between self and world, and heightened affectivity. Like aesthetic consciousness, these altered states are contrasted with a pragmatic, and logico-discursive orientation. However, a crucial distinction between aesthetic consciousness and, for example, meditative states lies in their respective aims. As I have stated, aesthetic consciousness is directed toward full experience of an aesthetic object. By contrast, a person in a meditative state aims at loss of ego, at fusion of self and world. In the trancelike state of absorption exemplified in the practice of Yoga, "the meditator experiences sinking into or becoming one with the meditation object, so that there is no longer an experience of being a subject meditating, merely the experience 'meditation is' " (Schuman, 1980, p. 335).

WERNER'S VIEWS ON AESTHETIC PHENOMENA

Although Heinz Werner never directly addressed himself to an aesthetic orientation or mode of experiencing, his views on aesthetic phenomena served as the starting point for the studies to be reported in this chapter.[3] Werner clearly assumed that the world does not present itself in identical fashion to all forms of life (see for example, Werner, 1934/1978, p. 153; Werner, 1940, p. 379). He assumed that human beings inhabit multiple phenomenal worlds—the play world, the mythic, the scientific, the aesthetic—all implicitly distinct from the mundane or everyday world. He assumed that these worlds become distinct in the course of development. For example, he stated that the young child "distinguishes only vaguely, or not at all, between aesthetic reality and that of everyday experience" (Werner, 1940, p. 393).

It is likely that Werner's insistence on the variety of experiential worlds was rooted in the climate of phenomenology pervasive in Germany and Austria in the first decades of the 20th century (Franklin & Barten, 1980; MacLeod, 1970; Spiegelberg, 1972). However, Werner's purpose was not so much to argue for a phenomenological stance as to provide evidence for a developmental approach to modes of experience. Thus, Werner stressed

---

[3]Werner clearly harbored a lifelong interest in aesthetic awareness and experience. Upon entering the University of Vienna, he planned to become a musicologist and composer, and his doctoral dissertation in 1916 concerned the psychology of aesthetic enjoyment. Shortly thereafter, he published a monograph on melodic invention in children. In 1924, Werner published *Die Uspruenge der Lyrik* (The Origins of Lyric Poetry), a work focused on the roots of lyric poetry in magic, song, and dance, and intended as the first volume of a developmental psychology of the arts. The second volume, never completed, was to have dealt with the origins of drama (see Werner, 1924, i). In *Die Uspruenge der Lyrik,* Werner elaborated a first version of his general developmental principles. Other early papers on rhythm and melody were followed by a series of studies on physiognomic speech, and on time and space in primitive art. Throughout these studies, Werner stressed that there was an empirical, psychological way of understanding aesthetic phenomena. Although biographical reconstruction is fraught with peril, it is quite possible that Werner's early interest in art, combined with his scholarly and empirical research in aesthetics and the roots of artistic form may have sensitized him to diffuse, syncretic, physiognomic modes of experience in all individuals. Perhaps Werner merely saw the world of the artist as an example of a more "primitive" world, one that must be contrasted with the psychologically more "advanced" world of logico-scientific thought. However, I am suggesting that Werner's deep understanding of aesthetic phenomena may have been the spark that led to the formulation of his general developmental theory.

that the "worlds" of the child, the psychotically regressed individual, or the pre-literate adult in non-western culture are more primitive than those of the "normal" western adult, and it can be argued that Werner's theory represents an early statement of developmental phenomenology. In a number of contexts, he stated that artists and poets are particularly gifted in the richness of their physiognomic awareness, and are therefore a source of information about this mode of experiencing the world. Werner (1957/1978) never conducted a systematic study of artists, and it was not until quite late in his career that Werner specifically addressed the issue of the genetic standing of aesthetic experience, stating:

> Though physiognomic experience is a primordial manner of perceiving, it grows, in certain individuals such as artists, to a level not below but on a par with that of 'geometric-technical' perception and logical discourse [p. 123]⁴

In Werner's view, the physiognomic mode of perception is closely tied to the aesthetic. As mentioned earlier, Werner believed that expressive forms, lines, and colors constitute the vocabulary of the artist. He asserted that a physiognomic mode of awareness was available to adults only in their experience of faces or gestures, but in a number of studies he showed that even non-artists are susceptible to physiognomic experience under certain conditions, for example, when asked to construe linear patterns as symbols or to consider words poetically (Werner, 1955/1978). However, Werner seemed to believe that no special instructions, conditions, or stimulus materials are required to elicit physiognomic apprehension in artists. The question not specifically addressed by Werner is whether the tendency to transcend or depart from the "everyday," the "geometric-technical," is a *general* characteristic of artists' experience, that is, even when they are not engaged in artistic creation. This question was the focus of my doctoral dissertation (Speier, 1960) and it taken up in the next section.

OBJECT DESCRIPTION IN ARTISTS AND SCIENTISTS

The study to be reported was undertaken to determine whether the divergent specialized orientations of artists and scientists lead these groups to experience everyday objects differently, and specifically, whether there is evidence for an aesthetic mode of consciousness in artists. I asked 16 male

---

⁴This statement is somewhat ambiguous. Its intent clearly was to deny that artists are less developed than non-artists. But it is not clear whether Werner means that artists refine and develop physiognomic experience as *they* themselves develop geometric-technical experience, or as fully as non-artists develop geometric-technical experience. In either interpretation, Werner saw that artists achieve a specialized orientation toward the world, one that cannot be understood under the assumption of a uniform progression towards logico-scientific thinking in all persons.

visual art students, enrolled in the Boston Museum of Fine Arts School, and 16 male graduate students in chemistry from Clark University and M.I.T. to describe eight common objects: an old stapler, a soup spoon, a twig, a small octagonal bottle, a locker key, a hand mirror, a pair of nail scissors, and a rock.[5] Instructions were to "describe" each object, to "tell what it looks like and also what other things it might look like or remind you of." I did not inform subjects that they were being studied as members of a particular group, in order to avoid instilling an aesthetic or scientific attitude or response bias. Nevertheless, some subjects may have construed the task this way, and the influence of subtle demand characteristics of the situation cannot completely be discounted. It can be argued that the instructions were not entirely open-ended and neutral in that they suggested the possibility of going beyond consensual object properties. However, instructions inevitably suggest *some* orientation, and our aim was to allow a range of modes of description and to stress that correctness and accuracy were not at issue.

In order to convey the distinctive flavor of artists' and scientists' descriptions, I present two rather typical responses for each group.

Description of bottle

Artist: Morandi (Italian painter). Sensuous. Feminine somehow. Heavy. Glass. Manmade but there's more beauty to it. Can hold something. Has mystery. It's part of something. Shiny. Smooth. Easier to look at than the key—more flowing lines. Gives strange images when you look through it. You can see a lot in it—lot of reflection. Breakable. If broken, its beauty would be lost. It has the shape of a bell. Tulip bulb. A muller to grind paints.

Scientist: I guess you'd call it a flask. 3'' in length. Made of glass. Inside diameter of the neck is about 3/4''; outside diameter about an inch; the neck—inside diameter about the same as the top. Outside diameter about 1/4'' smaller than the top; just below the neck it curves out to an outside diameter of about 2''. Inside diameter of about 1 1/2''; the outside of the neck is octagonal; same with the base. Each face is slightly concave; has a capacity of about 50ml. There's a—in the base—a circular portion with about 1 1/2'' radius. Looks something like an Erlenmeyer flask.

Description of twig

Artist: It looks like you picked this one because it looks like a hand. Looks like somebody clumsily floating through the air. Looks like a monkey—arms are up and it's falling. Has a nice wrinkly consistency—I want to peel it. Has a flamelike quality. Even something gothic because it's reaching to the sky, reaching to the sun for more life. Has scabs and pimples and sores. Doesn't look like it's dead—looks like it's dying because of the extreme motion in it. Seems alive, but it's so bare. Can't grow anymore, can't move. Still green—shrivelling up—not quite dead. Has a soft heart. From the front it's falling into despair. From the back it's—not quite

[5]I focus here on the task involving object description, omitting results of a second task aimed at determining divergent orientations towards word meaning. In general, the results for the words task indicate comparable stylistic differences between groups. (See Speier, 1960, for a fuller description of procedures and results.)

comedy. More sinister looking from the back. This would be the front—here's head. If you hold it flat, it seems more graceful—it seems to glide—there's a swooping motion to it. Looking at it from one end, it looks like a dead man stretched out—these are his arms and legs. This way it's the head of a spider with his head out to bite you: real vicious thing.

> Scientist: Twig of some sort. Looks like it's not off a tree—like it's off some sort of a flowering shrub. Also, apparently didn't have any leaves on it when it was broken off, but it was still alive. The branches or leaves seem to come out opposite each other on the stem. Not extremely strong wood, as most tree wood is. More like bushes—don't have to support much weight or force. Reminds me of biology class in high school—we used to figure out what kind of tree twigs came from. Probably make good kindling wood if it were dried out. Not much good for anything. Got pith down the middle so couldn't whittle much out of it.

Consonant with the assumption that aesthetic consciousness is less concerned with consensual classification and identification, artists gave half as many names as scientists (e.g. "a black stapler," "twig"). Further, when artists did mention the conventional name or category of the objects, it tended to come late in the description, whereas scientists generally gave the name first. Artists very rarely specified the objects in terms of standard geometrical properties ("elliptical," "triangular") and quantitative estimates of weight, size, number of parts, or volume, whereas this mode of description was quite frequent in scientists, perhaps one index of a scientific orientation. Also, significantly more of the scientists' descriptions were focused on physical qualities and functional attributes—"black," "long for a soup spoon," "made of plastic," "used for cutting." The high proportion of such qualitative physicalistic descriptions of color, shape, composition, and mode of functioning in *both* groups, however, suggests that both artists and scientists as functioning members of society must share the same everyday construction of objects for purposes of efficient action and communication. Artists greatly exceeded scientists in the number of physiognomic responses ("it limps," "impudent," "yawning," "about to jump") and metaphoric transformations ("double-edged ax" (for key); "a hand" (for twig); "German soldier's helmet" (for stapler); "voodoo object" (twig); "ballerina" (bottle). Frequently, these metaphors appear to be based upon perceived expressive properties of the objects. Almost 50%, on the average, of artists' responses included such physiognomic and metaphoric descriptions, as compared to only 15% in scientists. Finally, artists tended to couch their descriptions in non-neutral, evaluative terms, saying, for example, "this curve makes it kind of nice"; "it's a welcome thing in a room;" "ugly." (See Table 10.1 for a summary of the categories of object description and the relative frequencies of responses given by each group.)

A closer examination of the evaluative responses provides evidence of a group difference in degree of subject-object differentiation. Eleven of the 16 artists made at least one critical comment about four or more of the eight objects, as compared with only two chemists. (Artists' mean = 4.4;

TABLE 10.1
Examples and Mean Percentages of the Modes of Object Description
by Artists and Chemists

	Artists	Chemists	p*
Naming the whole: "a rock", "a black stapler."	8.0%	15.4	<.01
Quantitative-geometric specification: "it has 5 branches," "weighs about 6 ounces," "the holes for the fingers are elliptical."	.8	13.7	<.001
Qualitative-physicalistic predication: "used for cutting," "black," "long for a soup spoon," "made of plastic," "got a long handle."	33.0	53.4	<.001
Physiognomic predication: "it limps," "it's sad," "impudent," "yawning," "about to jump."	18.3	1.0	<.001
Metaphorizing: "something you squash vegetables with" (for bottle); "double-edged ax" (for key); "a hand" (for twig); "German soldier's helmet" (stapler); "a voodoo object" (twig).	29.9	13.8	=.01
Aesthetic or moral evaluation: "this curve makes it kind of nice," "it's a welcome thing in a room," "ugly."	10.0	2.7	<.01

*Based upon Mann-Whitney U-tests (Siegel, 1956).

Chemists' mean = 1.5.) The artists' criticisms tended to *fuse* object and self, e.g., "the color bothers me a lot," "this really is disturbing," "I like the way it's rusty," whereas the scientists were more likely to couch their comments in more objective terms, for example, "the edges should be more rounded," "interesting design." Another assessment of subject-object polarization was based upon analysis of the indirect or contextual object descriptions. These were of two types: (1) articulating the objective context, e.g., location, associated objects, or manner of construction; and (2) affective-motor reactions. The latter included statements such as "I want to punch it," "I feel like rubbing it," "I feel sad looking at the mirror." The fact that the chemists' indirect descriptions were predominantly articulations of objective contexts of the objects while only about half of the artists' descriptions were of this type (Chemists' mean = 75%; Artists' mean = 55%) again suggests greater externality and distance of objects as experienced by the scientists.

One objection that could be raised about this study is that it dealt only with impersonal objects. Several years ago, one of my students (Solomon, 1976) conducted a study to find out whether artists and scientists would differ in their descriptions of photographs of hands in various positions and performing various gestures. It is not necessary to transcend or relinquish a mundane, everyday orientation to see a hand as "relaxed," "open," "pointing," or "strong." Solomon therefore predicted that artists would not differ from scientists on this task. The results were extremely interesting and somewhat equivocal. The artists again gave a higher proportion of physiognomic descriptions than the scientists and tended to see the expressivity *in* the hand rather than as a characteristic of the owner of the hand. For example, artists tended to say "limp hand," "they show exuberance," "a sense of wonder and excitement," while scientists were more likely to say "an isolated or depressed woman," "someone who is very nervous." Also, as in the object description task, scientists gave a higher proportion of descriptions involving identification, physical properties, and realistic action or position ("looks like it's about to punch somebody," "a child reaching for the sky"). Although scientists on this task did give more physiognomic responses to the hands than had the scientists in my original study, they gave even *fewer* metaphoric transformations than had the scientists in the object description task. The artists seem less constrained to identify and locate the object in an intersubjective "world," sometimes even commenting on the transition from hand to non-hand in their experience, e.g. "the more I look at it, the less it looks like a hand," a sort of lapse of mundane meaning. Artists much more frequently described the hands in metaphoric terms, e.g. "a flower," "looks like an alligator," "the palm wrinkles look like a breeze blowing over water," "craters on the moon," "fingers look like sea creatures."

CONDITIONS FOR EXPRESSIVITY

As we have seen, many of the characteristics of aesthetic consciousness—The predominance of dynamic features, decreased subject-object polarization, attention to non-consensual properties—are found in free descriptions of objects and pictures by artists even when they are not explicitly directed toward artistic activity. The findings of the studies mentioned strongly the operation of a consistent, habitual orientation or mode of apprehending the world. The causal antecedents of the aesthetic mode of consciousness in artists constitute a fascinating area for longitudinal studies and can only be speculated upon. Does this style of relating to objects guide certain individuals into artistic activity, or does engaging in artistic activity refine and sensitize nascent artists' aesthetic consciousness? Undoubtedly, the answer will lie in a complex interplay of formative conditions, rather than a linear causal sequence. Surely such inquiry into determinants should be an important focus of investigation in the psychology of art.

However, a prior question can be raised: Do the obtained differences reflect *preferred* orientations or different *capacities* in artists and scientists? One may approach this question by attempting to induce an aesthetic orientation in non-artists. My dissertation research included a task that explicitly sanctioned violation of a central tenet of the mundane orientation, namely the different *locations* of physical and psychological attributes (see p. 181, above). In this task, the subjects were invited to match a set of animate attributes to the eight objects they had previously described. They were asked whether and how the objects could be seen as GAY, CLEVER, SAD, SOLEMN, LAZY, HUNGRY, BOLD, and STUPID. Within the mundane attitude, such attributes are used to describe people and animals directly, and only applied to objects metaphorically. As one might have expected, the artists assigned more than twice as many of the terms to objects than did the chemists (Artists' mean = 18.7; Chemists' mean = 8.4). Two chemists denied that *any* of the attributes could be used to describe the objects. These results may again be interpreted to indicate that artists more readily experience inanimate objects as possessing action and mood qualities than scientists. Qualitatively, the results were even more revealing. Subjects had been asked to state their reasons for assigning attributes to the objects, and these justifications can be classified under three broad categories: *direct attributions, indirect attributions,* and *metaphoric reinterpretations.* In direct attributions, the subject notes a physical or physiognomic property of the object itself (e.g. "the rock looks solemn because it has a sort of mystery and melancholy behind it"; "the bottle looks bored because it comes to a big lump and sits there"). Indirect attributions involve justifications in which the attribute is predicated of an associated agent (e.g. "I think of a gay young thing looking into a mirror"; "you could get gay out of a bottle"; "the stapler is clever because a clever person invented it"). Metaphoric reinterpretations involve shifting the meaning of the attribute so that it no longer connotes an animate property (e.g. "the twig is shy of leaves"; "the spoon has a bold design"). Only direct attributions clearly violate assumptions of the mundane attitude pertaining to the separateness of the animate and inanimate domains, and as can be seen from Table 10.2, the artists gave a preponderance of this form of justification. However, the scientists did produce a high proportion of such direct matches, in which they saw objects as possessing action, postural, mood, and conative qualities. Since physiognomic properties were much less frequent in chemists' free descriptions, it can be assumed that the capacity for physiognomic experience is not absent in them but is usually subordinated to a more "realistic" mode of apprehension.

TABLE 10.2
Mean Percentages of Attribute-Object Matches Based Upon
Each Attribution Mode

	Direct Attribution	Indirect Attribution	Metaphoric Reinterpretation
Artists	87%	8%	5%
Chemists	62	24	14

The foregoing analysis suggests that physiognomic experience results from a particular relationship between properties of objects and intentionalities of persons. It should, however, be emphasized that there is an interaction between habitual, preferred orientation and specific task demands: while scientists did produce many more physiognomic responses than they had in the free descriptions, the difference between artists and scientists on this matching task was dramatic in that artists gave so many more attribute-object matches. The sanction to depart from the mundane orientation thus attenuated but did not eliminate the divergence in habitual orientation.

In a study recently completed by Laura Schulman as part of a senior thesis at S.U.N.Y. Purchase (Schulman, 1981), yet another means of inducing a shift from a mundane mode of apprehending objects was investigated. Undergraduate non-artists were asked to describe a common, functional object (telephone receiver) and a less structured, nonfunctional object (large piece of driftwood) under two conditions: *looking* and *playing*. Subjects in the looking condition merely viewed the object as the experimenter slowly rotated it for them, whereas subjects in the playing condition were invited to take the object and pretend to play with it. Each subject described only one of the objects under both conditions. Analysis of the data revealed a greater preponderance of "transformative" descriptions than "realistic" descriptions for the driftwood than for the telephone. Subjects easily saw animals, faces, and expressive qualities in the driftwood, even when viewing it from afar. More significantly, there seems to be a difference between the looking and playing conditions only for the telephone, both in the number of transformative descriptions and in the type of transformation. Invited to play with the object, subjects gave more "enactive metaphors" (Winner, McCarthy, Kleinman, & Gardner, 1979), placing the phone on their heads and saying "horns", under their chin and saying "bowtie," or rocking it saying "seesaw"; they also produced more alternate uses that do not involve denial of the identity of the object, saying for example, "you could hammer a nail with this." One might conclude from these findings that the kind of object orientation that non-artists manifest in a pretend play condition is typical in artists even when they are not overtly manipulating or explicitly requested to pretend. Whether this indicates that the boundary between the imagined and the real is more fluid in artists than in non-artists is an intriguing question for further inquiry.

CONCLUSIONS

This chapter has addressed the nature and conditions for aesthetic experience, an orientation toward the world that dominates the experience of artists but is not exclusive to them. I should like to conclude with some thoughts about the psychology of art, and briefly to suggest some directions for further investigation. To date, "psychology of art" has encompassed three distinguishable, though not always mutually exclusive, areas of study: (1) the psychology of the artist; (2) the production and experience of works of art; and (3) the nature of aesthetic consciousness.

As part of differential psychology, the psychology of artists aims to reveal personality characteristics, cognitive styles, and biographical variables that differentiate artists from non-artists, or that differentiate some types of artists from others. MacKinnon (1962) and Barron (1958) typify this first approach; both attempt to uncover personality traits of architects, painters, and other artists. Hudson's (1966) work exemplifies the effort to determine in a longitudinal study the characteristics of "future" artists. Basically correlational, this approach tells us only what variables are associated with being classified as an artist. The psychology of the artist is generally a purely psychological theory, one that entails no explicit commitment to a particular theory of art. Therefore, by assuming that the definition of "artist" is nonproblematic, there is no way within this approach to determine whether good artists differ from bad ones or what it is to be an artist as against a craftsman. That is, studying artists in terms of correlated aspects of personality function at best may provide some knowledge of causal antecedents and predisposing personality features that lead some persons to become artists. This approach, however, will not go far toward deepening our understanding of art. In part, the study of the psychology of the artist is limited by the assumption that the investigation of artists (their history and personality) is quite apart from the specific activities, awareness, and works of art produced by them, that is, apart from an understanding of exactly those activities and aims which define them as artists. The second line of inquiry within the psychology of art, in contrast with the first, focuses on the perceptual and constructive activities of the artist working in a medium to create a work of art.

This second focus, whether from the standpoint of viewer or artist, stresses that artistic perception and activity are processes occurring within a medium. As Arnheim (1954) states:

> The artist's privilege is the capacity to apprehend the nature and meaning of an experience in terms of a given medium and thus make it tangible. The non-artist is left "speechless" by the fruits of his sensitive wisdom. He cannot congeal them in adequate form . . . In the moments in which a human being is an artist, he finds shape for the bodiless structure of what he has felt [p. 133].

Similarly, Cassirer (1942/1979) eloquently speaks for a definition of artistic process that, he says, cannot be considered in isolation from a given medium in which forms become art:

> Art is not only expression in general, in an unspecified manner, but expression in a specific medium. A great artist does not choose his medium as a mere external and indifferent material. To him the words, the colors, the lines, the spatial forms and designs, the musical sounds are not only technical means of reproduction; they are the very conditions, they are essential moments of the productive artistic process itself [p. 161].

According to Cassirer, art introduces us to the "world of pure forms," a world of emotions divorced from their material content.

The study of artistic process is, in part, the study of the way in which the medium is perceived and constructed. Psychologists need to conduct collaborative studies with artists, dancers, and musicians in order to clarify the manner of formulating experience within various art media, because this kind of analysis requires intimate familiarity with the vocabulary and conventions of each art form. One approach involves studying artists' introspections about their creative activity, (e.g., Kandinsky, 1913/1964; Klee, 1924/1964; Milner, 1973). A most promising avenue for investigating artistic process consists in examining the successive versions in the creation of a work of art. A prime example is Arnheim's (1962) analysis of the preliminary sketches and notebooks made by Picasso in the course of creating "Guernica."[6] Another important facet of this second approach deals with the perception and appreciation of art and dimensions of aesthetic preference (see Hogg, 1969).

While the study of creating and perceiving works of art will undoubtedly clarify our notions about the nature of aesthetic consciousness, experience of art and aesthetic consciousness must not be equated. Aesthetic consciousness, as a generic mode of experience, is not confined to art objects. As a particular kind of relation between subject and object, the aesthetic mode is not limited to particular subjects (e.g., artists) nor to particular objects (e.g., works of art).

I am suggesting that the psychology of art needs to be viewed as part of a

---

[6]More recent experimental attempts to monitor the process of creating poems, stories, and melodies may be found in Perkins and Leondar, 1977.

psychology of experience (Franklin & Barten, 1980). It is necessary to take a phenomenological stance and ask about the nature of the aesthetic "world" and the nature of aesthetic consciousness in order to develop a clearer understanding of the aesthetic process. To date, phenomenological analyses of art have been conducted mainly by philosophers (e.g., Cassirer, 1942/1979; Fingarette, 1963; Langer, 1957; Merleau-Ponty, 1964; Ortega y Gasset, 1975).

Such analysis in psychology must entail a broadened conception of perception, one less exclusively focused on accuracy and quantitative judgments but embracing qualitative differences in attentional style and modes of apprehending the world.[7] One area within perception that deserves further study is the experience of stimuli without conventional meaning, e.g. non-representational linear patterns. Early studies by Krauss (cited in Werner & Kaplan, 1963), Scheerer and Lyons (1957), and more recent studies reported by Werner and Kaplan (1963) suggest that when such visual material is viewed symbolically, dynamic and expressive properties begin to predominate.

Another avenue of research is the experience of musical and dance forms. How and under what conditions do "ordinary" sounds and "everyday" movements become transformed into music and dance in the experience of performer and audience? Does a shift in orientation toward these forms emphasize their expressive-dynamic character and cause us to stop classifying, identifying, and locating them within a functional or pragmatic context? How, in turn, are such orientations produced and sustained in and through music and dance?

Early in this chapter, I suggested that both as cause and as consequence of artistic training and activity, artists experience the world in a manner distinct from non-artists. Although it may be impossible to disentangle the causal variables, we should be able to observe the emergence and refinement of aesthetic consciousness in artists and non-artists. One of the difficulties in this enterprise is that we cannot assume that someone "has" an aesthetic orientation if it is not expressed in some form. A person unable to communicate aesthetic experiences probably has only a dim awareness of this orientation. While all human beings have the potential for an aesthetic mode of experience, perhaps those individuals who become artists learn to "incarnate" their experience in some external form and through this process develop and refine their aesthetic consciousness. In the words of Collingwood (1958, p. 312), the artist "will conceive himself as his audience's spokesman, saying for it the things it wants to say but cannot say unaided."

---

[7]For examples of a phenomenological approach to perception, see Alapack (1971), McConville (1978), Merleau-Ponty (1964).

ACKNOWLEDGMENTS

Many individuals helped me to shape the ideas elaborated in this chapter. Bernard Kaplan, as my dissertation sponsor at Clark University, first taught me the place of the aesthetic in human experience. Many of the ideas presented here were developed through conversations with Margery B. Franklin. Julie Barten, as a visual artist, was an invaluable sounding board for my thoughts on the artistic process.

REFERENCES

Alapack, R. J. The physiognomy of the Mueller-Lyer figures. *Journal of Phenomenological Psychology,* 1971, *2,* 27–47.

Arnheim, R. *Art and visual perception.* Berkeley: University of California Press, 1954.

Arnheim, R. *The genesis of a painting: Picasso's Guernica.* Berkeley: University of California Press, 1962.

Barron, F. Psychology and imagination. *Scientific American,* 1958, *199,* 150–166.

Cassirer, E. *The philosophy of symbolic forms, Vol. 3: Phenomenology of knowledge.* New Haven: Yale University Press, 1957.

Cassirer, E. The problem of the symbol and its place in the system of philosophy (1927). *Man and World: An International Philosophical Review,* 1978, *11,* 411–427.

Cassirer, E. Language and art I (1942). In D. F. Verene (Ed.), *Symbol, myth, and culture. Essays and lectures of Ernst Cassirer,* 1935–1945. New Haven: Yale University Press, 1979.

Collingwood, R. G. *The principles of art.* New York: Oxford University Press, 1958.

Deikman, A. Experimental meditation. *Journal of Nervous and Mental Disease,* 1963, *136,* 329–343.

Fingarette, H. *The self in transformation.* New York: Basic Books, 1963.

Franklin, M. B., & Barten, S. S. *Heinz Werner's contribution to a psychology of experience.* Paper delivered at the Eastern Psychological Association Meeting, Hartford, Conn., April, 1980.

Hogg, J. Ed. *Psychology and the visual arts.* Baltimore: Penguin Books, 1969.

Hudson, L. *Contrary imaginations: A psychological study of the young student.* New York:

Kandinsky, W. Reminiscences (1913). In R. L. Herbert (Ed.), *Modern artists on art.* Englewood Cliffs, N.J.: Prentice-Hall, 1964.

Klee, P. *The thinking eye.* New York: Wittenborn, 1961.

Klee, P. On modern art (1924). In R. L. Herbert (Ed.), *Modern artists on art.* Englewood Cliffs, N.J.: Prentice-Hall, 1964.

Langer, S. K. *Problems of art.* New York: Scribners, 1957.

MacKinnon, D. W. The nature and nurture of creative talent. *American Psychologist,* 1962, *17,* 484–495.

MacLeod, R. M. Psychological phenomenology: A propaedeutic to a scientific psychology. In J. L. Royce (Ed.), *Toward unification in psychology.* Toronto: University of Toronto Press, 1970.

Merleau-Ponty, M. *The primacy of perception.* Northwestern University Press, 1964.

Milner, M. *On not being able to paint.* New York: International Universities Press, 1973.

McConville, M. The phenomenological approach to perception. In R. S. Valle, & M. King (Eds.), *Existential-phenomenological alternatives for psychology,* New York: Oxford University Press, 1978.

Moncrieff, D. W. Aesthetic consciousness. In R. S. Valle, & M. King (Eds.), *Existential-phenomenological alternatives for psychology,* New York: Oxford University Press, 1978.

Ortega y Gasset, J. *Phenomenology and art.* New York: Norton, 1975.

Perkins, D., & Leondar, B. (Eds.), *The arts and cognition.* Baltimore: Johns Hopkins University Press, 1977.

Scheerer, M., & Lyons, J. Line drawings and matching responses to words. *Journal of Personality,* 1957, *25,* 251–273.

Schulman, L. *College students' realistic and transformative descriptions of objects: Differences between Look and Play orientations.* Senior thesis, SUNY, College at Purchase, 1981.

Schuman, M. The psychophysiological model of meditation and altered states of consciousness: A critical review. In J. M. Davidson, & R. J. Davidson (Eds.), *The psychobiology of consciousness.* New York: Plenum Press, 1980.

Siegel, S. *Non-parametric statistics for the behavioral sciences.* New York: McGraw-Hill, 1956.

Solomon, J. *The apprehension of objects by artists and scientists.* Senior thesis, SUNY, College at Purchase, 1976.

Speier, S. *A comparative analysis of verbal structuring of objects by groups differing in their habitual orientation.* Unpublished Ph.D. Dissertation, Clark University, Worcester, Mass., 1960.

Spiegelberg, H. *Phenomenology in psychology and psychiatry.* Evanston: Northwestern University Press, 1972.

Werner, H. *Die Urspruenge der Lyrik. Eine Entwicklungspsychologische Untersuchung.* Munich: Reinhardt, 1924.

Werner, H. Das Prinzip der Gestaltschichtung und seine Bedeutung im Kunstwerklichen Aufbau. *Zeitschrift fur angewandte Psychologie und Charakterkunde,* 1931, *59,* 241–256.

Werner, H. *Comparative psychology of mental development.* New York: Harper, 1940.

Werner, H. Unity of the senses (1934). Reprinted in *Developmental processes: Selected writings of Heinz Werner, Vol. 1.* S. S. Barten, & M. B., Franklin (Eds.), New York: International Universities Press, 1978.

Werner, H. A psychological analysis of expressive language (1955). Reprinted in *Developmental processes: Selected writings of Heinz Werner, Vol. 2,* S. S. Barten, & M. B. Franklin (Eds.), New York: International Universities Press, 1978.

Werner, H. The concept of development from a comparative and organismic point of view (1957). Reprinted in *Developmental processes: Selected writings of Heinz Werner, Vol. 1,* S. S. Barten, & M. B. Franklin (Eds.), New York: International Universities Press, 1978.

Werner, H., & Kaplan, B. *Symbol formation: An organismic-developmental approach to language and the expression of thought.* New York: Wiley, 1963.

Winner, E., McCarthy, M., Kleinman, S., & Gardner, H. First metaphors. In D. Wolf (Ed.), *Early symbolization. New Directions in Child Development,* 1979, *3,* 29–41.

11 Play as the Creation of Imaginary Situations: The Role of Language

Margery B. Franklin
Sarah Lawrence College

INTRODUCTION

> Each province of meaning—the paramount world of real objects and events into which we can gear by our actions, the world of imaginings and fantasms, such as the play world of the child, the world of the insane, but also the world of art, the world of dreams, the world of scientific contemplation—has its particular cognitive style. It is this particular style of a set of our experiences which constitutes them as a finite province of meaning (Schutz, 1962, p. 341).

Saying that play has to do with the creation of imaginary situations is not likely to evoke much controversy. However, if this idea is located in a theoretical context and its implications drawn out, it takes shape as a point of view that contrasts quite clearly with other ways of conceptualizing children's make-believe play. In the first part of this chapter, I draw on some ideas in Heinz Werner's work to provide grounding for a view of play as the creation of imaginary situations (or, more grandly, imaginary realities), indicating along the way the contrast between Werner's non-reductionist stance and other approaches. The central portion of the chapter focuses on the problem of how to conceptualize the role of language in play. Three paradigms are formulated, with primary emphasis given to the "reality creation paradigm"—a conceptualization of ways that language enters into the creation of imaginary situations. In a concluding section, I explore some questions about play, everyday reality, and developmental progression.

In *Comparative Psychology of Mental Development*, Werner (1957) uses the metaphor of "psychological worlds" to express the idea that realities experienced by different living creatures have their own distinctive shapes and do not simply mirror the external world. Werner employed the metaphor of different worlds to characterize the realities of animals as compared with humans, "primitive peoples" as compared with Westernized adults, schizophrenics as compared with "normals," and young children as compared with older children and adults.[1] He elaborated the world metaphor by talking about "spheres of reality" within worlds. In line with some other early developmentalists, Werner suggests that the young child lives in a relatively diffuse reality dominated by the "emotional-reactive" mode, a mode in which structurings and reactions are governed by actions, feelings, thoughts, and needs of the moment, and so-called "objective" features of objects and events are not apprehended or slip into the background. In this mode-of-being there is relative self-world fusion; what is inside and what is outside are not necessarily distinguished, the "subjective" and "objective are not cleary demarcated. Here, Werner is positing a primordial state out of which the spheres of "everyday reality" and what we might call "imaginal reality" emerge correlatively, being formed and differentiated in relation to one another. The emergence and development of differentiated spheres is marked (and in some sense formed) by the emergence of differentiated actions and attitudes that go along with distinctive ways of construing and responding to objects, persons, and events. As various spheres become differentiated with respect to one another, "there is at the same time an internal differentiation within the regions of each sphere." For example, within the everyday sphere, the school region and the home region become differentiated. Each has its own specific lawfulness and, accordingly, the child responds differently to the "same" external event. So, in Werner's words, a "plurality of milieus develops, above all because of a plurality of sets of behaviors in which the specific lawfulness for each region of reality is

---

[1]The concept of "spheres of reality" as it appears in Werner's work has a family relationship to Lewin's concept of "life space," Koffka's discussion of the child's world in *Growth of the Mind* and his later distinction between behavioral and geographic environments, and to the more general notion of "psychological field." In these conceptualizations, as in the work of other Gestalters and comparative psychologists such as von Uexküll, Buytendjik, and Klüver, the influence of phenomenological thinking is evident. These thinkers shared the conviction that psychology should go beyond recognition of discrepancies between the person's experience of something-out-there and the object defined "objectively" (within a physical world framework)—a recognition that stands at the center of traditional psychophysics—to a stronger and more holistic conception of psychological experience, a conception that views environment not as an assortment of stimuli but as a more-or-less integrated "world" and the organism not as an assemblage of faculties but as an integrated living creature whose activities (overt and covert) can be understood only through the attempt to discern the nature of its experience. In their attempts to go beyond "mere phenomenology" (as they often called it), to avoid being subjectivistic and to engage in the scientific enterprise as they conceived it, these theorists struggled to find an adequate conceptualization of relations between "psychological reality" and "objective reality." It is not clear that any of them achieved a consistent, coherent position on this issue.

present, more implicitly than explicitly, more emotionally and behaviorally than rationally'' (Werner, 1957, p. 402).

I want to note three interrelated themes in Werner's treatment of "spheres of reality.'' First, while Werner did not further develop the concept of "spheres of experience,'' his discussion in *Comparative Psychology* not only reflects a phenomenological orientation evident in some of his other work but suggests possibilities for developmental psychology.[2] A concept of development as the differentiation, progressive construction and integration of spheres within psychological reality provides an alternative to viewing mental development as a linear (or spiralling) progression directed towards adaptation to a pre-existing "external reality'' or towards the construction of a psychological reality dominated by a given mode of thought (such as the 'scientific'). Second, in Werner's discussion we find the idea that everyday reality and other realities emerge correlatively out of a relatively diffuse reality, a primordial state. This conceptualization differs markedly from those that posit a mundane, pragmatically ordered reality organized prior to the emergence of an "imaginal'' orientation. Piaget and Vygotsky appear to share the latter kind of view, although for different reasons. The third theme—Werner's view of play—will take us directly to the central portion of this paper.

Werner suggests, as indicated earlier, that initially the child does not clearly differentiate between "everyday reality'' and "make believe.'' Affective processes and relatively primitive forms of perceptual structuring permeate functioning overall. A playful, wish-governed mode may be manifest in non-play activities—as in the example of the two-year-old boy who pretended to butter a roll and then ate it, although a moment before he had professed to despise it. Gradually, the spheres of "make believe'' and everyday reality begin to differentiate. The child does not handle the doll as if it were a living creature (and would indeed be surprised if it moved); yet, at the same time, she imbues it with life. This process of endowing the inanimate with life seems to involve a flow of emotion from self to object—sometimes achieved at a distance but in play often mediated through actions on the object (for example, the piece of wood becomes a baby because it is handled like a baby). As the child grows older, awareness of the distinction between "make believe'' and "everyday reality'' becomes conscious: The spheres are now clearly demarcated.

Werner's characterization of different "spheres of reality'' resonates with Schutz' description of finite provinces of meaning. Such formulations lead us to view pretent play in a non-reductionist fashion, as a special kind of human activity, involving a distinctive orientation and having a

---

[2]Franklin and Barten (1980) have argued that Werner's work contains several phenomenological themes that Werner himself did not emphasize and perhaps did not fully recognize.

particular direction or telos: the creation of imaginary situations (cf. Vygotsky, 1978, pp. 93–95). This general orientation contrasts with the reductionistic approaches that figure in a good proportion of contemporary work. A few remarks will clarify the point at issue. One strong tendency in the study of play—whatever the form under consideration—is to view play as an indicator or reflection of something more basic, as an activity that provides a glimpse or measure of the child's underlying emotional life, knowledge, cognitive capacities, or social understandings. Another prevalent tendency is to view play—again specifying different forms—in terms of its functional significance, focusing on its role as a causal factor in the appearance or enhancement of some non-play activity or capacity, or on its role as a matrix for the development of a non-play activity or capacity.[3] While neither of these stances necessarily involves the classic form of reductionism—dissolving a phenomenon into constituent (and presumably basic) elements—they both reflect a reductionistic bias in viewing play primarily (and sometimes exclusively) in terms of what it tells us about something else (non-play). Such perspectives may be appropriate and useful for some purposes but by no means exhaust the possibilities of the phenomena. Studies of play necessarily involve assumptions about what play "is"—its essence or core meaning. While some work reflects interest in the idea of play as imaginative activity, the field has been dominated by inclinations to see play in terms of the more established categories of psychological functioning: personal-emotional life, cognitive-intellectual life, or social life. Here children's pretend play is viewed as belonging to the category of imaginative-expressive activities. And, in a non-reductionistic spirit, such activities are considered basic rather than derivative, drawing on and reflecting back upon the interrelated domains of emotional, intellectual, and social life.

In the play process, children create a medium of expression from the materials available to them. As many have noted, this medium involves the use of bodily actions of various kinds, objects made and found, the space between and around persons and props, and—in a large proportion of instances—language. A holistic approach requires, ultimately, conceptualizing the dynamic interactions among these aspects of the medium, and between the medium and that which it embodies or represents. Here, I focus on how language enters into the play process. Three paradigms of the role of language in play are delineated. As indicated earlier, the third—the "reality creation" paradigm—is part of the view of play as the creation of imaginary situations.

---

[3]Fein's (1981) recent review includes discussion of studies explicitly concerned with the functions and consequences of pretend play.

LANGUAGE IN PLAY: THREE PARADIGMS

In talking about language and play, it is important at the start to distinguish between a focus on language *and* play, and a focus on language *in* play. A clear sense of the distinction requires a brief glance at the language-and-play part of the domain. I then turn to discussion of three paradigms pertaining to language in play.

Language and Play

Three distinct streams can be discerned in the current literature on language and play. One of these has to do with play with language (Garvey, 1977). The two other streams are of more direct concern in the present context. First, there is growing interest in parallels or correspondence between the sequence of emerging patterns in language on the one hand, and symbolizing play on the other. Second, a number of investigators are currently working from the thesis that interactive play situations provide crucial settings for the child's acquisition of various aspects of language.

Literature bearing on parallels or correspondence between language and play is reviewed by Nicolich (1981) and Sachs (in press). Nicolich points to the distinction between studies more or less restricted to correlational analysis and those that attempt to uncover specific relationships between emerging patterns in play and in language. A good portion of this latter work takes off from the idea that pretend play and language may be rooted in the same cognitive abilities. Given a method of characterizing progression in each domain, investigators can raise questions concerning contingencies between progress in one domain and the other: Is progress in the language domain a prerequisite of (or precursor to) advance in symbolic play, or vice versa? Similar questions about parallels and possible contingencies between language and symbolic play were raised in another era, around issues concerning the so-called "disadvantaged child." Needless to say, any laying out of "levels" in the two domains stems from strong theoretical convictions about how to characterize the "stuff" in each domain—in terms of structures, functions, or some combination of these. The literature reflects a range of possibilities.[4]

The focus on play as a setting for language learning is linked to a more encompassing interest in the question of environmental input to language acquisition. It reflects, on the one hand, rejection of the Chomskian perspective concerning the "essence" of language and processes of acquisition and, on the other hand, rejection of behavioristic learning theory con-

---

[4]See for example, Bates (1979), Bloom (1974), Nicolich (1977; 1981), Roscianno (1979).

ceptualizations of both environment and language. Much of this literature (reviewed by Sachs, in press) is concerned with how patterns established in pre-symbolic or non-symbolic play (particularly with adults) contribute to the child's understanding and mastery of linguistic reference, conversational patterns such as turn-taking, and the combinatorial nature of language. There is also growing interest in possible contributions of symbolizing play to aspects of language acquisition (see Sachs, in press). It is suggested that the kinds of exchanges that occur in socio-dramatic play not only reflect what children already know but provide occasion for learning more about the structure and functions of dialogue. Children's role-enactment in pretend play may provide opportunity for trying out different "voices"—voices that vary in acoustic features but also in structure and content (what kinds of things one says to whom in what kinds of situations, and how). Moreover, play situations may provide a particularly good context for learning the narrative functions of language (Sachs, 1980). Sachs (in press) characterizes the emerging view as a "constructive interactive model" based on the idea that language is acquired in a "social, affective and linguistic environment that is supportive of language learning," and suggests that patterns of acquisition reflect "both the nature of the child and the nature of the social interactional setting in which language is used."

Given this brief excursion into the language-and-play part of the terrain, we may turn to the central focus of this section. The three paradigms of language in play that I delineate have in common the assumption that language—or, more accurately, speaking—plays a very important part (perhaps a central role) in the play process. Each of these paradigms has taken shape in the past ten years. Previously, there was a tendency to view the language of play merely as "indicator": a means for understanding what is going on. This latter approach pervades most psychoanalytic and cognitive approaches to symbolizing play. The three paradigms may be termed the self-guidance paradigm, the communicational paradigm, and the reality-creation paradigm.

The Self-Guidance Paradigm

The self-guidance paradigm of language in play puts at center stage the child playing alone or in the presence of (but not actively engaged with) another. Speech is viewed in terms of the self-guiding or self-regulatory functions it serves in organizing the activity of play for the player. These functions are assumed to be essential rather than peripheral to the meaning and course of play activity.

Many observers of child play note that children playing with others or by themselves engage in what Piaget (1926) called "egocentric speech"—speech that does not appear to be addressed to a listener. For

Piaget, such speech can be viewed as part of play or as an accompaniment to play, but is not seen as having a significant function in shaping play activity. An alternative conceptualization of "self-directed" speech, and therefore its potential role in play, is provided by Vygotsky (1962) who sees the child's early "egocentric" speech as serving several distinctive functions that are subsequently realized through the specialized form of inner speech. In Vygotsky's words, egocentric (and later, inner) speech "serves mental orientation, conscious understanding; it helps in overcoming difficulties; it is speech for oneself, intimately and usefully connected with thinking" (Vygotsky, 1962, p. 122).[5]

In his investigations and those of his co-workers, Vygotsky found grounds for suggesting variation in the relation of the child's egocentric speech to activity. Accidentally provoked utterances may influence subsequent action, as in the case of the child who remarks "It's broken" of a pencil and then goes on to draw a broken streetcar. In problem solving, the child moves from speech that describes or analyzes the situation to speech that has a "planful" character and often precedes the action. As Vygotsky says, "Now speech guides, determines, and dominates the course of action: the planing function of speech comes into being in addition to the already existing function of language to reflect the external world" (Vygotsky, 1978, p. 28).

We are familiar with the idea that for Vygotsky, in contradistinction to Piaget, the primary form of speech is social: language, speaking, and thought itself have their origins in the interpersonal matrix and their earliest forms reflect these origins. Early on, social speech differentiates into communicative speech proper (speech for and with others) and egocentric speech (on the way to inner speech). The development from social to egocentric to inner speech represents the gradual internalization (and transformation) of interpersonal, collaborative forms of behavior (Wertsch, 1979). It is worth pointing out, finally, that in Vygotsky's view, the two forms of speech—for oneself and for others—come to have increasingly differentiated forms subserving different functions.

The paradigm under discussion conceptualizes children's talk to themselves in play not as "egocentric" in the Piagetian sense or as "social" in the sense to be described below, but as self-directed, realizing the functions Vygotsky ascribed to egocentric and inner speech: serving mental orientation and conscious understanding, guiding and determining the course of action.

One exemplification of this paradigm appears in Luria and Yudovich (1959). Contemporary exemplifications are found in the work of Rubin

---

[5]See Fein (1979) for discussion of Piaget's and Vygotsky's views regarding relations between language and play.

(1979) and Fuson (1979). Rubin brought individual children to a playroom with an array of toys and materials and let them play freely for ten minutes. Private speech was coded in terms of a category set that singles out analytic statements (reasoning out what is required), comments about materials and own activities, and directions to the self, among other types of utterances. Rubin assessed the frequency with which utterances of each type occurred prior to, during, or at conclusion of the activity—thus aiming to get a glimpse of the extent to which verbalizations served planning functions. Like Rubin, Fuson began with a focus on private speech which she studied initially in relatively circumscribed situations and subsequently in free play—the child playing alone at home. Her category scheme is based on the idea that private speech serves three main functions: a regulating function, an emotional/expressive function, and a fantasy/role playing function. Only the first is directly related to the self-guidance paradigm.

In my view, these contemporary exemplifications of the self-guidance paradigm represent a narrow (and perhaps inaccurate) interpretation of Vygotsky's views of language, taking as central the effects of one type of activity (speaking) on another type of activity (carrying out the play sequence).[6]

The Communicational Paradigm

As the self-guidance paradigm places at center stage the child playing alone, so the prototypical case for the communicational paradigm is two or more children playing together. (Here, again, I am speaking of make-believe or pretend play).

The communicational paradigm conceptualizes pretend play as a social interactive process that reflects (and perhaps enhances) children's understandings of the world and of social relations in particular. In this view play is not "social" merely in a general sense but is *au fond* a social activity established and carried out through the exchange of communicational statements (typically, if not exclusively, in linguistic form). Emphasis on the interactive structure of play, sustained or embodied in the exchange of "messages," is not limited to discussions of language. However, the communicational paradigm being articulated here focuses on language as the medium of communication. The paradigm contains a distinction between

---

[6]On the issue of Vygotsky's views, see Glick (this volume). My point is that current exemplifications of the self-guidance paradigm rest on the version of Vygotsky that Glick designates as Vygotsky II. As will be seen, the reality-creation paradigm draws on the version that Glick designates as Vygotsky I. It should be pointed out that current exemplifications of the self-guidance paradigm do not appear to have a view of pretend play as unique, clearly demarcated from other kinds of activity. The categories for analyzing speech stem primarily from work on "private speech" in the context of tasks like bead-stringing and putting puzzles together (see Zivin, 1979).

communications that establish "context" and those that form the "text" of play. Both kinds of communications help to establish the play as "make believe," demarcated from other kinds of activity. Exemplifications of this paradigm tend to use a concept of "situated action"; perhaps this should be included as a component of the paradigm.

One source of the communicational paradigm lies in the work of Bateson (1956, 1972). Interested in issues of communication, Bateson sought to clarify the idea that meaning of a particular action or utterance depends on the "frame" or "context" of the activity. How one creature takes the behavior of another, and therefore the ability to engage in successful communication, depends on shared frames or context. According to Bateson, animals engaged in mock fighting are sending each other messges indicating "This is play" so that while the activity simulates fighting, the participants do not confuse it with the real thing. The analogy to children's make-believe play is remote at best.

Goffman's (1974) development of the concept of framing contributes to the concept of play as rule-governed transformational activity that is agreed upon by the participants. Drawing on phenomenological formulations (in particular Schutz' concept of finite provinces of meaning), Goffman goes beyond Bateson in elaborating the idea of framing as a *human* activity that has to do with socially shared understandings. This leads to a concept of "make believe" as a particular type of "keying" that the participants regard as an "avowed, ostensible imitation or running through of less transformed activity, this being done with the knowledge that nothing practical will come of the doing," and that is not to be taken at face value: It is understood as a representation of something other and in this sense as nonliteral.

Another important source of the communicational paradigm lies in developmental psycholinguistics. Within the past ten years or so, there has been a marked departure from formalistic analyses of child language (with emphasis on syntax and aspects of semantics) to a more functionalist view that emphasizes language-in-context and places the communicative origins and uses of language at center stage. In this move towards a more context-based, pragmatic view of child language, the "speech act" dethroned—at least to some extent—the sentence. And with the growing interest in communicative interchange, the speech act assumed its place as a unit within discourse. For some theorists, the type of discourse called dialogue has become the prototypical form of human interaction. Work on infancy that conceptualizes early behavior in interactional terms (involving concepts of focused attention, joint action, turn-taking) supports the view of the child as turned towards others, and as involved—from the beginning—in rule-governed communicational exchanges that both reflect and extend the range of intersubjective understandings.

A very clear exemplification of the communicational paradigm is found in the work of Schwartzman(1978, Ch.8). Drawing explicitly on Bateson, Schwartzman adopts a "view of play characterized by its production of paradoxical statements about persons, objects, activities and situations." (The "paradox" refers to Bateson's recognition that in play, entities have a dual meaning. They are what they are and at the same time "stand for" something other). Being an anthropologist, Schwartzman did what relatively few psychologists have done in the past thirty years: She ventured into the classroom and observed children engaging in pretend play in their natural habitat, over an extended period of time. The aspect of her work that bears most directly on the communicational paradigm is reflected in the category scheme for classifying communicative statements. The nine categories encompass contextual and textual statements and are readily applicable to the kinds of things children say while playing, but they could as readily be applied to many other kinds of social interactive situations. For example, formation statements (in play: "Let's play house") occur in many situations where one is trying to engage another in joint activity; similarly, rejection statements ("You can't play here") and acceptance statements ("o.k. now I'm eating it") occur in a wide variety of circumstances other than pretend play. Perhaps most important for a consideration of play, Schwartzman's category of definition statements covers a wide range of communications that Garvey and Berndt (1977), Sachs, Goldman, Chaille, and Seewald (1980) and others (including myself) have thought it essential to differentiate when talking about the language of play—for example, the statements "I'll be the princess," "I'm cooking dinner," "This is rice."

A study by Sachs et al. (1980) considers the range of communications in play—from those that signal and explicitly negotiate pretend play to unambiguous role-enactment statements. Aspects of Garvey's work (Garvey, 1974, 1979) represent another exemplication of the communicational paradigm. Garvey (1974) is concerned with how children communicate to each other the reality-play distinction, with the identification and working out of themes, and with the kinds of rules that govern interactions in the play process. A distinction is made between general procedural rules (for example, those that govern turn-taking) and rules pertaining to specific enactments or situations (for example, maintaining consistency in mother-appropriate behavior). In other work, Garvey (Garvey & Berndt, 1977) considers a wider range of communicative statements and presents a category scheme that attends to interacting aspects of the play process: negation of pretend, play signals (markers of play orientation), procedural or preparatory behaviors, and explicit mention of pretend transformations; the latter contains subcategories pertaining to assignment of roles, making plans, and transforming of objects. Here, it seems that Garvey is working as much within the reality-creation paradigm as within the communicational paradigm. However, the communicational paradigm is clearly present and perhaps paramount: "The social conduct of pretending was shown to rest on extensive and diversified communicative behaviors."[7]

The Reality-Creation Paradigm

For this paradigm of language in play, the child playing alone and children playing together are equally prototypical situations. Like the other two paradigms delineated, it assumes that "private" activities and in fact individuality itself take form in a social matrix—not just the social matrix of "culture" but in day-to-day interactions with other persons. Further, it assumes that pretend play activity (like most of what we do) rests on some base of intersubjective understandings and that assumptions as well as questions about this understanding figure prominently in play situations (Wolf, 1981). The reality-creation paradigm subsumes or incorporates aspects of the self-guidance and communicational paradigms but in its emphasis on play as the creation of imaginary situations, it raises to a position of prominence the distinction between "make believe" and non-pretend activity. Related to this, it views pretend play *au fond* as symbolizing activity, and the language of play—by virtue of its status as a symbolizing medium—as serving both constitutive and integrative functions in the context of play. In other words, this paradigm takes as basic the idea that symbolizing does not—in its basic form—merely reflect or communicate what is already known but is formulative, meaning-creating. The direct source for this conceptualization is Werner and Kaplan (1963). It is important to note the extent to which the idea of symbolization as "radical metaphorizing" (Kaplan, 1962) or "radical interaction" differs from versions of symbolizing extant in the psychological literature.

This paradigm is termed the "reality creation" paradigm with the understanding that "reality" here does not refer to pre-given reality but to imaginative realities that are created in play. In the background is the idea that large portions of psychological functioning can be understood in terms of contrasts or tensions between two forms of realities, both of which we

---

[7]Another clear exemplification of the communicational paradigm is Gearhart's (1979) study of preschoolers playing "store." Particular attention is given to the way children interact in pre-planning their joint play. A subsequent presentation (Gearhart, 1980) also concerns play-text and negotiational statements over the course of play, with attention given to the uses of language in establishing and playing out social roles. In a study recently reported, Wolf (1981) describes the emergence and developmental course of different kinds of verbalizations of a young child engaged in pretend play with an adult. The conceptualization of this study seems to reflect the communicational paradigm, but the category scheme for classifying types of verbalizations—like that of Garvey and Berndt (1977)—is, in part, suggestive of the reality-creation paradigm.

create: those which (at a given time in our lives) we take for granted as more or less enduring stable frameworks and which we do not experience ourselves as creating—it takes a psychologist, philosopher, or anthropologist to suggest that life-spaces, frameworks, or world-views are created—and the realities that we experience ourselves (or someone like us) as making up and often call "imaginary" or "fictional." These latter realities can be momentary or more enduring. The present paradigm pertains to both the creation of imaginary situations that are relatively short, circumscribed episodes and the creation of imaginary "worlds" that are sometimes created by children over extended periods of time.

Whether communicating with others or talking to herself, the child at play is involved—according to this paradigm—in reality-creation. In such activity, some things are "taken for granted" at the outset; others are problematic and have to be "settled" (for the self as much as interpersonally) before things can go on. Further, what is taken for granted in one sphere may be problematic in another. Thus, what the young child takes as "given" in the everyday sphere may have to be established anew in play.

This paradigm is exemplified in a set of categories developed a few years ago (Franklin, 1977),[8] initially applied to classroom observations and then to videotapes of pairs of children in a lab playroom.

What has to happen for a play episode to take place? First, there is the range of activities that have to do with *establishing, specifying,* and *maintaining* the sphere of play. Second (although not in a temporal sense), *entities in play must have identities*; we can designate the entities of play as *objects, persons,* and *places.* Third, in all but the most rudimentary symbolizing play, episodes (or sequences of episodes) take place—clearly there is a set of processes that has to do with *creating and organizing events and sequences.*

Establishing, specifying, and maintaining the play sphere.   The first subcategory here is *differentiating play from everyday reality.* The classic form in interpersonal situations is "Let's pretend." A young two-year-old, being invited by his teacher to engage in pretend play, was heard to say, "This is fafa? Right?" ("Fafa" was the child's made-up word for pretend activities.) Another two-year-old who liked playing with plastic fruit often put it in her mouth. One day, as she picked up each piece of fruit, she addressed each and said, "Not for real . . . . not really (pear) . . . . not really real . . . ."

Exchanges about specifics among older children also reflect efforts to

---

[8]As noted earlier, category sets developed by Garvey and Berndt (1977) and Wolf (1981) may also serve as exemplifications of this paradigm, although not explicitly formulated in these terms.

establish and/or maintain the distinction between pretend and real. For example, two four-year-olds at play:

> Standing by a shelf near the housekeeping corner, J grasped small round rubber pieces; then she let them fall into a plastic dish. C skipped over to join her. After grabbing two of the rubber circles, J commented, "These are pennies. Let's be owners of the store." C looked at her questioningly, and replied, "But I'm not an owner, and those (pointing to the rubber circles) are rubber pieces." J responded, "Yes, but we're just pretending. They're really black rubber pennies."

It is interesting to note here J's compromise, presumably motivated by a wish to get C involved in the play.

The next sub-category is *establishing specific play spheres*. Two-year-olds tend to do this by getting involved themselves with specific materials, or inviting another child to join them in a particular play activity: "Let's take a ride on the firetruck." Older children often designate the proposed activity in more generic terms: "Let's play house." Or, in somewhat less direct ways indicate the specific sphere, as in the above example ("Let's be owners of store"). Another sub-category, *transitions and blendings,* encompasses verbalizations that have to do with shifting from one type of play to another: "I'm tired of playing house. Let's play school now . . ."

Establishing identities for objects.   In the course of pretend play, a considerable portion of statements are concerned with *assigning identities to objects*. Interestingly, two-year-olds (and occasionally older children) often name realistic objects—life-size or miniature replicas—sometimes apparently talking to themselves and at other times vaguely addressing or directly querying a by-standing adult. For example:

> N take a plastic chicken from the table and puts it into the childcraft refrigerator. Turning to the observer, she says: "A chicken."

> G holds a baby doll, puts a bottle in its mouth, rocks the baby back and forth . . . Puts the bottle down on a nearby table, and says (quietly) "bottle," then picks it up and puts it back in doll's mouth. Gets her mother's attention by saying "Mommy," shows her doll and says "Doll with bottle."

In many instances such as these, we have reason to believe that the child would not be naming the objects outside of the context of play, suggesting that when you are just learning about transporting items across sphere boundaries, there may be special need to mark identities.

The *naming of realistic objects* wanes but naming subsequently (and quite early, see Wolf, 1981) appears in the context of *object transformation* (see Matthews, 1977). In the reality-creation paradigm, it is assumed that such naming does not simply reflect perceptual and enactive restructurings of objects (see Winner, 1979) but—at least sometimes—plays a crucial role in the transformational process. A child hands another a wooden disk and says "Have a chocolate chip cookie"; another child tears up little pieces of paper, places them in a row on the table, and says to her co-player: "These are our medicines." These two examples illustrate the fact—noted by many—that object designation can occur *within* play (as a text statement), or as a statement *about* some aspect of play (as a contextual statement, e.g. "These are our medicines").

There are also numerous examples of naming used in the context of *creating imaginary objects*. This is often supported by gestural enactment and the availability of other objects. A three-year-old walks across the room with a string of beads trailing behind her, and says (to no one in particular), "I have a kitty cat . . . ." And, then, as she continues walking, turning in the direction of her "pet": "Here, kitty . . . here, kitty." (The game and related verbalizations continue.) Often, particularly among somewhat older children, this kind of statement occurs in the context of a play sequence, in the absence of gestural or object support.

Establishing identities for persons.   Young children beginning to engage in pretend activities like feeding the baby are not necessarily assuming "roles"; they may be simply acting themselves in relation to some creature (doll, stuffed animal) that they have endowed with life through acting in relation to it, and—interestingly—through talking to it. In much early play, there is the sense of a transitional phase in which the child is not just "being herself" and, on the other hand, has not assumed any definable role. Somewhat later, children are actively involved in games—by themselves but more often with others—where character identities and other aspects of role are more-or-less clearly established (see Garvey & Berndt, 1977; and Garvey, 1979). This is mediated by language in two ways: First, by *explicit role assignment* (where one gives oneself or another a role: "I'm the baby"; "You be the daddy"; "I'm a fireman," etc.); second, through *character speech,* talking in character.

> Two three-year-olds are playing in the kitchen corner. They have just completed a perfunctory meal. One says to the other, "Listen, sweetie, I'm going shopping, I'll be right back." The other responds, "I'm going too," and the first says, "No, you wait here."

Clearly, explicit role assignments are "outside" the play proper: They establish aspects of context. Character speech is within the play, part of (and sometimes the entire) text of play. Speaking is also used extensively to argue matters of role assignment, or to signal changes in role: "I don't want to be the Daddy anymore. Can I be the dog?" It should be clear that character speech not only serves the function of establishing role but may function simultaneously to construct the events of play (as in extended dialogue between two characters).

Establishing the setting.   To my knowledge, relatively little work has been done on how children transform the real space of the environment into the imagined space or setting of play. In the play of two-year-olds and in older children's play with miniature toys, a lot of the work of establishing setting is strongly supported by props and action but even in these situations—and clearly in the sociodramatic play of fours and fives—speaking appears to play a formative role in establishing general locale or giving identities to specific parts of the environment.

The following example (from the play of older two-year-olds) shows some disagreement about what is and what is not part of the "play space":

> Four children are rocking in a play boat and singing "Row, row, row your boat." When the rocking slows down, C starts to climb out of the boat. A becomes quite agitated and says to her, "You're in the water! Get back in the boat! There's sharks!" C gazes at him and says calmly, "No, it's plastic" (there is a plastic sheet on the floor). A responds: "No, no, it's the water!" C shakes her head solemnly and does not move. A grabs her hand and tries to pull her back into the boat. Getting back into the boat, C says, "Oh, yes, it's the water . . . ."

Another example illustrates the difference between being inside and outside the imaginary setting of play. (This also provides an example of dialoguing, to be discussed below.) Two four-year-old girls are sitting on play cars with steering wheels, turning the wheels back and forth as if driving.

N: We're going to Florida.
L: We'd better stop and get some gas soon.
N: Okay, I'll look for a station.
L: There's one! (spoken loudly as child points to her left).
N: (leaning to one side): Fill it up.
L: I'm going to the bathroom (gets off car and runs to other side of room, where
      she stands in corner, hands on hips).
S: (approaching L): What are you doing?
L: You'd better not stand here. You're in the girls' bathroom!
S: I think you're crazy!
L: (getting back in car): Let's go!

The generic category of *creating and organizing events* will be briefly discussed in terms of three sub-categories: *planning, describing/explaining,* and *narrating/dialoguing.*

Planning.   Role-assignment and establishing a specific play sphere before play begins ("Let's play house") serve planning functions. These and a more specific type of planning statement that announces what is going to be done precede action (see Gearhart, 1979, 1980). These statements can be very brief ("I'm going to set the table so we can play dinner") but, on occasion, the beginning of a story-line is spelled out, as when one four-year-old said to another as they climbed on the cars: "Are we going to the gas station, and then fill it up with gas and then pick up my sister?"

Here is the exchange of two four-year-old girls who have just arrived in a lab playroom; while only some of these are strictly planning statements, the exchange provides a typical example of "getting started" in play. The two children sit down at a table on which are arranged little dolls, doll furniture, blocks, and other toys.

> B: Let's set it up like a house.
> P: (Takes the chairs and sets them around the table, picks up baby): He needs a seat.
> B: We need a high chair for him. Looking at the baby (holding it up for other child to inspect).
>   What is this? A bed? (holding up bed)
> P: Yes. And this (holding up other bed) is another bed.
> B: Wait, wait (arranges blocks around furniture) . . . This could be the bedroom . . .
> P: Here's the baby bed. This is the bed where the baby sleeps.
> B: And, look, here's the bathtub.
> P: Yes, pretend . . . o.k. Wanna pretend it's night-time and everyone is having supper?
> B: O.K.

In play with miniature toys as in sociodramatic play, children move in and out of "frame" to make plans, although often—particularly if there are no problems—the sequence develops without explicit planning statements.

Here is another example of two four-year-old boys playing with blocks and wooden airplanes in the classroom:

> N puts his plane on the floor and is joined by D. Each child loads his arms with an assortment of blocks; they put their blocks on the floor. N. says: "D, we need a waiting room right here," and points to the floor in front of him. They proceed to build. D then says (apparently to himself): "To make the road to the airport" (as he lays out a line of blocks). Continuing to build, D says: "There, now the cars can get into the parking lot." At this point, they begin to play—flying the airplane, taking turns. When the wooden plane slips off the runway, N says, "It's still too small. We need more." And both D and N reach for more blocks which they add to the construction. Play proceeds.

Describing/explaining. Children at play often talk about what they are doing while they are doing it; sometimes these statements are clearly addressed to a co-player or by-standing adult, sometimes to no one in particular; often, they appear to be self-directed. Many of these statements are like planning statements, but they accompany the play or come at its conclusion rather than precede it, and have a more ambiguous status with regard to the context-text distinction.

> In the large block area, B begins to take some blocks from the stack to the middle of the room; she selects one at a time and then arranges them. To the teacher standing nearby, she says: "See, this is the step. I'm making a house." Another child joins her. As they begin to play, B describes the parts of the structure.

A three-year-old playing alone builds a block structure with compartments and picks up, one by one, a series of small animals. As he places each one in a compartment, he says, "And this one goes here . . . and the horse goes in here . . . and the mommy and baby cows are together here . . . and now they're having supper."

Narrating/dialoguing.   Narrating is observed in elaborated play with blocks and/or miniature toys. (It is virtually impossible to narrate socio-dramatic play if you are one of the actors.) While many instances are ambiguous, some of the talk that accompanies play seems to be thoroughly embedded in the play activity—to be clearly textual—as contrasted with the type of talk just characterized as "describing."

A four-year-old is playing with miniature houses, cars and trucks in a lab playroom. A non-participating adult is present. Moving the fire engine across the table, the child talks (without turning toward the adult, and in a low voice): "Well, the fire engine goes up the street, up the street . . . (turning fire engine around) . . . and it goes to put out the fire at this house . . . he's putting out the fire now . . . (gestures) . . . spfft . . . spfft . . . The fire is out . . . See, now it turns around . . . and it goes back, back to the fire house . . . and into the fire house. But then the guy remembers, there was another fire, he forgot, and he gets back with the other guys and off they go . . ." (play continues for a brief period).

Dialoguing in sociodramatic play has already been illustrated (in the trip to Florida). Here is a final example, from two five-year-old girls playing in the lab playroom. An assortment of little dolls, doll furniture, vehicles, and blocks is on the table.

M: I'll be her (picking up one of the little dolls).
C: I'll be her also. (Reaches for doll held by other child, who does not hand it over).
   I mean I'm not going to be him. I'll be her (picking up girl doll). And I'll be the baby also.
M: Darling, it's time for your bath (uses mother-like voice).
C: Yes, ma-am (uses a babyish voice).
M: O.K. I won't let her drown (adjusts baby in tub). I'll fix us some nice supper (marches doll to the refrigerator).
C: (standing up girl doll):   Like what?
M: Um, scrambled eggs or something (dolls stationed to look in refrigerator).
C: Scrambled eggs for dinner? (in an emphatic, high-pitched voice).
M: No, o.k. we're going to have quiche.
C: Quiche, yuk!
M: Well, what *would* you like to eat?
C: Chicken or steak.
M: O.K. let's see if we have any chicken or steak (doll is moved back to "look" again into refrigerator) . . . we have some chicken.
C: O.K. I'll have some chicken.
M: But we don't have any steak. Tomorrow I'll buy . . . I'll buy lots of things cause we're running out of food.
C: O.K. Time for dinner (seats her doll at table) . . . all finished.

M: You have your . . . you have your chicken . . . (C gets up and goes to other side
      of table, looks at other toys) a . . . Hey, this is cute, why don't we play with
      this, C?

With this sample of happy domestic life, we come to a temporary stopping place. In sum, the first generic category described pertains to
statements directed toward establishing, maintaining and specifying the
sphere of play; the next set of categories to establishing identities for objects, persons and places; and the final set of categories pertains to providing
temporal structure as events are created and organized in play. Clearly,
many of the utterances in play are multifunctional. While this presents
problems for the researcher, it is inherent in the complexity of the language
of play.[9]

CONCLUDING COMMENTS

Play and Reality

One of the questions that recurs in the literature on pretend play concerns
the "resources" of play and the way that such resources are used by the
child in constructing play episodes. Most would agree with Garvey (1979)
that children at play draw on resources at their command—"motion . . . objects and object attributes, language, social constructs, and rules or limits."
However, if Werner is on the right track, we need to consider that these
"resource" entities may not always have the kinds of identities attributed
to them in the everyday orientation. The child who picks up a corkscrew
and whizzes it through the air, calling it "a bird," did not necessarily apprehend it as a corkscrew prior to the moment of imaginative construction.

Recognition that in play children often appear to be re-presenting—with
relatively slight modification—scenes from everyday life has led to a focus
on the schemata (Garvey & Berndt, 1977), formats (Garvey, 1974) or scripts
(Nelson & Gruendel, 1979)—presumably abstracted from everyday
life—that may serve as organizing plans in pretend play. Several questions
may be raised here: Is the "everyday" world the only source of schemata,
or do some originate in other regions? What is the relation of schemata
(assuming they exist) to play activity? Do they lie in the background and inform play in some subtle way, or do they serve as blueprints for action?
Certainly we find instances of play that can be readily viewed as "scripted,"
but a good deal of play seems to have a genuinely *improvisational* char-

---

[9]See Garvey and Berndt (1977), Sachs (1980) and Wolf (1981) on developmental changes in
the use of language in play.

acter—whether or not it deals with subject matter lifted directly from the child's everyday life.

Discussion about whether the relation of play to non-play everyday reality should be construed as replication, reconstruction, or transformation continues (Rubin, 1980; Sutton-Smith, 1979, pp. 115–121). As indicated, much current work focuses on "reality based" play but interest in the wilder regions of fantasy as a source of play is also evident. In this connection, it can be suggested that there are two primary tendencies inherent in pretend play—leading to the construction of worlds of different kinds. One is the tendency toward realism, the other toward the fantastical. Much play embodies both tendencies while some exemplifies one tendency almost to the exclusion of the other.

In realism, the intent is the re-construction (with modification and elements of invention) of aspects of everyday life. We find the familiar themes of feeding baby, having dinner, going on a trip enacted with striking verisimilitude. In my view, such play is not replication but it may be described as reality-oriented (and may have something in common with "realism" in the novel or other art forms).

In fantastical play, children construct happenings that run *against* everyday reality, that in some sense violate day-to-day conscious experience. This play too is organized by some kind of schemata but the prevalence and forms of such play suggest that we need to look beyond the mundane in search of the child's schemes for organizing experience and activity. Instances of play that embody defiance of the "rules" of the everyday world are myriad. Magical thinking is everywhere in evidence. More elaborated forms of such play may involve rules that provide specific permutations of everyday reality. One continuing saga in which I participated was called "The Fancy Ladies of North Poo-Poo"—the title itself embodies the theme of contradiction or paradox around which this game was structured. These two ladies did everything in a fashion we considered "opposite" to our own experience: They laughed when they should have cried, they entered subways via windows rather than through doors, and so forth. With the principle of "opposites" we generated countless novel, reality-inverting situations that gave us great enjoyment and, no doubt, satisfied all kinds of unconscious wishes.

Some Questions of Development

In this chapter, I have not considered—except in passing—issues concerning developmental patterns or trends in pretend play or in play more generally. The empirical and theoretical literature bearing on such issues is vast; most of it reflects implicit or explicit concern with the "telos" of play closely linked to ideas about the relation of play to other aspects of psychological functioning or other types of human activity.

With the growing interest in symbolic processes, there has been considerable focus on aspects of play such as the transition from presymbolic action and object use to symbolic representation, subsequent trends in object transformation and role enactment, and related phenomena. For most investigators, a conceptual framework informs empirical work, but quite often the forest gets lost for the trees and aspects of play (such as object transformation) are considered out of context. A recent paper by Uzgiris (1981) represents the kind of integrative work that is sorely needed in the field.

Looking at developmental patterns in pretend play, many authors note increasing flexibility, decontextualization, and introduction of imaginary elements in play, but at the same time emphasize a trend towards "realism." Werner and Kaplan (1963)—here in agreement with Piaget— say:

> As the child enters the sphere of make-believe play and distinguishes this sphere from that of serious action, there is a growing trend towards realism; the play content becomes less 'subjective,' 'fantastic,' 'idiosyncratic,' and more directed towards the depiction of events and objects of everyday life. The child, having distinguished his play from the sphere of "reality," increasingly shapes his make-believe play for the representation of this sphere of "reality." [p. 94].

Many observers of children's play note the heightened interest in representing reality that seems to emerge around six or seven years of age: the highly "realistic" though stylized enactment of real-life situations such as that which occurs in playing school or house; the child's pleasure in toys that are exact replicas of the real thing: vehicles, dolls with real hair, dollhouses, fire-stations, and so forth. I have just suggested that this is only part of the story. During this same period, many children are also developing an interest in fairy-tales or modern-day fantastical sagas, a penchant for elaborated fantasy that—in play—often takes the form of using very realistic materials in the context of developing narratives that are marked by a clear departure from the constraints of everyday life.

I do not find compelling evidence for the idea that, overall, there is a trend toward increasing "realism" in pretend play. Rather, it seems to me that there is a trend toward greater *inner coherence* in both reality-oriented and fantastical play (as well as in mixed forms). Tendencies toward consistency—in role enactment, in attending to matters of scale and style (for example, not mixing toys of markedly different size or type), in observing imaginary boundaries (the water's edge) can be understood as part of the movement towards inner coherence that marks all forms of world-making.

Many discussions of pretend play locate it in a developmental sequence that begins with the child's early exploration of objects or playful rule-governed interactions with others and culminates in conventionalized games with rules (ranging from ringolevio to chess). Piaget (1951) and Vygotsky (1978) provide strong arguments for such a sequence. I suggest that we take a critical look at this picture of evolution. It is true that these forms of play follow each other ontogenetically, that each involves some shift from a purely pragmatic mode, and a set of rules governing activity. But in other respects this line of development is hard to discern, particularly if one sees pretend play as imaginative work, involving complex interweavings of realistic and fantastical elements, basically creative rather than codified, directed toward the creation of new realities. In this respect, the dramas of childhood play would seem to have much more in common with myth-making, literary works, and even scientific theory-building than with conventionalized rule-governed games.

Imaginative World-Making

For many children, the creation of imaginary situations in play evolves into something grander: the creation of imaginary worlds. A particular cast of characters, certain thematic elements and rules of conduct become the basis for a continuing saga. Sachs' daughter (at ten) explained to her mother that it was "very hard to use her model horses in play with new friends because they did not know the characteristics of each horse and the history of the herd" (Sachs, 1980). Cobb (1977) talks about the world-making of the Brontë children who constructed two imaginary kingdoms, Angria and Gondal, populated by characters with names like "Sneaky" and "Bravy." I have vivid memories of several continuing sagas—in addition to the Fancy Ladies of North Poo-Poo—that were an important part of my own childhood. With few exceptions, I do not recall specific episodes but the characters, scenes, and atmosphere of these worlds are as clear to me now as any events or scenes of the "everyday reality" that I inhabited, and in some ways much more coherent, like well-defined islands in memory.

To my knowledge, this aspect of children's pretend play has not been explored. It seems a fertile field. Parents and teachers can catch glimpses of such world construction. As Drucker (1981) suggests, therapists are often in a position to observe close-up the extended metaphoric constructions that children develop in play in treatment situations. And now that autobiography is becoming legitimate data in psychology, we could undertake retrospective studies that would cast light not only on the prevalence and nature of such world-making but on our sense of its place in our lives.

One other thought: We talk about the "worlds" created by artists but do not always recognize the significance of the metaphor. Consider the difference between viewing one or two paintings by Chagall, and seeing a retrospective show. To enter the world created by a painter, photographer, or sculptor, one has to see a series of works. The single work is a snapshot: It is difficult to construct a world from a single glance. By contrast, with art work that contains temporal ordering and an indication of place—novels, plays, and films—one enters a world effortlessly and often experiences a palpable sense of loss when the fiction comes to an end. All of these comings and goings involve fundamental shifts in orientation, departures from the "everyday" and, I suggest, can be most fully described within a phenomenological framework that provides grounding for the concept of imaginative world-making.

ACKNOWLEDGMENTS

Some of the ideas in this chapter come out of collaborative work with two colleagues: Sybil S. Barten and Jan Drucker. I want to express my appreciation to them and to former and present students who took verbatim records of classroom play: Alysson Ames, Diana Barnum, Patricia Gildea-Dial, and Arieta Slade; Patricia Gildea-Dial also worked on transcription and categorization of videotape material. This work was done at the Sarah Lawrence College Early Childhood Center, with the helpful cooperation of head teachers.

REFERENCES

Bates, E. *The emergence of symbols: Cognition and communication in infancy.* New York: Academic Press, 1979.

Bateson, G. The message "This is play." In *Group processes: transactions of the second conference.* New York: Josiah Macy Jr. Foundation, 1956.

Bateson, G. *Steps to an ecology of mind.* New York: Ballantine Books, 1972.

Bloom, L. *Language and play as developmental correlates.* Paper presented at American Psychological Association meetings, New Orleans, 1974.

Cobb, E. *The ecology of imagination in childhood.* New York: Columbia University Press, 1977.

Drucker, J. *Discussion: Panel on cognitive and affective aspects of children's fantasy-making.* Paper presented at American Orthopsychiatric Meetings, New York, 1981.

Fein, G. Echoes from the nursery: Piaget, Vygotsky, and the relationship between language and play. In *New Directions for child development, No. 6,* 1979. E. Winner, & H. Gardner (Eds.), Fact, fiction and fantasy in childhood.

Fein, G. Pretend play in childhood: An integrative review. *Child Development,* 1981, *52,* 1095–1118.

Franklin, M. B. *Functions of language in play.* Paper presented at the meetings of the National Association for the Education of Young Children, Chicago, 1977.

Franklin, M. B., & Barten, S. S. *Heinz Werner's contribution to a psychology of experience.* Paper presented at Eastern Psychological Association Meetings, Hartford, Conn., 1980.

Fuson, K. C. The development of self-regulating aspects of speech: A review. In G. Zivin (Ed.), *The development of self-regulation through private speech.* New York: Wiley, 1979.

Garvey, C. Some properties of social play. *Merrill Palmer Quarterly,* 1974, *20,* 163–180.

Garvey, C. Play with language and speech. In S. Ervin-Tripp, & C. Mitchell-Kernan (Eds.), *Child Discourse*. New York: Academic Press, 1977.

Garvey, C. Communicational controls in social play. In B. Sutton-Smith (Ed.), *Play and learning*. New York: Gardner Press, 1979.

Garvey, C., & Berndt, R. *Organization of pretend play*. Catalogue of Selected Documents in Psychology, November, 1977, Vol. 7, 107. Ms. 1589.

Gearhart, M. *Social planning: Role play in a novel situation*. Paper presented at Society for Research in Child Development Meetings, San Francisco, 1979.

Gearhart, M. *Dramatic play: Children as directors and actors*. Paper presented at conference "The Language of Young Children: Frontiers of Research," Brooklyn College, 1980.

Goffman, E. *Frame analysis*. Cambridge, Mass.: Harvard University Press, 1974.

Kaplan, B. Radical metaphor, aesthetic and the origin of language. *Review of Existential Psychological and Psychiatry*, 1962, *2*, 75–84.

Luria, A. R., & Yudovich, F. la. *Speech and the development of mental processes in the child*. Baltimore: Penguin Books, 1959.

Matthews, W. S. Modes of transformation in the initiation of fantasy play. *Developmental Psychology*, 1977, *13*, 212–216.

Nelson, K., & Gruendel, J. M. At morning it's lunchtime: A scriptal view of children's dialogues. *Discourse Processes*, 1979, *2*, 73–94.

Nicolich, L. McCune Beyond sensori-motor intelligence: Assessment of symbolic maturity through analysis of pretend play. *Merrill-Palmer Quarterly*, 1977, *23*, 89–101.

Nicolich, L. McCune Toward symbolic functioning: Structure of early pretend games and potential parallels with language. *Child Development*, 1981, *52*, 785–797.

Piaget, J. *The language and thought of the child*. London: Routledge and Kegan Paul, 1926.

Piaget, J. *Play, dreams and imitation*. London: Wm. Heinmann Ltd., 1951.

Roscianno, L. *Object play and its relation to language in early childhood*. Unpublished doctoral dissertation, Columbia University, 1979.

Rubin, I. H. The impact of the natural setting on private speech. In G. Zivin (Ed.), *The development of self-regulation through private speech*. New York: Wiley, 1979.

Rubin, K. H. Fantasy play: Its role in the development of social skills and social cognition. In *New Directions for Child Development*, No. 9, 1980: K. H. Rubin (Ed.), Children's Play.

Sachs, J. The role of adult-child play in language development. In *New Directions for Child Development*, No. 9, 1980: K. H. Rubin (Ed.), Children's Play.

Sachs, J. Children's play and communicative development. In R. Schiefelbusch (Ed.), *Communicative Competence: Acquisition and Intervention*. In press.

Sachs, J., Goldman, J., Chaille, C., & Seewald, R. *Communication in pretend play*. Paper presented at the American Educational Research Association Meetings, Boston, 1980.

Schwartzman, H. *Transformations: The anthropology of children's play*. New York: Plenum Press, 1978.

Sutton-Smith, B. (Ed.) *Play and learning*. New York: Gardner Press, 1979.

Schutz, A. *Collected papers*, Vol. I. The Hague: M. Nijhoff, 1962.

Uzgiris, I. *Representation in symbolic play*. Paper presented at the meetings of the Society for Research in Child Development, Boston, Mass., 1981.

Vygotsky, L. S. *Though and language*. Cambridge, Mass.: M.I.T. Press, 1962.

Vygotsky, L. S. *Mind and society*. Cambridge, Mass.: Harvard University Press, 1978.

Werner, H. *Comparative psychology of mental development*. New York: International Universities Press, 1957. (First edition in English, 1940.)

Werner, H., & Kaplan, B. *Symbol formation*. New York: Wiley, 1963.

Wertsch, J. V. From social interaction to higher psychological processes: A clarification and application of Vygotsky's theory. *Human Development*, 1979, *22*, 1–22.

Winner, E. New names for old things: The emergence of metaphoric language. *Journal of Child Language*, 1979, *6*, 469–492.

Wolf, D. *Playing along: Shared meaning in pretense play*. Paper presented at Society for Research in Child Development Meetings, Boston, 1981.

Zivin, G. (Ed.) *The development of self-regulation through private speech*. New York: Wiley, 1979.

12 Concept and Symbol Formation by Infants

Jonas Langer
University of California at Berkeley

Determining the initial developing relations between language and thought is a problem for all major theories of cognitive development (Piaget, 1926/1955, 1951; Vygotsky, 1934/1962; Werner, 1948; Werner & Kaplan, 1963). It is worth taking up this problem again at this time for two related reasons. Previous theoretical analyses were based on data in which conceptual developments are confounded with symbolic developments. The microanalytic data generated in our studies of cognitive development provide new findings on children's initial conceptual constructions. Moreover, these cognitive data are independent of those on infants' developing symbolic activity.

While our findings range across the ages 6 to 60 months, the developments at age 18 months are crucial to the present concerns since this is the age period when researchers of varying theoretical persuasion agree that children's cognition is becoming representational. Yet to be determined is *how* representational cognition develops during this age period and *what* its structural organization is.

So, the present analyses focus on our findings on conceptual development, symbolic development, and their structural developmental relations at age 18 months. Our findings on conceptual development from ages 6 to 18 months have been reported in detail elsewhere (Langer, 1980, 1981, 1982, in preparation). Here, therefore, I review only those findings on conceptual development by age 18 months necessary for the subsequent analyses of symbol formation at this age.

Conceptual development takes two basic forms. These forms are developments in part-whole operations that characterize logicomathematical cognition, and developments in means-ends functions that characterize physical cognition.[1] These are reviewed in the next two sections.

The method used to study these two forms of conceptual development during infancy and early childhood is simple in form, if complex and elaborate in execution. Subjects are presented with small collections of different objects such as rings, columns, and spoons. They are made out of nonmalleable material (e.g., wood), malleable Play-Doh, and combinations of the two. The data include quantitative measures of subjects' spontaneous manipulations of and constructions with these objects, as well as exhaustive qualitative observations. The results of experimenter-provoked manipulations and counterconditions supplement these measures.

This research strategy elicits both part-whole and means-ends transformations; although, as intended, the former predominate. To illustrate the former, the part-whole relations of a malleable Play-Doh object may be transformed from one form of object into another such as from a ring into a solid or from a solid into a ring or both. To illustrate the latter, the means-ends relations between two adjacent nonmalleable objects may be transformed from nondependency to dependency when infants try to stack one on the other.

OPERATIONS

The organization of logicomathematical cognition that I have proposed comprises three sets of foundation structures. These are structures of part-whole transformations that subjects generate in interacting with their environments. They are: (1) combinativity operations, which include composing, decomposing, and recomposing; (2) relational operations of addition, subtraction, multiplication, and division; and (3) conditional operations of exchange (e.g., commutativity), correlation (e.g., one-to-one correspondence), and negation (e.g., reciprocity). Their constructive products are equilvalence, ordered nonequivalence, and reversible relations between elements, sets, and series.

The development during infancy that I have proposed comprises two progressive levels in the organization of logicomathematical cognition. The first year of infancy is dominated by the formation of first-order combinativity, relational, and conditional operations. While first-order operations continue to progress during the second year, they begin to lose their primacy

---

[1]Elsewhere I have referred, more precisely, to these two basic forms as proto-operations and protofunctions. Here I will sacrifice precision for stylistic fluency without, however, in any way implying that the discussion is about anything more advanced than proto-operations and protofunctions.

in cognitive development. The shift in structural development is directed toward the formation of second-order combinativity, relational, and conditional operations.

First-order operations construct elementary equivalence, nonequivalence (iterative ordering), and reversible relations between elements and within single sets and single series. Objects are composed so as to form single sets; sets are not related to each other to form binary compositions; objects are added to and subtracted from each other to produce single ordered series; objects are exchanged within single sets to maintain consecutive equivalence between quantities; and both ordered nonequivalence and unordered equivalence relations are negated to produce elementary reversibility. These constructions constitute some of the central structures of first-order operations.

So, to illustrate, by age 18 months infants consistently unite as many as four nonmalleable objects into compositions. They also consistently reunite these compositions into derivative recompositions. Some of these infants reunite their four-object compositions into derivative four-object recompositions by pragmatic replacement, substitution, and commutativity. All these exchange operations produce quantitative equivalance between compositions and derivative recompositions. Many are featured by inverse reversibility.

The main developments in first-order operations from ages 6 to 18 months are twofold. Their application is expanded to ever larger numbers of objects within single sets and single series; and these constructions become progressively reversible by negation. Still, all first-order operations are limited to producing equivalence, ordered nonequivalence, and reversibility between elements and within single sets or series that infants do not relate to or coordinate with any of their other constructions.

Progressive coordination distinguishes first- from second-order operations. First-order coordinations are limited to elements and single sets or series. Second-order operations coordinate infants' first-order operations into new and more powerful constructions. In effect they constitute coordinations of elementary coordinations. Their most apparent behavioral manifestation is that they apply to two sets or series at the same time or in partial temporal overlap.

To illustrate, by age 18 months infants consistently unite a small number of objects into two separate but related compositions. With rare exceptions, all infants construct two sets of two objects in one-to-one correspondence, such as by building two parallel stacks of two blocks (cf., Sugarman, 1982). Infants also consistently reunite these binary compositions into derivative binary recompositions. For instance, almost half of these 18-month-old infants reunite their binary compositions by pragmatic substitution. Many of these exchange derivations are featured by inverse reversibility. The products of these second-order exchange operations are derivative quantitative equivalences or equivalences of equivalences. In contrast, as noted earlier, the products of first-order exchange operations are only elementary quantitative equivalences.

These findings illustrate a general point about the organization and development of logicomathematical cognition during infancy. Both the constitutive (coordinations) and the constituted (products) structural developments of second-order operations are continuous with and discontinuous from the first-order operations out of which they evolve and which they, in turn, integrate. The constitutive structures of second-order operations are already relatively complex pragmatic computations. Their constituted structures are already relatively powerful logicomathematical derivations of equivalence, ordered nonequivalence, and reversibility.

FUNCTIONS

Parallel developments are expected in the organization and development of physical cognition. In brief, I have proposed that by age 18 months (a) infants develop advanced first-order functions, and (b) the structural dominance is shifting to forming second-order functions.

Both proposals are confirmed by our findings on infants' constructions of causal means-ends transformations. Causal transformations are central to the formation of infants' initial conceptions of physical phenomena.

Two rudimentary but basic forms of first-order causal functions are already generated by infants at age 6 months. One form consists of constructing, minimally replicating, and observing effects that are directly dependent upon causes. For instance, infants use one object as a means to push another object repeatedly while observing their causal constructions. The other complementary form consists of anticipating and observing effects that are dependent upon causes. For instance, infants use one object as a means to block and stop another object that is rolling in front of them while observing the effects of their causal predictions and constructions.

By age 18 months infants semisystematically vary actions and objects when constructing first-order causal functions. They generate ordered series of causal actions in order to produce differential results. For example, they push objects harder and harder; and carefully monitor and replicate the differential results. Infants also vary the causal objects in order to control the effects. For example, they push only one kind of object so that they predetermine the results.

First-order causal functions are elementary dependency relations between means and ends. Formally, they constitute direct ratio relations between independent and dependent causal semivariables, such as "Moving Further is a function of Pushing Harder.'' The functions only relate semivariables because the causes and effects are only partially and semisystematically varied. For instance, infants usually push one of the two kinds of objects presented to them without trying out and determining the differential effects of pushing the other kind of object.

Second-order causal functions coordinate the elementary means-ends transformations of first-order functions. Formally, they constitute proportional relations between independent and dependent causal semi-variables, such as "Moving is a function of Pushing as Stopping is a function of Blocking.'' So 18-month-old infants begin to covary the dependency relations in their means-ends transformations. For instance, they use one object as an instrument with which to push another dependent object; when the effect is that it rolls away, they transform the instrument into a means with which to block the dependent object; and so on.

Thus, infants begin to covary the dependencies between causal means and ends in second-order functions. Ends depend on means and means depend on ends in first-order functions but they are not coordinated with each other. Second-order functions coordinate means-ends relations by proportional covariation.

Like second-order operations, then, second-order functions are coordinative constructions that produce new and more powerful cognitions. Here, too, the constitutive (e.g., coordination by proportional covariation) and the constituted (e.g., equivalence semivariables) structural developments of second-order functions are both continuous with and discontinuous from the first-order functions out of which they evolve and which they, in turn, integrate.

REPRESENTATION

The literature on symbol formation, including linguistic development, offers sparse guide to determining its semantic and syntactic organization when infants' cognition begins to be representational at around age 18 months. The list of unanswered fundamental questions is long. Is the initial underlying structure of symbolization, including language, semantic, syntactic, or both? Are semantics and syntax different organizations at the initial symbolic and linguistic stages? Is there any difference between deep and surface structures of grammatical relations, such as ''subject of,'' during the initial linguistic stages? Are grammatical relations even part of children's early language? What, if any, are the initial relations between the structures of cognitions and those of the semantics and syntax of symbolization, including language? It is to this last question that I address myself.

To the extent that concept and symbol formation interact to produce

representational cognition at about age 18 months, the predominant influence, I would propose, is that of conception upon symbolization. This
proposal applies to both the semantics and syntax of developing symbolization.

Our working hypothesis is that first- and second-order operations and
functions provide the initial stages of symbolization, including early
language, with a rich and developing conceptual foundation. This conceptual organization is exploited only in part as semantic features for the initiation of symbol formation.

This is the sense in which infants' conceptual structures have implications
for the semantic organizations of their symbolic structures in different
media (e.g., gesture, imagery, and speech). The interactions hypothesized
are not causal but implicatory. Independently developing semantic structures (a) select from the background significances constructed by operations
and functions, and (b) make these selected significances figural in
transformed expressive symbols in various media. The rules governing
selection and figural expression are inherent structural properties of symbolic systems that, as such, are independently developing structures.

The findings reviewed in the previous sections support the claim that the
conceptual structures that have developed by age 18 months include
relatively complex second-order constructions, such as proportional causal
functions. In comparison, any accompanying symbolic expressions are
most limited. Usually infants only symbolize a feature of the causal event
(*18BB* and *18PC*), or the object used in the causal construction (*18KM*), or
the action involved in the causal transformation (*18SO*):

> 5. BH knock over Red Cylinder 1, Red Cylinder 2, Blue Hexagonal Column
>   3, and Blue Hexagonal Column 2   subject: "Boing."
>   (*18BB*, page 60)
> 31. LH pushes Car   subject: "Vroummmm..."
>   (*18PC*, page 12)
>   3. RH rolls VW4 back and forth, twice   subject: "Car."
>   4. RH touches VW3
>   5. RH rolls VW3 back and forth, twice   subject: "Car."
>   (*18KM*, page 22)
> 20. RH tries to put Car 1 in LH
> 20a. C1 falls   subject: "Drop."
> 21. RH picks up C1 and tries again to place C1 in LH
> 21a. C1 falls again   subject: "Drop."
>   (*18SO*, page 58)

These symbolic productions are typical. At this age causatives are usually
limited to onomatopoetic or one-word utterances. Only one infant (out of
12 subjects tested) produced more advanced linguistic causatives; they all
accompanied her decompositions of Play-Doh objects:

9.	BH pull Left Piece into two	subject:	"Broke it.
			I broke it."
16.	LH puts Piece down she just pulled off Circular Ring 1	subject:	"I broke."
17.	LH pulls Piece 1 off Ball 3	subject:	"Peel."
23.	LH pulls Piece 3 off B3	subject:	"Peeling."
62.	LH pulls Piece 4 off Ball 1	subject:	"Doo. Ball."

(*18SO*, pages 28–31)

This is the most sophisticated linguistic behavior produced by any subject at this age. Subject *18SO* verbally describes her decompositions by three causative phrases (i.e., "I broke it," "Peeling," and "Doo. Ball."). Still, even this most advanced set of causative expressions does not approach or exploit as semantic elements the complexity of infants' causal significances, which, we have seen, include rudimentary second-order functions. Infants generate much more complex causal cognitions than one could ever suspect from examining only their symbolic causative productions. This is why it is possible for infants' linguistic comprehension to exceed their linguistic production.

Our working hypothesis on initial syntactic development parallels that on semantic development. First- and second-order operations and functions constitute a developing structural grammar of elementary cognitions that prepares infants for producing and comprehending both pretense and arbitrary but governing rules of communication. As such they provide the required foundations for and may facilitate infants' acquisition of symbolic syntax. Only part of this foundational grammatical knowledge, however, is exploited by the syntax of any given symbolic medium, such as language, at its inception.

At age 18 months the grammar of infants' elementary cognitive activity includes planned constructions using all objects, as long as they are few in number, within brief time spans and small spatial frameworks. They usually involve binary and ternary mappings (action-to-object relations) that are well differentiated and sequentially integrated with each other. The results are relatively well-designed routines:

19.5.   RH picks up Yellow Cup and sets it down upright on table
19.5.   LH holds Red and Yellow Spoons
21.   LH again inserts RS in YC and moves RS up and down inside of YC rapidly many times, hitting the edge of YC; while LH also holds YS outside of YC
21a.   YC is knocked over
22.   LH presses RS inside YC; while LH holds YS outside of YC
22a.   YC presses against subject's body
23.   LH raises both spoons; inserts YS into Red Cup and moves YS up and down inside of RC rapidly many times, while LH also holds RS outside of RC

24. LH continues motion with both spoons as in No. 23 but over table—
    not into either cup and not hitting against table
25. LH inserts RS into RC; while LH holds YS outside of RC
26.5. LH removes RS from RC as also continues to hold YS as placing YC
    upright with RH
26.5. RH sets YC upright
28.5. LH places RS in RC while holding YS outside of RC
28.5a. RC falls over
28.5. RH touches YC

(*18MK*, pages 6–7)

These well-organized routines represent but a small fragment of *18MK*'s systematic transactions. They are preceded and followed by many repetitions and variations on a basic theme: successively setting up the two cups with one hand, such that the other hand can then insert (i.e., place, move, hit, or press) one spoon into one cup while simultaneously holding another spoon outside of the cup.

At the time of construction, the only apparent link is that the transactions are generated simultaneously (lines 26.5.–28.5.). Shortly, however, it becomes evident that the subject has prepared the conditions for successive operational coordination:

34. LH inserts Red Spoon into Yellow Cup, not looking; while LH holds
    Yellow Spoon outside of YC
35. LH moves RS up and down inside of YC, not looking; while LH holds
    YS outside of YC
35a. YC is knocked over

(*18MK*, page 7)

The results are successive and reproductive insertions of the same spoon into the two different cups; thereby forming reversible correspondences coordinated with reversible substitutions.

Two developments mark infants' syntax of action at age 18 months. The first consists of elaborating a small set of relatively new mapping forms, such as "inserting." Some of these new mapping forms are marked by conventional or semiconventional symbolic features (e.g., *18MK*).

The second advance consists of combining elementary mapping forms into small but coordinated mapping routines; such as "pick-up then transfer and collect" and "inserting while holding and uprighting." Sequential integration into rule-governed forms begins by coordinating a very small number of elementary mapping forms into brief but well-designed combinations, that is, short protosyntactic routines. They are often reproduced many times such that they become fairly well practiced rule-governed routines; and they are applied to all the objects as long as the number is small.

Infants' mapping routines do not exhibit many features that mark fully syntactic constructions; for instance, they lack hierarchic organization. Yet these routines are already marked by other features of syntax, such as interruption that is clearly and repeatedly evident in *18MK*'s mapping routines (cf., Goodson & Greenfield, 1975). Although rule-governed, these routines are only protosyntactic because they are constructed by the individual and may (e.g., insert spoon into cup) or may not (e.g., pick up, transfer, and collect all objects) also conform to conventional or semiconventional rules of symbolic behavior. Moreover, the enactments of protosyntactic routines are less permanent and probably much less constrained (or have many more degrees of freedom) than fully syntactic productions. As such they are more idiosyncratic constructions and less efficient as potential communicative systems than are fully syntactic symbolic systems. Consequently, they are less amenable to the social feedback necessary for them to be elaborated into fully communicative symbolic systems.

A consequence of these protosyntactic transactions is that the semantic domain constructed by infants is expanding exponentially, to the second and sometimes third degree. Infants no longer construct the semantic domain of transactions as simply representing elementary forms, such as "pushables" and "holdables." The semantic domain is elaborated by infants to include protosyntactic combinations of elementary forms, usually taken two-at-a-time but sometimes already three-at-a-time. Such rudimentary mapping routines entail minor reconstructive and anticipatory extensions of immediate into mediate representations by infants. Thus, they constitute the necessary structural developmental conditions whereby here-and-now protosymbolic mappings are initially transformed into not-here-and-not-now symbolic systems or languages.

The semantic domain remains protosymbolic insofar as the representations constructed by infants at this stage are not yet fully detached from the objects of their transactions, are not yet arbitrary constructions, and are not yet fully conventional communicative systems. Yet, the semantic domain is becoming symbolic as a function of infants' progressive flexibility in combining mapping forms into small routines marked by rudimentary protosyntactic, reproductive, and anticipatory features.

Conventional and semiconventional symbolic features progressively mark (a) mapping forms that are already generated sometimes at previous stages as well as this stage (*18BB*), and (b) new mapping forms that are never generated at previous stages (*18KM*):

    6.   RH brushes her hair (from front to back) with back of Brush for about 15 seconds, as laughs and smiles

  10.   RH brushes her hair (from front to back) with back of Mirror

  14.   RH brushes her hair (from back to front) for about 8 seconds

  18.   RH brushes her hair with bristle side of B

  33.   RH holding Spoon waves or brushes through her hair

                                            (*18BB*, pages 1–5)

    7.   RH scoops briefly, twice, in Receptacle 2 with Spoon 2

    8.   LH picks up Spoon 1 and scoops briefly in Receptacle 2

                                            (*18KM*, page 16)

Subject *18BB* substitutes conventional (a brush) and semiconventional (a mirror, a spoon, her hand, and her arm) objects as functional equivalent means with which to brush her own hair in a variety of conventional and semiconventional (backwards) ways. Subject *18KM*'s scooping transactions are entirely conventional.

Protosyntactic constructions also mark new mapping forms:

19.   RH takes out Green Doll in upside-down position from Orange Cup 2 which is the top cup in previously constructed stack of OC2/Yellow Cup 2/Yellow Cup 1/Orange Cup 1
20.   BH turn GD right-side up in air
21.   BH put GD down on table right-side up to the right of the stack of four cups
22.   RH holds edge of OC2 and extracts OC2 from stack of four cups
23.   RH brings OC2 close to self and tilts OC2
24.   looks in OC2 as BH hold OC2 tilted close to self
25.   mouth makes drinking motion on OC2 held tilted by BH
26.   BH withdraw OC2 from face
27.   BH hold OC2 over table
28.5. RH tilts OC2 over GD as if pouring on GD, as smiles
28.7. LH picks up GD (one-half way through RH's pouring action with OC2)
28.8. LH holds GD closer to lip of "pouring" OC2 held tilted by RH
31.   RH places OC2 upright on table
32.   LH places GD inside of OC2
33.   RH raises OC2 with GD inside
34.   RH tilts OC2 with GD inside toward face and looks inside

(18BB, pages 33–34)

The protosyntactic routine generated by *18BB* is as complex and well-designed as any found at this stage. It includes preparatory adjustment (lines 19–24), pretend drinking from (line 25), and pretend pouring on a doll (lines 26–28.8.). Such protosyntactic routines, then, include large elements of flexible pretense. For instance, this routine includes transforming pretending to drink liquid from an empty cup into pretending to pour liquid from the same empty cup on a doll.

These constructions are transitional between protosymbolization and true symbolization. Some, as we have just seen, involve playful substitution which is one way of constructing mappings of mappings (cf., Werner & Kaplan, 1963). Playful mapping routines (such as pretending to pour liquid from an empty cup onto a doll) begin to stand for or represent real mappings (such as actually pouring liquid from a container onto an object). They are marked by first-order substitutions (e.g., an empty cup for a full cup). Some of these playful protosyntactic rountines just begin to substitute and match (by one-to-one correspondence) arbitrary objects and prototypical objects (cf. Fein, 1975):

11.5. RH brushes hair (front to back) with Triangular Column 4 for 10 seconds

11.5. LH brushes hair (front to back) with Triangular Column 3 for 10
seconds

(18BB, page 68)

Playful mapping routines even begin, on rare occasions and in rudimentary ways, to substitute organs for conventional instruments (cf., E. Kaplan, 1968; Overton & Jackson, 1973). Recall, as an illustration, that *18BB* uses her hand and her arm (perhaps together with a spoon) as substitutes for a brush (lines 14 and 33 presented on page 229).

These semisymbolic constructions, we have seen, are marked by two important features. First, they are protosyntactic. They comprise rule-governed sequentially ordered mapping routines. On the one hand, these mapping routines are marked by regularity of reproduction. Their repetitions are constrained to fairly exact copies. On the other hand, these mapping routines are marked by some flexibility and minor arbitrariness. For instance, different means may be substituted for each other (such as mirrors, spoons, and cylinders for brushes) within a given mapping routine. These objects are transformed into an equivalence class of "Brushes" by first-order functions. Thus, they are progressively detached as protosymbolic forms.

The second important feature marking semisymbolization is the conventionalization of mappings. On the one hand, these mapping forms are generated by infants in accordance with their own operational and functional level of cognition. On the other hand, the mapping forms progressively conform to properties of conventional usage, such as pretending to eat or mix with a spoon.

REPRESENTATIONAL COGNITION

The syntax of symbolization in action (e.g., *18BB*'s pretend drink from and pour on routines) is at least as complex as the potential syntax of symbolization in words during this age period; although there may be some rare exceptions to this structural developmental asynchrony, as noted below. The mean length of linguistic utterances at age 18 months is just about one word (e.g., Brown, 1973) and their meanings are holophrastic (Werner & Kaplan, 1963). Agent, action, and object are differentiated and coordinated (serially but not hierarchically) by symbols in action routines while this is not possible, semantically or syntactically, by one-word utterances.

The syntax of symbolization in words catches up with, overtakes, and outstrips that of symbolization in action during late infancy and early childhood. Precisely how and when this developmental reversal between symbols in action and symbols in words takes place are unsolved problems that require much theoretical analysis and empirical investigation. One hypothesis about the process is that primitive symbolization in words begins by "piggybacking" on more advanced symbolization in action. This might solve the problem of how verbal syntax catches up with action syntax. But it could not account for how verbal syntax eventually outstrips action syntax. This would required postulating the emergence of a mechanism that is, as yet, indeterminate. On this hypothesis, totally different processes would have to be proposed to account for the "catching up" and the "outstripping" phases of linguistic development. While possible, this is an inelegant and nonparsimonious theoretical solution.

The only verbal production we found at age 18 months that is comparable to the symbols in action level of grammatical complexity was generated by only one infant, *18SO* (see protocol fragment on page 227). Producing phrases such as "Broke it. I broke it." and "I broke." is much more complex than that usually found at this age (e.g., Braine, 1963; Brown, 1973). Moreover, current linguistic analyses are unable to determine whether the underlying structures of such verbal productions reflect semantic rules about agent, action, and patient, or syntactic rules about subject, verb, and object, or neither semantic nor syntactic rules (e.g., Bowerman, 1978). In any case, such unusually sophisticated linguistic phrasing by one infant does not exceed the grammatical complexity of the symbols in action routines that are generated by almost all infants at age 18 months.

We must also not overlook the fact that the structure of second-order functions already encompasses relatively complex conceptual relations between constructed agents, actions, and objects. Their relations, as wc have seen, are already governed by proportional schemes. Neither our own data nor any I know of in the literature even hints at the possibility that symbolization at age 18 months is governed by syntactic rules that approach the complexity and semisystematicity of rudimentary proportionality. Symbol formation in all media, including language, shows no evidence of being able to exploit the products of such advanced concept formation during this age period.

Notice, further, that the structures of physical cognitions are of a piece; they constitute a unified organization of one fundamental form—functions. Similarly, logicomathematical cognitions take one fundamental form—operations. In contrast with the unity of concept formation, symbol formation varies, often radically, with the medium of expression; from the highly graphic and motoric (as in gesture and drawing) to the ever more arbitrary and stipulated (as in speech and, especially, mathematics). This one-to-many relation between concept and symbol formation accounts, at least in part, for the initial lag of symbol formation behind conceptual development.

Four interactive relations between concept and symbol formation are possible when infants begin to be representational in the age period under consideration. The first two possible relations are symmetrical. Concept and symbol formation may be dependent systems of structural development that influence each other mutually and equally. Alternatively, they may be totally independent structural systems that have no implicatory relations to each other. Between these two extremes are two possible asymmetrical relations between concept and symbol formation. In both instances the structural systems are independent; but concept formation may have implicatory consequences for symbol formation and/or symbol formation may have implicatory consequences for concept formation.

Our data are consistent with the third and fourth possibilities only. As we have seen, the development of elementary (first- and second-order) logicomathematical operations and physical functions is not dependent upon the development of symbolic activity. Correlatively, we have found no evidence to indicate that elementary symbol formation is dependent upon concept formation; although our data do not bear as directly and comprehensively upon this possibility.

While elementary concept and symbol formation are independent structural systems, the development of one has implications for the development of the other. We have observed, for instance, how the construction of elementary physical concepts develops independently of symbol formation. Indeed, developing physical cognition precedes symbol formation about physical phenomena. This permits cognition to provide symbolization with a growing conceptual organization of the significance of physical phenomena, such as the covariation between causal and dependent semivariables. The semantic and syntactic organization of early language, and other symbolic media, exploits only a subset of infants' conceptual organization. And since, by hypothesis, conception precedes symbolization, then the formation of physical symbols (such as causatives) is expected and found to be more primitive than physical concepts (such as causal functions) during this formative stage of representational cognition.

The development of elementary symbolization has implications for concept formation as well. Symbolization may be exploited by infants to facilitate and expand elementary operations and functions. For instance, we have observed that playful pretense permits substitution of present and arbitrary (e.g., a column) for nonpresent and prototypic (e.g., a brush) objects. Symbolization thereby expands the computational range of operations and functions. It does so in at least two basic ways. First, it multiplies the constant given elements of operations and functions. Second, it increases the problem space to which operations and functions apply.

Our results, then, support the hypothesis that the transformation of first- into second-order operations and functions initiates the structural development of elementary representation. Symbolization expands elementary representation by extending it to the not-here and the not-now. Thus we are beginning to determine how representational cognition develops and what is its structural organization.

ACKNOWLEDGMENT

The research reported was supported, in part, by funds provided by the Institute of Human Development, University of California, Berkeley.

REFERENCES

Bowerman, M. Structural relationships in children's utterances: Syntactic or semantic? In L. Bloom (Ed.), *Readings in language development*. New York: Wiley, 1978.

Braine, M. D. S. The ontogeny of English phrase structure: The first phrase. *Language,* 1963, *39,* 1–13.

Brown, R. *A first-language: The early stages.* Cambridge: Harvard University Press, 1973.

Fein, G. A. A transformational analysis of pretending. *Developmental Psychology,* 1975, *11,* 291–296.

Goodson, B., & Greenfield, P. The search for structural principles in children's manipulative play: A parallel with linguistic development. *Child Development,* 1975, *46,* 734–746.

Kaplan, E. *Gestural representation of implement usage: An organismic developmental study.* Unpublished doctoral dissertation, Clark University, 1968.

Langer, J. *The origins of logic: Six to twelve months.* New York: Academic Press, 1980.

Langer, J. Logic in infancy. *Cognition,* 1981, *10,* 181–186.

Langer, J. From prerepresentational to representational cognition. In G. Forman (Ed.), *Action and thought*. New York: Academic Press, 1982.

Langer, J. *The origins of logic: One to two years.* In preparation.

Overton, W. F., & Jackson, J. P. The representation of imagined objects in action sequences: A developmental study. *Child Development,* 1973, *44,* 309–314.

Piaget, J. *Play, dreams and imitation in childhood.* New York: Norton, 1931.

Piaget, J. *The language and thought of the child.* New York: Meridian, 1926/1955.

Sugarman, S. Transitions in early representational intelligence. In G. Forman (Ed.), *Action and thought*. New York: Academic Press, 1982.

Vygotsky, L. S. *Thought and language.* Cambridge: MIT Press, 1934/1962.

Werner, H. *Comparative psychology of mental development.* New York: International Universities Press, 1948.

Werner, H., & Kaplan, B. *Symbol formation.* New York: Wiley, 1963.

13 Figurative Action from the Perspective of Genetic-Dramatism

Leonard Cirillo
Bernard Kaplan
Clark University

INTRODUCTION

Genetic-Dramatism seeks not only to delineate how we human beings work in conflict and cooperation to form ourselves and our world, but also to improve the ways in which we and others go about living with each other and ourselves (Kaplan, this volume). The dramatistic aspect of our approach focuses, in detail, on the ways that human beings act in context by employing various means to realize their ends (Burke, 1945, 1972). Specifically, dramatism stresses the pervasive role of symbolic action in human affairs, highlighting the ways in which human beings act, speak, gesture, and produce things to express who they take themselves to be; to define and redefine the scenes in which they operate; to sanctify or condemn their actions; to form and reform their goals.

The "genetic" or developmental aspect of our approach emphasizes not only that human beings are "goaded by a spirit of perfection" (Burke, 1966), but also that human beings ought to work to perfect themselves and to help perfect others (Kaplan, this volume). We are, therefore, not concerned with the varieties of symbolic action merely for their own sake, as a purely theoretical or taxonomic enterprise. We wish to know how symbolic action works so that we may (1) discern and resist those forms of symbolic action noxious to human welfare, and (2) determine how best to intervene symbolically in our own lives and in the lives of others, so as to promote those "functions of reason" to which Whitehead (1929) alluded in his famous book—to live, to live well, and to live better.

This practical interest has directed us to those situations in which symbolic actions radically alter the customary ways in which individuals envisage themselves and their worlds and thereby transform the ways in which individuals act in the world. Some believe that such radical transformations may be brought about by pellucid logical argument and the adduction of facts. Such a belief is based on the assumption, or the hope, that symbolic actions are univocal, constant in meaning and reference, fixed in connotation and denotation. Some even insist on this myth of "proper meaning" in hopes of achieving or enforcing perfect communication. To the contrary, we maintain that all symbolic action is constructive or creative (Cassirer, 1944; Kaplan, 1962, this volume) and inherently open to multiple interpretation. In our view, literality is the result of the tacit establishment of a community, all of whose members see the world only in a certain way and talk about it only in a certain way. Within such a shared orientation, there may be clear univocality, literal fact, logical argument, straightforward request, and the like. But this depends on a customary way of envisaging oneself and one's world; it cannot be presupposed as the means of radically transforming the orientation of someone who does not already participate in the scheme of orientation.

Where symbolic actions based on such presuppositions fail, other actions that may seem to provide neither information nor argument may exert enormous power: a story, a witticism, a melody, an allusion, a certain smile. Such symbolic actions we have called *figurative,* borrowing a term usually reserved for certain speech acts. Figurative actions, then, are those symbolic actions which may radically transform one's orientation; rather than presupposing a shared vision of reality, they seemingly pertain to one orientation toward the world, but simultaneously pertain to one or more others, thereby transcending a conventional orientation.

Of course, we are all conventional in certain domains and at certain times, forgetting that our structuring in the world is but one among many. Only in the clash of perspectives, where one individual or group challenges another and seeks to influence the other to see the world in a new way and to act in a new way, does the creative (mind-molding) character inherent in all symbolic action stand out. It is for this reason that special attention is merited by those transactions in which one is trying to shake another out of his/her "dogmatic slumbers" or persuade another that his/her customary way of envisioning the world is hazaradous to his or her health. Politicians, priests, and promoters of new paradigms in science are clearly among those most likely to engage in obvious figuration action. So, too, poets and advertisers. Although we shall, now and then, consider some specimens from these sources, because of our special interest, we draw most of our illustrations here from psychotherapeutic transactions.

SPEAKING METAPHORICALLY

Relatively early in their work, both Heinz Werner and Kenneth Burke concerned themselves with what both took to be a central function of metaphor, a revolutionary one. In his book on the origins of metaphor, Werner took himself to be investigating the power "to break through customary ways of thinking" (1919, p. 6). And Burke, in his justly famous discussion of metaphor as perspective by incongruity, considered metaphor to be a "shattering on fragmentation" of an old orientation "by the merging of categories once felt to be mutually exclusive" (1954, p. 69). Both thought of "metaphor" in a very broad sense, going far beyond the intrusion of alien words or phrases in proper sentences.

Now, the bulk of psychological research on figurative speech, at least until recently, has emphasized the "merging of categories" occurring within a single, decontextualized metaphoric utterance (cf. Honeck & Hoffman, 1980), that trick in a phrase or sentence which Beardsley (1962) dubbed the *metaphorical twist*. For example, when Marx commented that government was "the executive committee of the bourgeoisie," he was breaking the bounds of convention and trying to reform our conceptions both of government and the middle class. For some researchers, it is these kinds of internally anomalous utterances that are taken as paradigmatic of figurative language and figurative action generally.

Yet it is clear that the experience of incongruity that leads one to think that such an utterance is metaphorical may take place in transactions involving utterances that are in no way semantically anomalous. Phrases and sentences perfectly proper in terms of some received view of syntactic and semantic propriety may, as symbolic actions, function figuratively because, in the scenes in which they occur, they evoke some sense of incongruity or insinuate into the concrete context of their occurrence another imagined dramatic scenario that may transform the ways in which we see ourselves and our situation.

Consider a subtle example from the hypnotist, Milton Erickson (Haley, 1973, pp. 189ff). Erickson's 3-year-old son had suffered profuse bleeding from a split lip and a displaced tooth. After verbally reflecting his son's pain and the desire for the suffering to stop, Erickson turned to his wife to comment on the large quantity of blood on the pavement, and asked her to check whether it was "good, red, strong blood." They agreed that it seemed to be, but that this could better be determined against the white background of a sink. Once there, they and the no longer sobbing boy could observe that his blood "mixed properly with water," and gave it a "proper pink color." Further inspection showed the boy's mouth to be "bleeding right" and "swelling right." Having satisfied himself aloud of his son's "essential and pleasing soundness in every way," Erickson told the boy that although he would have stitches in his lip, it was doubtful that he could have as many as he could count up to; he might not even have ten, though he could count to twenty. It was too bad that he could not have seventeen like his sister, Betty Alice, or twelve, like his brother, Allan; but he could have more than Bert, or Lance, or Carol. The boy counted the stitches as they were taken, and expressed disappointment when only seven were required.

To Erickson's own comment that his son was never given a false statement, we would like to add that he was never given a metaphorical one either, not in the "literal" sense of that term. Yet, despite the absence of any semantic anomaly, each aspect of the situation that would conventionally be interpeted in terms of injury, pain, and suffering came *also* to signify rightness and soundness. The sutures themselves were not simply means to close his split lip, but emblems of his new status among his older sibs. The surgeon, catching on to the scene-shifting operation, pointed out that the suture material was of a new and better kind than had been used with the sibs, and informed the boy that the scar would form the letter of his daddy's college! In this merging of categories ordinarily taken to be mutually exclusive, a scene of accidental suffering and injury is compensated by a narcissistic distinction. What would normally be taken in one way is, through Erickson's symbolic action, looked at from another perspective and transvalued almost into a scenario in which one is rewarded and elevated in status for valorous action. Despite the absence of a figurative utterance, in the "literal" sense, we submit that symbolic actions such as Erickson's are figurative actions.

From our perspective, figurative utterances in the "literal sense" are simply special cases within an "autonomous linguistic medium" (Werner & Kaplan, 1963, pp. 52–62) of the kinds of incongruities between agents and actions, actions and scenes, etc. that occur all the time in everyday life, when one would normally not even think of the operation of metaphors, metonymies, and other tropes. Just as "matter out of place" becomes "dirt," a symbolic action in the "wrong scene" or by the "wrong agent" becomes figurative action.

THE THERAPY OF POLITICS AND THE POLITICS
OF THERAPY

Those adopting a conservative stance toward symbolic action are convinced that figurative action does not transform reality but obscures the true nature of things. They believe that there is one way things are or ought to be and that it is possible through symbols unambiguously to designate the facts. But from our viewpoint, figuration is the means of creating new visions and of uncovering realities invisible to the corporeal eye. Literal language reflects the vision of those who already see eye-to-eye and mistake a limited convention of vision and of thought for nature unadorned. Since one is liable to suffer from eyestrain and nausea in considering several perspectives at once, it is not surprising that we are all literalists, to varying degrees, and much of the time. However, when we manage to step back and consider the possibilities from different angles, we may conclude that figurative action has the power to redefine reality because symbolic action defined it in the first place.

In the *Philosophy of Literary Form,* Burke (1973) remarked that:

> The magical decree is implicit in all language, for the mere act of naming an object or situation decrees that it is to be singled out as such-and-such rather than as something-other. Hence . . . an attempt to *eliminate* magic, in this sense, would involve us in the elimination of vocabulary itself as a way of sizing up reality [p. 4].

Thus, we are not in a situation where the choice is between magic and non-magic. Our choice is between one magic or another. Only an "infinite, omniscient mind" can achieve a completely accurate sizing up of reality.

That we work magic with words becomes obvious when we contend to rework our realities with other words. When acts that are obviously *treasonous* to some become *revolutionary* for others, when one group's obvious attempt to *save the nation* is another's *insurrection,* then the competing vocabularies tell us that events become what they are by virtue of the stance we take toward them and our attitude toward events both generates our verbal strategies and is reshaped by them. Political examples highlight the power aspects ingredient in any social intercourse: Any utterance may be viewed as an attentuated political act insofar as it exercises power over the definition of situations.

In a paper on hidden value judgments, Felix S. Cohen (1954) remarked that the value system shared by those within a group becomes embodied in a code and that the code reinforces the implicit standards of the group. He says,

> These codes become particularly important in a political campaign. Our candidates may *inspire;* they never *inflame* as do the other fellow's candidates. Our candidates may *demonstrate;* only their opposing candidates *allege.* Our candidates may *clarify;* only their opponents will *admit error.* Our candidates may *discern, enlighten, assist, serve, catalyze, counsel* or *cooperate.* On no account will they *theorize, propagandize, abet, interfere, instigate, incite, or conspire* [p. 553].

So also with regard to clashing evaluations of our words and theirs: We speak out openly and honestly, they manipulate the language to secure their narrow ends; we describe what is real, they distort it. Those who are identified with one another hear the ring of truth in their utterances; their enemies hear the Siren's call and lash themselves to the mast.

Burke (1954) discusses psychoanalytic therapy in the light of these powers of speech, likening cures to conversions and rebirths, and dubbing as "exorcism by misnomer" any use of a vocabulary of conversion to transform the frightening into the harmless. Following Bentham, he distinguishes such conversions downward (making molehills out of mountains) from conversions upwards (making a silk purse of a sow's ear). He suggests that two features characterize the conversion techniques of the various psychoanalytic schools: One is converting the patient's distress downward by means of an incongruous terminology, and the second is developing a substitute terminology providing the patient with a brand-new rationalization of motives.

Contemporary proponents of strategic therapies call similar reorientations *reframing*—changing the meaning of a situation by changing its viewpoint or setting (Watzlawick, Weakland, & Fisch, 1974), or *relabeling*—reframing by verbal means (Weeks & L'Abate, 1979). Among the tactics involving a vocabulary of conversion are: substituting *steadfast purpose* for *rigidity, taking care of oneself* for *withdrawal, sponatneous* for *impulsive, protection from hurt* for *avoiding intimacy* (Weeks & L'Abate, 1979), and so forth. The examples need not be multiplied since they completely parallel those offered by Cohen (1954) from political and legal domains, and they equally well illustrate his point that "almost any human characteristic may be described either in honorific or pejorative terms" (p. 552). Further, every such description may both express a value of the describer's and regulate an attitude of the listener's. Those descriptions that seem to us literally true are descriptions that conform to our "customary ways of thinking."

THE POWERS OF FIGURATIVE ACTION

From our perspective, figurative actions may be viewed as having two, connected, powers of organization. One is patent. When we name or characterize a situation in one or another way, we automatically, by virtue of the generalizing power of names to which Vygotsky (1962) among others has pointed, group that situation as a member of the same class as other situations thus named. Simultaneously we distinguish it from all others. The action of naming is not a mere labeling of a content that remains otherwise unmolested. The content is seen under a special illumination or through a certain set of spectacles—and one responds to that content as if it were what it was called. A figurative way of characterizing something newly unites that something with other states of affairs or entities with which it now seems naturally to belong and concurrently separates that something from other states of affairs or entities from which it now seems essentially to differ. Figurative action is therefore the power through which we reclassify and reorganize what there is.

But figurative actions possess a second reorganizing power. They concurrently serve to unite and divide *us* as we concur in or contest definitions of situation. Each figurative defining of a situation newly unites or identifies us with all those sharing the position or perspective from which that definition appears natural. And each such definition newly separates us from all those others defining the situation otherwise, that is, all those we view as distorting the situation and approaching it from some aberrant position or perspective, perhaps from "out in left field" or from "outer space." Every figurative action, then, reorganizes not only our worlds but also ourselves.

For example, when a court begins an opinion on an Indian property case by referring to Indians *roaming, wandering,* or *roving,* one can be fairly certain that the property rights claimed by the Indians are about to be rejected, for these are terms commonly used to describe the movements of buffalo, wolves, and other subhuman animals devoid of property rights; to ourselves, we would apply terms connoting social actions that are distinctively human, such as *traveling, vacationing,* or *commuting* (Cohen, 1954). Words shape reality and they do so in correspondence with social purposes. When a property court uses relatively indeterminate verbs to characterize the Indians' activity, the court separates them from the rest of us, and groups them with roving animals.

Similarly, when the family or group therapist renames or misnames an individual's actions honorifically, upgrading them from sins to virtues, from curses to blessings, the therapist at one and the same time is reclassifying the action so named and healing a division between the group and the pariah. So, for example, rather than view a child's problem behavior as an individual aberration or as a function of the child's role in a family conflict, we may view the problematic behavior as an attempt to help others in the family and view the child as a benefactor who is protecting others (Madanes, 1980, 1981). Then, the little devil is revealed as a fallen angel: The child has the best of intentions, only the means are ill-adapted to realizing those high purposes. Among the high purposes of apparently "low" behaviors may be: distracting others from their worrisome preoccupations, interrupting hostilities between others, sacrificing oneself so that another may go free, revealing defects so that another may seem whole, and so forth. These ways of recharacterizing symptoms are also ways of rehabilitating outcasts.

The therapist's renamings are directed not only toward rehabilitation of the outcast but also toward his or her own acceptance by the group. Some therapists who perceive certain families to "counter the therapist's every move with monolithic attack or resistance . . . shift quickly to some form of positive interpretation, praising the family and members and trying to reduce their resistance through ascribing the most noble of intentions to their actions" (Stanton, 1981). Positive interpretation of the actions of the members of an intimate group repairs division within the group and fosters acceptance of the interpreter as one with the group, at least in spirit.

Neither the therapist identifying both himself and the black sheep with the family nor the court disaffiliating the Indians represented these social purposes in explicit words. The court did not say that since the Indians are essentially different from us human beings they cannot have property rights. The therapist did not say that all of us, little Johnny and me too, have the family's best interests at heart, so let's all work together. Or, at least they did not say so directly, and the indirect ways in which they did say so are more typical of the ways we maintain and transform our relationships with one another.

Even these examples are notably transparent because those making the statements directly characterize those from whom they want identification or distance. The therapist characterizes the actions of the family members; the court characterizes the actions of the Indians. More commonly, however, people show one another by their garb and gestures, by their talk and tone, that they belong together or that they are divided. And these expressions of unity and division become means of bringing about unity and division where there was none. The catalogue of those ways in which we join and separate while speaking of other matters can not be summarized here (cf. Burke, 1966, 1973; Goffman, 1959, 1979; Perelman & Olbrechts-Tyteca, 1969), but we can attend to these matters in arenas closer to home.

THE HOME FRONT

Surely, we are now convinced, if we needed convincing, that people are constantly engaged in applying new names to old situations or old names to new ones, in order now, to maintain the status quo, now, radically to alter it. It would, of course, be an egregious error to conclude that such word-magic, such "displacement of concepts" (Schön, 1963) affects only the gullible and the guilty, or is exploited only by professional priests, practitioners, and politicians. It would reflect that "certain blindness in human nature" were we to conform to that law of human transactions: the greater probability of seeing the mote in the eye of another than the beam in one's own.

Rather, let us heed the suggestion of a philosopher (Schwayder, 1965) that psychologists might find it more informative in studying human nature to reflect critically on their own actions involved in defining their field, defining their subject-matter, defining their "findings," rather than merely to report the results ostensibly derived from an unbiased study of "other ones." For example, one might find it more profitable to examine our "construction of the child" than the "child's construction of reality"; our "construction of the development of the child" rather than "the child's development"; our "construction of the patient" rather than "the patient's aberrancies"—our ways of constituting any subject-matter or object prior to our "studying or investigating" the subject-matter or object. The philosopher, of course, was merely invoking the Socratic dictum, "Know thyself" before thou pretendest to know anything else. Doubtless, he was proposing that we envision our field in ways different from those to which we had become accustomed.

Consider how we struggle over the definition of our "field," our professional scene(s) of action. "What is 'psychology?' " is as much an object of contention as "what is justice?" or "what is scientific method?" (Black, 1954) or "What is an experiment?" And the same struggle takes place over the definition and boundaries of the several "states" of our "nation"; "What is clinical psychology?" "What is developmental psychology?" "What is cognitive psychology?" "What is experimental psychology?" We may avoid some friction and make a show of tolerance, by constituting "cities," "towns," or even "communities" in the states and the nation, small enclaves of those who wear the same clothes, walk in the same way, talk in the same way, think in the same way; still preserving our national identity ("we are all psychologists") while designating our distinctiveness and separateness. Some, of course, disgusted with it all, may become migrants or expatriates, identifying themselves with another "nation," with more congenial and correct ways of talking, seeing, thinking.

It would be nice to believe, despite all this contentiousness, that we respect each other's rules, regulations, ways of being, and ways of thinking, just as the states within our country respect each other. It would be nice to believe that we value equality of opportunity and equal access to resources. And we might adopt that posture in times of affluence, all living harmoniously under the same roof. Graciously, we might concede that no state, city or community is privileged or central; that no way of talking (Burke's "terministic screen") is literal; that no way of acting or thinking is the right way.

But is not this "show of tolerance," and respect for the perspectives of others, ideal though it may be, a mask? Given the expulsion from the Garden of Eden or the "fall," are we not, covertly in times of affluence, overtly in times of retrenchment, likely to take our "community" as the center (cf. Eliade, 1959)? Our Way (met-hodos) as the true way? Our "construction of reality," even our construction of others' "constructions of reality" as, somehow, given by God or inherent in Nature? Indeed, do not even those of us who value "decentering," take our state or community as the center, and characterize all other realms on the map—allies, neutral, enemies—in terms of their relations to us? And if someone else challenges, by word or gesture, our position in the center, are we not moved to strike back, construing their action as "obstructionist," "petty," "pedantic," "motivated by self-interest," and in terms of all the other pejoratives to which Cohen (1954) refers?

Obviously, in characterizing what we do in "political language," and in terms "properly" belonging to the description of "cults," we have used figurative action. And such usage is intended to provoke in the reader a perspective by incongruity; to transform, if only transiently, a way of orienting oneself in the world. Some may angrily insist that we have misrepresented the way things are. Others may both accept and reject our attempt, characterizing it as "mere" metaphor. Still others may accept this view of what takes place among a group of academics, and come to classify our transactions quite naturally with other political and religious transactions, thereby enlarging the proper scope of application of political and religious terminology and, at the same time, instigating "reflective abstraction" (see Melito, 1980).

Those who insist that we have misrepresented may claim that they are able to provide a neutral, literal characterization of what goes on. But surely by now we realize that there is no such beast in the zoo. All attempts to describe what is, including this one, are symbolic actions from a certain perspective, and all classifications, including those used by psychologists to mark off areas, functions, processes, etc., are classifications in the service of certain ends. They are symbolic actions. And if we, or the classifiers, or both, recognize them as "metaphors," they are then figurative actions, in the sense in which we are using that expression.

MUNDANE ALLEGORIES

Besides speaking the literal truth and finding that the literal truths of others contradict our own, we may ourselves say one thing and mean one or more other things besides. The full-blown exemplars come from the literature of allegory—*The Divine Comedy, Pilgrim's Progress,* and so forth. In a letter, Dante speaks of "the truth hidden under a beautiful lie." Such hidden truths depended upon a special view of the cosmos, common to medieval writers (Dunbar, 1929/61; Grandgent, 1933; Wimsatt & Brooks, 1967) but not restricted to them (cf. Lovejoy, 1936; Tillyard, 1959). Allegorical, tropological, and anagogical meanings built on and alongside the literal, resonated in souls accustomed to hermeneutic exegeses of the scriptures and accustomed to viewing the natural world as God's symbolic book.

To minds so constituted, the cosmos is inspired by hidden affinities, and the depths of meaning to be unveiled in literary works are mundane reflections of celestial visions. We are more likely to reduce the heavenly to the earthy as, for example, in inferring bodily urges behind or beneath other activities. Yet, we may be no less likely to govern our actions in harmony with latent correspondences.

When Milton Erickson treated a couple having sexual problems not being discussed directly, he would choose an aspect of their lives analogous to the sexual and, by discussing that aspect, he would seek to influence their sexual relations as well. He might, for example, prefigure changes in sexual relations by contriving to talk

> with them about having dinner together and draw them out on their preferences. He will discuss with them how the wife likes appetizers before dinner, while the husband prefers to dive right into the meat and potatoes. Or the wife might prefer a quiet and leisurely dinner, while the husband, who is quick and direct, just wants the meal over with. If the couple begins to connect what they are saying with sexual relations, Erickson will "drift rapidly" away to other topics, and then he will return to the analogy. He might end such a conversation with a directive that the couple arrange a pleasant dinner on a particular evening that is satisfactory to both of them (Haley, 1973, p. 27).

Perhaps the meal would turn out like the one in the motion picture, *Tom Jones*.

In psychoanalytic treatment, it is orthodox to take the patient's unconstrained speech as allegorical. So, under certain conditions, reporting dreams, narrating early memories, commenting on world events, and the like will be taken as also addressing the relationship to the therapist and indirectly characterizing and attempting to transform that relationship.

For example, a patient who was often quiet or speaking superficially was undergoing pressure from his parents to go into group therapy, presumably as a supplement to his individual therapy. When the therapist confronted the patient about his silence, the patient reported a thought about a ballplayer who was recently traded from one team to another. The therapist commented that a ballplayer cannot play for two teams at once and that the patient's thought of entering group therapy was at the same time a flight from individual therapy. In the subsequent session, after deciding not to enter group therapy, the patient reported a dream in which he was attacked by the dog. The dog could be the therapist, said the patient, but he was unsure. The dog was one that had been loitering around because the patient's roommate had a dog in heat. In the next session, the patient reported almost not coming because of illness and searching for his old medication for stomach upsets; he spoke again of entering group therapy. The therapist commented that the patient saw himself in therapy like his roommate's dog: taking in things from the therapist frightened him and he had to push the therapist away to protect himself. The patient then remembered that the dog had gotten pregnant, been given an injection, and aborted. He went on to talk about his father's ways of prying and getting secrets that the patient kept from him (Langs, 1973, pp. 456–458).

Here, a current event from the newspaper, dream imagery, and a series of events involving dogs are synthesized into an indirect reference to the feared closeness to the therapist whose interventions are experienced as sexual intrusions and from whom distance is being sought.

Sentiments of fear and loathing appear to motivate the indirection of the discourse in the case of the analytic patient, a constellation akin to the connection between metaphor and taboo that was focused on early by Werner (1919; Barten & Franklin, 1978). Similar modes of action can be studied under other conditions by, for example, asking people to do the following. Consider an early event in one's life, say, learning to ride a bicycle. If a client were to describe such early memories in therapy so as to comment indirectly on the relationship to the therapist, what aspects of the relationship might the client be symbolizing? Further, what transformations in the relationship might the client be aiming for? Do the same with any memory, with any current event (shooting of the Pope, marriage of Prince Charles, etc.) or with any fantastic state of affairs, akin to dream imagery. That is, given an image from any source, ask for the range of patient-therapist or two person encounters that one may take the image symbolically to transform.

Consider approaching the same kind of indirect communication the other way around; take a particular encounter or relationship between patient and therapist, say a vacation or a temporary separation; conjure up imagery from some other context to symbolically cope with it. What early memory, what current event, what fantastic constellation of events might represent the episode and imaginatively transform it?

This way of studying mundane allegories can be extended quite generally. The description of any concrete set of events may be used to comment on and transform our relationships with one another. Such interpersonal allegories, in their small way, parallel the moral and anagogic import of the classic literary examples.

SECULAR RITUALS

"Words are also actions, and actions are a kind of words" said Emerson. Although we have mostly emphasized, up to now, figurative words, parallel considerations apply to nonverbal actions. Take an example that is parasitic on verbal discourse. Suppose yourself to be discussing your position on some issue and your interlocutor waves goodbye to you. If the wave is not accompanied by the usual leavetaking, then this conventional act clashes with the current context and provides a metaphorical twist that might be verbally paraphrased, "I am no longer with you on this issue; we have come to a parting of the ways." If, instead, the interlocutor had given a tilt of the head, a twisted smile, and waved by flapping the hand open and shut, you might get the message that he was not waving goodbye to an equal, but was waving "bye-bye" to an inferior. What Firth (1973) called "bodily symbols of greeting and parting" offer rich possibilities for such figurative exploits since they ritually connote joining and separating, elevating and lowering, as social fact.

The participation of nonverbal figurative actions in transforming individuals and groups is particularly familiar from those forms of psychotherapy utilizing dramatic methods; psychodrama (Moreno, 1946), group "games" (Lewis & Streitfeld, 1972; Schutz, 1967; Stevens, 1971), Gestalt therapy (Perls, 1969, 1973; Van de Reit, Korb, & Gorrell, 1980), some forms of family therapy (Bloch, 1973; Madanes, 1981; Selvini-Palazzoli, 1974; Selvini-Palazzoli, Boscolo, Cecchin, & Prata, 1978), and child analysis (cf. Ekstein, 1966).

One of the most provocative of these techniques is prescribing a family ritual. Selvini-Palazzoli and her colleagues conceive of rigid patterns of interaction within a family as grounded in a family myth (Ferreira, 1963) which may have evolved over generations and regard a family ritual as a way

> to change the rules of the game, and therefore the family epistemology, without resorting to explanations, criticism or any other verbal intervention (Selvini-Palazzoli et al., 1978, p. 95).

They believe that a ritual occurring on the level of action is more powerfully transforming than any form of verbalization can hope to be because it is a collective experience in which the behavior of each participant is directed toward a common goal so that new group norms silently replace old ones.

For example, five brothers and their southern Italian families migrated to the city to begin a construction business; their family had been tenant farmers for generations. In the city, they attempted to preserve the myth that the survival and dignity of each member of the extended family depends upon the undifferentiated communion of the whole—"he who separates is lost." As a scenic expression of the myth, the families each moved into an apartment in the same building, but the doors to the apartments were always kept open for the unannounced visits of the others. At the time of therapy, the 15-year-old daughter of one of the families was anorexic (she was five feet nine inches tall and weighed seventy pounds) and was behaving psychotically. She attempted suicide, apparently because the family rule requiring each to speak only well of the others had been violated when she had been struggling to exclude all acrimony from her relations to one of her cousins.

Part of the successful treatment was the prescription of a ritual. The family was told that the emerging hostility toward the clan endangered the group; it was vital to follow the prescription and to allow no hostility to escape the family into the clan. Therefore, for two weeks, every other night, after dinner, the front door was to be locked and bolted. The four family members were to clear the dining room table of everything but a clock. In order of seniority, each was to speak or be silent for fifteen minutes, the others maintaining strict silence during this period and making no expressive gestures. No negative word about any member of the clan was to be uttered outside the ritual context; rather, they were to redouble their courtesy and helpfulness.

This ritual was an enactment of a different set of regularities than those customary in the family. It differentiated the nuclear family from the rest, substituting explicit but private criticism of clan members for total silence; it established the right of each member of the nuclear family to express his/her perceptions without contradiction or disqualification. Two weeks later the members of the nuclear family were openly sharing criticism of the clan as well as guilt over the criticism (Selvini-Palazzoli, 1974, pp. 236–239; Selvini-Palazzoli, et al., 1978, pp. 83–97). So, the ritual simultaneously served two structural (Aponte & Van Deusen, 1981; Minuchin, 1974) purposes: the differentiation of the nuclear from the extended family and the differentiation of the members of the nuclear family.

In such rituals, verbal action is only one component and this component may itself be reduced in character to that of a magical incantation, whether diffuse or formulaic (Evans-Pritchard, 1937; 1967; Malinowski, 1948; 1950). For instance, a 6-year-old boy diagnosed as minimally brain damaged and being medicated was permitted to behave like a maniac at home—kicking at mother's face, pouring soup on her, lunging at family members with a table knife, and so forth. The family, according to a prescribed ritual, walked in a procession to the bathroom after supper, the father carrying all the child's medicine bottles. He told his son that the doctors had instructed him to throw all the medicines away because the boy was perfectly well, simply a normal child; they would no longer put up with all his nonsense. Then, with great ceremony, the father poured the contents of each bottle down the toilet, solemnly intoning each time, "You are perfectly well; you are perfectly well." Despite the mother's fear that her son would kill her without his sedatives, his aggressive behavior disappeared (Selvini-Palazzoli, 1974, pp. 236–237).

With the elimination of aggression we appear to be nearing our destination—perfection—so we may now return to the ideal end of the figurative acts we have illustrated.

FIGURATIVELY FREE

The development of figurative action may be defined as the progress toward perfection of multiple meaning. On the expressive side, the control and modulation of speech and gesture to convey allegory, irony, and satire "at will" is one manifestation of developed figurative action. It is of course, not surprising that the most developed agents of figurative action are artists, poets, humorists, and so on. On the receptive side, development is manifested in interpreting hidden or oblique meanings in verbal and nonverbal expressions, in seeing signs as the embodiments of references and allusions invisible to others until they are revealed.

Clearly, the expression and apprehension of multiple meaning is not enough. For not only do psychoanalysts, literary critics, and religious apologists skillfully unearth levels of meaning; so, too, do lovers uncertain of reciprocated affection and paranoids certain of the opposite. Diverse meanings must be integrated into a coherent whole. Otherwise, we are left with an unrelated or a warring plurality of meanings.

It has been remarked (Grandgent, 1933) that no one but a child would be interested in the literal story of Bunyan's *Pilgrim's Progress,* and we can recall as children reading *Gulliver's Travels* as though it were simply amusing fiction, just as naive adults once thought it a faked travel book. When we finally grasp it as multi-layered (Ingarden, 1974; Wellek & Warren, 1956), both it and we are transformed—*Gulliver's Travels* is then ironic and we are then capable of irony. We can simultaneously apprehend the consciousness of the ethnocentric Gulliver and, behind his back, that of the implied author with whom we exchange knowing glances (Booth, 1961). As the figurative action becomes more fully and richly a multiplex unity, we learn to speak with and to hear many voices and to interweave them in harmony and in counterpoint.

Perhaps the systematically ambiguous or equivocal calls for us to articulate and synthesize our own multiple possibilities. Perhaps even as a figurative action is pressed in pursuit of a special, sometimes nefarious, purpose by means of its particular character, it also fosters the free play of the imagination by virtue of its general form. Those actions that can be taken as figurative invite us to see the gaps in what we thought was seamless and to grasp the connection where we suspected only division. Whatever their special aims, they playfully help to free us from limited visions and narrow identifications.

In some traditions, "folktales" are said to be recited so that, in accordance with the social context and the dispositions of the listeners, they may provide spiritual nourishment to feed individuals on their journeys toward perfection (Shah, 1973). These tales are said to be multiform in their potentialities of interpretation, at once responsive to the potentialities of the listener and transforming them. Some of the stories are able figuratively to comment on their own transforming purposes, as is this one with which we conclude, the story of the merchant and his parrot (Shah, 1970, p. 189; Whinfield, 1975, p. 28):

> A merchant who kept a parrot in a cage, being about to visit the parrot's homeland, asked if he had any message to be delivered to his kinsmen. The parrot asked him to announce his captivity to the free birds in the jungle there. The merchant did so, and no sooner did he than a wild bird just like his own fell dead from a tree. Upon returning, he told his parrot that one of his relatives fell dead upon hearing of the parrot's

captivity. As soon as the words were spoken, the parrot, too, fell dead to the floor of his cage. Sorrowfully, the merchant went to dispose of the corpse, which miraculously recovered life, flew to a nearby branch, and said:

"Now you know that the message you thought was disaster was good news for me, and that the suggestion of how to behave in order to free myself was transmitted through you, my captor." And he flew away, free at last.

REFERENCES

Aponte, H. J., & Van Deusen, J. M. Structural family therapy. In A. S. Gurman, & D. P. Kniskern (Eds.), *Handbook of family therapy.* New York: Brunner/Mazel, 1981.

Barten, S. S., & Franklin, M. B. (Eds.) *Developmental processes: Heinz Werner's selected writings* (2 vols.). New York: International Universities Press, 1978.

Beardsley, M. C. The metaphorical twist. *Philosophy and Phenomenological Research,* 1962, *22,* 293–307.

Black, M. The definition of scientific method. In M. Black (Ed.), *Problems of analysis.* Ithaca, N.Y.: Cornell University Press, 1954.

Bloch, D. (Ed.) *Techniques of family psychotherapy: A primer.* New York: Grune & Stratton, 1973.

Booth, W. C. *Rhetoric of fiction.* Chicago, Ill.: University of Chicago Press, 1961.

Burke, K. *A grammar of motives.* New York: Prentice-Hall, 1945.

Burke, K. *Permanence and change* (2nd rev. ed.). Los Altos, CA: Hermes, 1954.

Burke, K. *Language as symbolic action: Essays on life, literature, and method.* Berkeley, CA: University of California Press, 1966.

Burke, K. *Dramatism and development.* Worcester, MA: Clark University Press, 1972.

Burke, K. *The philosophy of literary form* (3rd ed.). Berkeley, CA: University of California Press, 1973 (originally published, 1941).

Cassirer, E. *An essay on man: An introduction to a philosophy of human culture.* New Haven: Yale University Press, 1944.

Cohen, F. S. The reconstruction of hidden value judgments: Word choices as value indicators. In L. Bryson, L. Finkelstein, R. M. Maciver, & R. McKeon (Eds.), *Symbols and value: An initial study.* New York: The conference on science, philosophy and religion in their relation to the democratic way of life, Inc., 1954.

Dunbar, H. F. *Symbolism in medieval thought and its consummation in The Divine Comedy.* New York: Russell & Russell, 1929/61.

Ekstein, R. *Children of time and space, of action and impulse.* New York: Appleton-Century-Crofts, 1966.

Eliade, M. *The sacred and the profane: The nature of religion.* New York: Harcourt, Brace & World, Inc., 1959.

Evans-Pritchard, E. E. *Witchcraft, oracles, and magic among the Azande.* London: Oxford University Press, 1937.

Evans-Pitchard, E. E. The morphology and function of magic: A comparative study of Trobriand and Zande ritual and spells. In J. Middleton (Ed.), *Magic, witchcraft, and curing.* Garden City, N.Y.: The Natural History Press, 1967.

Ferreira, A. J. Family myth and homeostasis. *Archives of General Psychiatry,* 1963, *9,* 457–473.

Firth, R. W. *Symbols: Public and private.* Ithaca, N.Y.: Cornell University Press, 1973.

Goffman, E. *Presentation of self in everyday life.* Garden City, N.Y.: Doubleday, 1959.

Goffman, E. *Gender advertisements.* Cambridge, MA: Harvard University Press, 1979.

Grandgent, C. H. *La Divina Commedia di Dante Alighieri* (Rev. ed.). New York: D.C. Heath, 1933.

Haley, J. *Uncommon therapy: The psychiatric techniques of Milton H. Erickson, M.D.* New York: Norton, 1973.

Honeck, R. P., & Hoffman, R. R. (Eds.). *Cognition and figurative language.* Hillsdale, N.J.: Lawrence Erlbaum Associates, 1980.

Ingarden, R. *The literary work of art.* (G. G. Grabowicz, trans.). Evanston, Ill.: Northwestern University Press, 1974.

Kaplan, B. Radical metaphor, aesthetic and the origin of language. *Review of Existential Psychology and Psychiatry,* 1962, *2,* 75–84.

Langs, R. J. *The technique of psychoanalytic psychotherapy* (Vol. 1). New York: Jason Aronson, 1973.

Lewis, H. R., & Streitfeld, H. S. *Growth games.* New York: Harcourt Brace Jovanovich, Inc., 1972.

Lovejoy, A. O. *The great chain of being.* Cambridge, MA: Harvard University Press, 1936.

Madanes, C. Protection, paradox and pretending. *Family Process,* 1980, *19,* 73–85.

Madanes, C. *Strategic family therapy.* San Francisco: Jossey-Bass Publishers, 1981.

Malinowski, B. *Magic, science and religion, and other essays.* Garden City, N.Y.: Doubleday, 1948.

Malinowski, B. *Argonauts of the Western Pacific.* New York: E.P. Dutton & Co., 1950.

Melito, R. *Studies of literal and metaphoric comprehension.* Unpublished doctoral dissertation, Clark University, 1980.

Minuchin, S. *Families and family therapy.* Cambridge, MA: Harvard University Press, 1974.

Moreno, J. L. *Psychodrama* (Vol. 1). New York: Beacon House, 1946.

Perelman, C., & Olbrechts-Tyteca, L. *New rhetoric: A treatise on argumentation.* Notre Dame, In.: University of Notre Dame Press, 1969.

Perls, F. S. *Gestalt therapy verbatim* (Ed., J. O. Stevens). Moab, UT: Real People Press, 1969.

Perls, F. S. *The Gestalt approach and eyewitness to therapy.* Palo Alto, CA: Science & Behavior Books, 1973.

Schön, D. *Displacement of concepts.* New York: Humanities Press, 1963.

Schutz, W. C. *Joy: Expanding human awareness.* New York: Grove Press Inc., 1967.

Schwayder, D. *The stratification of behavior.* London: Routledge & Kegan Paul, 1965.

Selvini-Palazzoli, M. *Self-starvation: From the intrapsychic to the transpersonal approach to anorexia nervosa.* London: Human Context Books, Chaucer Publishing Co. Ltd., 1974.

Selvini-Palazzoli, M., Boscolo, L., Cecchin, G., & Prata, G. *Paradox and counterparadox.* New York: Jason Aronson, 1978.

Shah, I. *Tales of the Dervishes.* New York: E.P. Dutton & Co., 1970.

Shah, I. The teaching story: Observations on the folklore of our "modern" thought. In R. E. Ornstein (Ed.), *The nature of human consciousness.* San Francisco: W.H. Freeman & Co., 1973.

Stanton, M. D. Strategic approaches to family therapy. In A. S. Gurman, & D. P. Kniskern (Eds.), *Handbook of family therapy.* New York: Brunner/Mazel, 1981.

Stevens, J. O. *Awareness: Exploring, experimenting, experiencing.* Lafayette, CA: Real People Press, 1971.

Tillyard, E. M. *Elizabethan world picture.* New York: Random House, Inc., 1959.

Van de Riet, V., Korb, M. P., & Gorrell, J. J. *Gestalt therapy: An introduction.* New York: Pergamon Press, 1980.

Vygotsky, L. S. *Thought and language.* (E. Hanfmann & G. Vakar, Ed. & trans.) Cambridge, MA: M.I.T. Press, 1962 (originally published, 1934).

Watzlawick, P., Weakland, J. H., & Fisch, R. *Change: Principles of problem formation and problem resolution.* New York: Norton, 1974.

Weeks, G. R., & L'Abate, L. A compilation of paradoxical methods. *American Journal of Family Therapy,* 1979, *7,* 61–76.

Wellek, R., & Warren, A. *Theory of literature.* New York: Harcourt, Brace & World, Inc., 1956.

Werner, H. Die Ursprunge der Metapher. *Arb. Z. Entw.-Psychol.* (Krueger), III. Leipzig: Engelmann, 1919.

Werner, H., & Kaplan, B. *Symbol formation.* New York: Wiley, 1963.

Whinfield, E. H. *Teachings of Rumi: The Masnavi.* New York: E. P. Dutton & Co., 1975.

Whitehead, A. N. *The function of reason.* Princeton, N.J.: Princeton University Press, 1929.

Wimsatt, W. K., & Brooks, C. *Literary criticism: A short history.* New York: Vintage Books, 1967.

Epilogue

The principal aim of this volume is to suggest, through the presentation of papers by former colleagues and students of the late Heinz Werner, that the Wernerian schema for a developmental psychology is not only alive, but worthy of deep consideration by those who are searching for a psychological approach to human nature and human destiny that begins scholarly inquiry and practical intervention with the following presuppositions:

1. That the development of human beings is something to be promoted and attained, not something that simply occurs as a function of chronology.

2. That the development of human beings is something more than intellectual or cognitive development, and includes the perfection of diverse modes of operation (e.g., aesthetic, moral) that are not reducible to or derivable from strictly cognitive development.

3. That the cultural institutions and collective representations established by human beings in their transactions with each other and with their surroundings are relevatory of mental functioning, reflect different levels of mental development, and are active forces in influencing, for good or ill, the development of individual human beings.

4. That human beings are not merely or mainly the products of causes or conditions that necessitate their modes of action and collaboration with each other, but that they have the capacity (however constrained or limited by certain conditions) to shape their own formation and transformation, their own development.

5. That developmental psychology itself ought to be a practicotheoretical discipline whose explicit aim is the promotion of human development.

6. That a developmental psychology so conceived has intrinsic linkages to all other disciplines and to all domains of human practice, and will serve to promote goal-directed interdisciplinary or transdisciplinary work.

It is important to emphasize that as much as we have admired Werner and profited from his vision, we have no vested interest in sacralizing his name. There are many movements—e.g., Marxist and neo-Marxist, Freudian, Piagetian, and Vygotskian—which share in varying degrees the kind of vision that Werner had: a comprehensive attempt to understand all human actions and institutions from a developmental point of view. Werner would have been the last one to argue for a closed system. Although he was in principle bound to a developmental perspective of sufficient generality and scope to encompass all domains of human and even infrahuman activity, he sought always to be responsive to the concrete phenomena in the different areas of human functioning and to look for methods—e.g., naturalistic, phenomenological, hermeneutic, experimental—appropriate and adequate to their investigation.

We, who have absorbed his vision and sought to extend it, have, in general, a commitment not only to understand processes of development in different spheres of performance and personality formation, but also to work toward the developmental advances in human functioning. This enterprise takes us beyond a psychology narrowly defined and links developmental psychology, as we construe it, to all of the disciplines in the University and to many modes of activity outside of the University.

In sum, our aim as developmentalists in the Wernerian tradition is to promote human development in historical social orders, to have this aim govern our research inquiries—conceptual and empirical—and to use findings from such research to promote the betterment of humankind. This is what we mean by a holistic developmental psychology: obviously an infinite task and a task requiring the collaboration of all people of good will and with a commitment to human progress.

Author Index

A

Abrams, M. H., 101, *108*
Adorno, T., 107, *108*
Ainsworth, M. D., 121, *130*
Alapack, R. J., 193, *194*
Albert, M. S., 145, 148, 151, 152, 153, *155*
Allen, P. M., 28, *32*
Aponte, H. J., 248, *250*
Apter, D., 125, *130*
Arber, A., 63, *71*
Argyris, C., 91, *93*
Aristotle, 65, 70, *71*
Arnheim, R., 75, *93*, 181, 191, 192, *194*
Aronoff, J., 165, *176*
Asch, S. E., 165, *177*
Aune, J., 134, *140*

B

Bakan, D., 56, *71*
Baker, A. H., 159, *176*
Baker, E., 146, *156*
Barron, F., 191, *194*
Barry, J. R., 137, 138, *141*
Barten, S. S., 172, *175*, 183, 193, *194*, 199, *218*, 246, *250*
Bates, E., 35, *52*, 201, *218*
Bateson, G., 205, *218*
Beardsley, M. C., 237, *250*

Beck, L., 56, 58, *71*
Begnini, L., 35, *52*
Bentley, A. F., 100, *108*
Berkeley, G., 173, *175*
Berndt, R., 206, 207, 208, 210, 214, *219*
Bernstein, R. J., 56, *71*
Bevan, E., 60, *71*
Birren, J. E., 135, *140*
Black, M., 61, 71, *71*, 243, *250*
Bloch, D., 247, *250*
Bloom, L., 201, *218*
Boas, F., 97, 98, *108*
Boas, G., 101, 105, *108, 109*
Booth, W. C., 64, 65, *71, 72*, 249, *250*
Boscolo, L., 247, 248, *251*
Bower, T. G. R., 172, *175*
Bowerman, M., 232, *234*
Boyd, W., 97, *108*
Bradford, G. E., 134, *140*
Braine, M. D. S., 232, *234*
Brent, S. B., 7, 8, 9, 18, 19, 21, 25, 26, 28, 31, *32, 33*
Bretherton, I., 35, *52*
Brissett, D., 56, 61, *72*
Brooks, C., 244, *252*
Brown, R., 231, 232, *234*
Brown, R. H., 82, *93*
Bryant, P. J., 9, *33*
Bryant, S. V., 9, *22*
Bryson, L., 67, *72*

Buchler, J., 71, *72*
Buckley, H. D., 125, *130*
Bunzel, R., 98, *108*
Burke, K., 54, 55, 56, 57, 61, 63, 64, 65, 67, 69, *72,* 100, 107, *108,* 115, *130,* 235, 237, 239, 242, *250*
Burrell, D., 69, *72*
Bushnell, E. W., 173, 175

C

Calhoun, J. B., 29, *33*
Camaioni, L., 35, *52*
Carlin, G., 96, *108*
Casey, E., 100, *108*
Cassirer, E., 56, 61, 67, *72,* 103, *108,* 116, *130,* 179, 192, 193, *194,* 236, *250*
Castaneda, A., 122, *131*
Cecchin, G., 247, 248, *251*
Chaille, C., 206, 217, *219*
Chodak, S., 84, *93*
Ciottone, R., 56, 64, *74,* 113, 119, *131*
Cirillo, L., 159, *176*
Cobb, E., 217, *218*
Cohen, F. S., 68, *72,* 239, 240, 241, 243, *250*
Cohen, M. M., 171, *176*
Cohen, S. B., 56, *74,* 113, 123, *130, 131*
Collingwood, R. G., 60, *72,* 101, *108,* 193 *194*
Cope, J., 56, 61, *72*
Crocker, C., 61, *73*
Cronholm, B., 134, *141*
Crowell, M. F., 134, *141*

D

Dalziel-Duncan, H., 56, *72*
Deikman, A., 182, *194*
Dewey, J., 56, *72,* 100, *108*
Drucker, J., 217, *218*
Dunbar, H. F., 244, *250*
Duncker, K., 170, *176*
Dunn, E., 87, *93*
Durkheim, E., 84, *93*

E

Eckerman, C. O., 121, *131*
Edelman, E., 125, *130*
Edgley, C., 56, 61, *72*
Eigen, M., 32, *33*
Ekel, T. M., 133, *142*

Eklund, J., 134, *140*
Ekstein, R., 247, *250*
Eliade, M., 243, *250*
Evans-Pritchard, E. E., 248, *250*

F

Fein, G., 200, 203, *218,* 230, *234*
Fergusson, F., 56, 61, 65, *72*
Ferreira, A. J., 247, *250*
Ferris, S. H., 134, *141*
Feyerabend, P., 71, *72*
Field, J., 172, *176*
Fingarette, H., 100, *108,* 193, *194*
Finkelstein, L., 67, *72*
Firth, R. W., 246, *250*
Fisch, R., 240, *251*
Fischer, D. H., 66, *72*
Fletcher, A., 65, *72*
Foucault, M., 35, *52*
Franklin, M. B., 183, 193, *194,* 199, 208, *218,* 246, *250*
Freeman, J. T., 133, *140*
French, V., 9, *33*
Freud, S., 30, *33*
Fry, R. J. M., 133, *141*
Frye, N., 65, *72*
Fuson, K. C., 203, *218*

G

Gardiner, W., 32, *33*
Gardner, H., 190, *195*
Garfinkel, H., 84, *93*
Garvey, C., 201, 206, 207, 208, 210, 214, *218, 219*
Gasseling, M. T., 133, *141*
Gearhart, M., 207, 211, *219*
Geertz, C., 41, *52,* 96, *108*
Gershon, S., 134, *141*
Geschwind, N., 154, *155*
Gibbs, J. T., 125, *130*
Gibson, J. J., 167, 168, 171, *176*
Giorgi, A., 128, *130*
Goffman, E., 63, *72,* 205, *219,* 242, *250*
Goldman, J., 206, 217, *219*
Goldstein, K., 134, *141*
Gombrich, E. H., 63, *72,* 175, *176*
Goodglass, H., 148, 149, 151, 154, *155*
Goodman, N., 61, 67, *72*
Goodson, B., 229, *234*
Gorrell, J. J., 247, *251*

Grandgent, C. H., 244, 249, *250*
Graybiel, A., 170, *177*
Greenfield, P., 229, *234*
Gropius, W., 83, *93*
Gruendel, J. M., 214, *219*

H

Haley, J., 237, 245, *251*
Hall, P., 86, *93*
Hallpike, C. R., 98, *108*
Hardison, O. B., 71, *72*
Hardy, L. H., 139, *140*
Hayflick, L., 133, *141*
Heinrich, A., 134, *141*
Heyn, J. E., 137, 138, *141*
Himwich, H. E., 134, *141*
Himwich, W. A., 134, *141*
Hoagland, H., 67, *72*
Hoffman, R. R., 237, *251*
Hogg, J., 192, *194*
Holliday, R., 134, *141*
Honeck, R. P., 237, *251*
Hooper, H. E., 147, *155*
Horkheimer, M., 107, *108*
Hornstein, G. A., 128, *130, 131*
Hudson, L., 191, *194*
Hughes, H. S., 56, *72*
Hukami, K., 139, *141*
Hyman, S. E., 56, *73*

I

Ichikawa, H., 139, *141*
Ingarden, R., 249, *251*

J

Jackson, J. P., 231, *234*
James, W., 172, *176*
Jantsch, E., 84, *93*
Jencks, C., 80, *93*
Jenneret, C. E., 80, *93*
Joad, C. E. M., 100, *108*
Johnson, M., 61, *73*
Johansson, G., 168, *176*

K

Kagan, J., 173, *176*
Kairis, M., 134, *141*
Kandinsky, W., 179, 192, *194*

Kanizsa, G., 158, *176*
Kaplan, A., 71, *73*
Kaplan, B., 6, *6*, 54, 55, 56, 64, 67, 69, *73, 74*, 97, 98, 103, 106, *108, 109*, 111, 113, 116, 117, 123, *130, 131, 132*, 152, 156, 158, 174, *176, 177*, 193, *195*, 207, 216, *219*, 221, 230, 231, *234*, 236, 238, *251, 252*
Kaplan, E., 145, 146, 148, 149, 151, 152, 153, 154, *155*, 231, *234*
Kawakami, G., 139, *141*
Kerenyi, K., 59, *73*
Kearsley, R. B., 173, *176*
Kennedy, J. M., 158, *176*
Kinsbourne, M., 148, *156*
Klee, P., 179, 192, *194*
Kleinman, S., 190, *195*
Kluckhohn, C., 96, 107, *108, 109*
Köhler, W., 103, *109*
Kohn, H. I., 133, *141*
Korb, M. P., 247, *251*
Kroeber, A., 96, 107, *109*
Kuhn, T. S., 35, *52*
Kuppers, B., 32, *33*

L

L'Abate, L., 240, *251*
Lackner, J. R., 171, *176*
Lakoff, G., 61, *73*
Langer, J., 221, *234*
Langer, S. K., 67, *73,* 100, *109,* 179, 182, 193, *194*
Langs, R. J., 245, *251*
Lashley, K. S., 164, *176*
Lee, J. A., 136, 137, 138, *141*
Leondar, B., 192, *195*
Leopold, I. H., 136, *141*
Lesher, S., 133, *141*
Lester, G., 169, *176*
Levander, S. E., 134, *141*
Leveton, L. B., 121, 125, *131*
LeVine, R., 96, *109*
Lewis, H. R., 247, *251*
Leyhausen, P., 30, *33*
Liepmann, H., 154, *156*
Linn, S., 134, *141*
Louch, A. R., 104, *109*
Love, J., 6, *6*
Lovejoy, A. O., 55, *73,* 101, *109,* 244, *251*
Lucca-Irizarry, N., 122, 123, *130*
Luria, A. R., 203, *219*
Lyons, J., 193, *195*

M

MacIver, R. M., 67, *72*
MacKinnon, D. W., 191, *194*
MacLeod, R. M., 181, 183, *194*
Madanes, C., 241, 247, *251*
Madden, E., 71, *73*
Malinowski, B., 248, *251*
Mandelbaum, M., 55, *73*
Margenau, H., 100, *109*
Marsh, G. R., 134, *142*
Matthews, W. S., 209, *219*
Maynard, L. A., 134, *141*
McCarthy, M., 190, *195*
McCay, C. M., 134, *141*
McConville, M., 193, *194*
McDonald, R. A., 133, *141*
McGrew, J. F., 139, *141*
McKeon, R., 61, *73*
McNeil, O. V., 126, *130*
Mead, G. H., 56, *73*
Melito, R., 244, *251*
Merleau-Ponty, M., 182, 193, *194*
Milner, M., 179, 182, 192, *194*
Mindus, P., 134, *141*
Minuchin, S., 248, *251*
Mitchell, N. B., 139, *141*
Moncrieff, D. W., 179, 182, *195*
Morant, R. B., 165, 167, 169, 175, *176*
Moreno, J. L., 247, *251*
Murray, H. A., 107, *108*

N

Needham, R., 96, *109*
Nelson, K., 214, *219*
Newman, O., 81, *93*
Nicolich, L. McCune, 201, *219*
Niven, J. I., 170, *177*
Norberg-Schulz, C., 76, *93*
Northrop, F. S. C., 59, *73,* 106, *109*

O

Olbrechts-Tyteca, L., 68, *73,* 242, *251*
Orgel, L. E., 134, *141*
Ortega y Gasset, J., 193, *195*
Overton, W. F., 35, *52,* 231, *234*

P

Pacheco, A. M., 122, 123, *131, 130*
Palladio, A., 77, *93*
Palmer, E. P., 146, *156*
Pate, R. H., 125, *131*
Pepper, S. C., 35, *52,* 65, *73,* 104, *109*
Perelman, C., 68, *73,* 242, *251*
Perkins, D., 192, *195*
Perls, F. S., 247, *251*
Pevsner, N., 76, *93*
Piaget, J., 202, 217, *219,* 221, *234*
Pick, H. L., 174, *176*
Pines, M., 134, *141*
Polanyi, M., 101, *109*
Pollack, R. H., 136, 137, 138, 139, *141, 142*
Prata, G., 247, 248, *251*
Prigogine, I., 28, *33*

Q

Quirk, M., 119, *131*

R

Radin, P., 98, *109*
Ramirez, M. III, 122, *131*
Rand, A., 83, *93*
Rand, G., 139, *140*
Redfield, R., 99, 106, *109*
Redondo, J. P., 121, 122, *131*
Reese, H. W., 35, *52*
Reiner, J. R., 125, *131*
Reisberg, B., 134, *141*
Rheingold, H. L., 121, *131*
Ricoeur, P., 63, *73,* 100, *109*
Riegel, K. F., 135, *140*
Rierdan, J., 125, *130, 132*
Risch, T. J., 125, *131*
Rittler, M. C., 139, *140*
Robinson, D. W., 125, *131*
Roheim, G., 100, *109*
Roscianno, L., 201, *219*
Rubin, I. H., 203, *219*
Rubin, K. H., 215, *219*
Rubner, M., 133, *141*
Russell, B., 173, *176*
Rykwert, J., 79, *93*

S

Sack, R., 6, *6*
Sachs, J., 201, 202, 206, 214, 217, *219*
Sanglier, M., 28, *32*
Sapir, J., 61, *73*
Saunders, J. W. Jr., 133, *141*
Saunders, L. C., 133, *141*
Schalling, D., 134, *141*
Scheerer, M., 193, *195*
Schmitt, V., 121, *131*
Schneider, D., 107, *108*
Schön, D., 91, *93*, 242, *251*
Schouela, D. A., 121, 125, *131*
Schulman, L., 190, *195*
Schuman, M., 183, *195*
Schuster, P., 32, *33*
Schutz, A., 58, *73*, 197, *219*
Schutz, W. C., 247, *251*
Schwartz, D., 137, *141*
Schwartzman, H., 206, *219*
Schwayder, D., 242, *251*
Seewald, R., 206, 217, *219*
Selvini-Palazzoli, M., 247, 248, *251*
Serlio, S., 79, *93*
Shah, I., 249, *251*
Shock, N. W., 133, *141*
Shumaker, W., 6, *6*, 65, *73*
Siegel, S., 187, *195*
Siegler, R. S., 45, *52*
Silberberg, M., 134, *141*
Silberberg, R., 134, *141*
Simon, Y., 60, *73*
Skoff, E., 139, *142*
Sohal, R. S., 133, *142*
Solomon, J., 188, *195*
Solomon, P., 158, *176*
Speier, S., 184, 185, *195*
Spiegelberg, H., 183, *195*
Stanton, M. D., 241, *251*
Steadman, P., 75, *93*
Steinberg, L. M., 121, 125, *131*
Steiner, I., 28, *33*
Stevens, J. O., 247, *251*
Stokes, A., 76, *93*
Straus, E., 61, *73*
Strauss, L., 97, *109*
Streitfeld, H. S., 247, *251*
Sugarman, S., 223, *234*

Sun, A. Y., 134, *142*
Sun, G. Y., 134, *142*
Sutton-Smith, B., 215, *219*

T

Taylor, C., 56, *73*
Tanabe, S., 139, *141*
Thompson, L. W., 134, *142*
Thorndike, L., 71, *73*
Thurstone, L. L., 55, 63, *73*
Tillyard, E. M., 244, *251*
Toffler, A., 81, *93*
Trotsky, L., 66, *73*
Tuchman, B., 30, *33*
Turbayne, C., 61, *73*

U

Urban, W., 67, *73*
Uzgiris, I., 216, *219*

V

Van de Riet, V., 247, *251*
Van Deusen, J. M., 248, *250*
van Scott, E. J., 133, *142*
Velhagen, K., 139, *142*
Vickery, J., 61, *74*
Volterra, V., 35, *52*
von Bertalanffy, L., 65, *74*
Vygotsky, L. S., 43, 46, *52*, 200, 203, 217,
    219, 221, *234*, 240, *251*

W

Walk, R. D., 174, *176*
Warren, A., 249, *252*
Wapner, S., 6, *6*, 56, 64, *74*, 113, 117, 119,
    121, 122, 123, 125, 126, 128, *130, 131, 132*,
    159, 164, 165, 172, 173, *176, 177*
Watkins, M., 128, *131*
Watzlawick, P., 240, *251*
Weakland, J. H., 240, *251*
Wechsler, D., 144, 146, *156*
Weeks, G. R., 240, *251*
Weinstein, C., 146, *156*
Weintraub, S., 148, *156*
Wellek, R., 249, *252*

Werner, H., 24, *33,* 37, *52,* 54, 67, *74,* 83, *93,* 97, 98, *109,* 111, 117, *131, 132,* 134, *142,* 143, 144, 152, *156,* 158, 159, 164, 165, 172, 173, 174, *176, 177,* 181, 183, 184, 193, *195,* 197, 199, 207, 216, *219,* 221, 230, 231, *234,* 237, 238, 246, *252*
Werkmeister, W., 63, *74*
Wertsch, J. V., 203, *219*
Wheelwright, P., 53, 68, *74*
Whinfield, E. H., 249, *252*
White, H., 66, *74*
White, L., 96, 97, *109*
White, S., 59, *74*
Whitehead, A. N., 61, 64, *74,* 101, 107, *109,* 235, *252*
Whiteside, T. C. D., 170, *177*
Whorf, B., 65, 67, *74*
Wimsatt, W. K., 244, *252*

Winkler-Oswaitsch, R., 32, *33*
Winner, E., 190, *195,* 209, *219*
Witkin, H. A., 165, *177*
Wittig, B. A., 121, *130*
Wittkower, R., 77, *93*
Wofsey, E., 125, *132*
Wolf, D., 207, 208, 209, 214, *220*
Wolfe, T., 81, *93*
Wolff, K., 134, *142*
Wright, F. L., 83, *93*

X,Y,Z

Yudovich, F., 203, *219*
Zelazo, P. R., 173, *176*
Zivin, G., 204, *220*
Znaniecki, F., 64, *74,* 104, *109*

Subject Index

A

Adaptation in visual perception, 160–167
Aesthetic consciousness, 179–193
  and agent's intentionality, 180
  and altered modes of consciousness, 182
  and mundane consciousness, 180–183
Aftereffects, 160–171
  body position, 160–166, 169–171
  visual tilt, 160–167
Aging, 133
Allegory, 244–246 (*see also* figurative action,
    figures of speech)
Apparent movement in perception, 169–171
Apraxia, 154
Architecture and psychology, 75–82
  practice and planning, 84–92
Art (*see also* artists, aesthetic consciousness)
  medium, 191–192
  and phenomenology of experience, 193
  production and experience of, 191–192
  psychology of, 183, 189, 191–193
Artists, 179–193 (*see also* aesthetic
    consciousness, art)
  experience of world, 193
  habitual experience of, 180, 190
  psychology of, 191
Audiogyral illusion, 168–169
Auditory localization, 166, 169

B

Brain injury
  gestural representation in, 151–153
  immediate memory in, 150–151
  naming in, 148–149
  process oriented diagnosis of, 143f(f)
  sequential strategy in, 153–154
  visuo-spatial performance in, 144–148

C

Camouflage, 136–139
Classroom structure, 10–30
  attentional model of, 26–28
  efficiency of, 11, 13–21
  formats of, 13–21
  group processes in, 13–16
  growth in, 7–33
  hierarchical forms in, 15–16
  informational models of, 26–28
Conflict in figurative action, 236–244
Context of play, 198, 205, 210
  text statements in, 205, 210, 213
Critical transitions, 112–114, 116–119
  application of orthogenetic principle to,
    117
  cultural specificity of, 113–114, 116–118
  defining characteristics of, 113

developmental aspects of, 114, 119
Cultural relativism, 69, 99

D

Development, 55f(f), 68, 96f(f) (see also
    genetic dramatism)
  and architectural form, 82–84
  and critical transitions, 114–119
  and ethnocentrism, 97f(f)
  and extrinsic causation, 55(f)
  and means-ends relationships, 55, 66
  and ontogenesis, 54(f), 57, 60
  and orthogenetic principle, 54, 60, 117
  and primitivity, 55f(f), 97f(f)
  and specialization, 60
  and stages (levels), 55, 60
  and teloi, 62f(f)
  as descriptive, 69, 100f(f), 105
  as freedom, 248–250
  as normative (ideal), 59f(f), 97f(f)
  in adults, 133
  of figurative action, 248–250
Developmental psychology, 54, 57
  and architectural form, 75, 93
  and architectural practice and planning,
    84–92
  and systems theory, 82f(f)
  need for reorientation of, 1f(f), 54f(f), 57
Developmental theory, 36–39
  conceptual object of, 37–39
  natural object of, 36–37
Differentiation, 24–26, 159, 174 (see also
    orthogenetic principle)
  and figurative action, 240–242, 248
Dramatism, 54, 56f(f), 66f(f)
  categories of, 56, 61–65
  definitions of situations in, 61–68

E

Embedded figures test (EFT), 136–139
Expression, 179–180 (see also physiognomic
    properties, expressivity)
  and aesthetic image, 179
Expressivity, 182
  and aesthetic orientation, 189
  conditions for, 188–191

F

Field dependence, 137
Figurative action, 235–250
Figure-ground segregation, 136–137
Figures of speech, 236
  honorific and pejorative speech, 239–240,
    243
  irony, 238–239
  metaphor, 237–238, 244, 246

G

Genetic-Dramatism
  development in, 57f(f)
  motivation in, 56
  and organismic-developmental
    psychology, 56
  sources of, 54f(f)
Gestural representation, 151–153
Gesture, 188

I

Imagination (see also play, spheres of reality)
Immediate memory, 150–151
Information and organization in classroom,
    7–33
  and channels of transmission, 11, 27–28
Integration and figurative action, 237–238,
    240–242, 247, 249–250
Intersensory (intermodal) coordination, 168,
    172–174

L

Labyrinthian stimulation, 169–171
Language (see also speech)
  in play, 200–214
  narrative functions, 202, 213
  paradigms, 201–214

M

Metaphoric transformation, 188–190 (see
    also object description, figures of
    speech)
Microgenesis, 158, 165–166

Migration, 114, 122–124
　characteristics of, 122
　conditions facilitating, 123–124
　developmental aspects of, 122–123
Models, 61, 70
　and metaphors, 61, 70
　and terministic screens, 61
Multiple worlds, 120–129

N

Naming in brain injury, 148–149
Normalization in perception, 166–167

O

Object (*see also* object description)
　and self, 187
　contemplative, 181
　mundane, 180–181
　subject-object polarization, 181–182
Object description
　evaluative, 186–187
　in artists and scientists, 184–188
　metaphoric, 186–187
　naming, 186–187
　physiognomic, 186–187
　under *look* and *play* conditions, 190–191
Object transformation in play, 199, 206,
　209–210
Objects
　aesthetic, 180–182
　assigning attributes to, 189–190
　externality of, 187
　preferred orientations toward, 189
Oculogyral illusion, 168–171
Operations, 221–228, 232, 233
Organic structures, 8–11, 16–18, 23–25 (*see also* organizational form)
Organismic-developmental viewpoint,
　112–117 (*see also* genetic-dramatism)
　contrast with other perspectives, 116–117
　extensions of, 56f(f), 111–112
Organizational form in classroom structure
　cohesiveness of, 18–26
　destabilization, 8
　development of, 24–26
　differentiation, process of, 24–26

efficiency of, 7–11, 17, 21–26
　integration, focus on, 23–25
　intended function of, 7
　levels of analysis, 8–11, 13, 17–18
　reorganization, spontaneous, 8, 11, 17
　stability of, 7–8, 17
Organizational form, characteristics of,
　7–11 (*see also* organic structures)
Orthogenetic principle, 54, 60, 158–159,
　174–175

P

Perception
　and memory traces, 167
　and representational art, 175
　developmental aspects, 157–175
　in infancy, 171–175
　of the straight-ahead, 159, 169–170
　of the vertical, 160–166
　phenomenological unity of, 171–175
　qualitative differences in, 193
Perspective, 53f(f), 65f(f)
　and metaphor, 70
　and terministic screens, 61, 65
　of genetic dramatism, 53f(f), 67
Phenomenology
　developmental, 184
　influence of, 198–199, 205
　in Germany, 183
　of art, 193
　of perception, 193
Physiognomic experience, 183–184 (*see also* expression)
　and geometric-technical experience, 184
Physiognomic properties, 180–181, 188–189
　(*see also* expression)
Piaget's theory, 39–43
　evolution, 41–42
　logical form, 40–41
Play, 197–218 (*see also* play episodes)
　and reality distinction, 206–209, 214, 215
　as precursor for language, 201–202
　as social, 204–207
　as symbolizing activity, 207
　developmental trends in, 215–217
　fantastical, 215–216
　imaginary worlds and, 215–218

imaginative-expressive, 200, 207
inner coherence of, 216–217
realistic, 215–216
Play episodes (*see also* play)
creating and organizing event sequence,
211–214
establishing identities for objects and
persons, 209–210
establishing the playsphere, 208–209
establishing the setting, 211
Population size in classrooms, 7–33
Prism rearrangement, 160–168
Process and achievement, 134, 139, 143f(f)
Process oriented diagnosis in brain injury,
143f(f)
Psychological worlds (*see also* spheres of
reality)
metaphor of, 197–198, 207–208, 217

R

Regression, 133–139
Representation, 225–231, 233–234
Representational cognition, 221, 231–234
Retinal flow pattern, 163, 168, 170–171
Retinal image theory, 168, 175
Ritual, 246–248
and myth, 247–248
Rod and frame test, 165

S

Saturation in classroom situations, 17–21, 30
Sensory-motor
responses, 159, 160
sub-systems, 166, 168, 171, 173
Sensory-tonic theory, 158–160, 164–165
Sensory unity (*see also* perception,
phenomenological unity of)
Sequential strategy, 153–154
Speech (*see also* language)
egocentric, 202–203
inner, 203

planning functions, 203–204
social, 203
Spheres of reality, 198–199, 207–208, 217
Starting position effects, 165
Stories and figurative action, 249–250
Structure, 8–9, 31–32
Supersaturation, 20–26
Symbolic action (Symbolicity), 60, 62, 67f
Symbolism (*see also* figurative action)
non-verbal, 246–248
symbolizing, 207

T

Terministic screens, 61, 101, 105f(f) (*see also*
perspective therapy)
and political language, 238–240
by prescribing rituals, 247–248
non-verbal methods, 246–248
psychoanalytic, 239–240, 245–246
renaming in, 240, 241–242
Tilted room effect, 165
Transitions
from high school to college, 114, 124–127
from home to nursery school, 114, 119–121
from one culture to another (migration),
114, 122–124
from work to retirement, 114, 127–129

V

Virtual objects, 172–173
Visuo-spatial exemplars in brain injury,
144–148
Vygotsky's theory, 43–47
different versions of, 43–47
inner and external speech, 46–47
socialization of knowledge, 43–45

W

Werner's theory, 47–52